BREAST CANCER

CURRENT CLINICAL ONCOLOGY

Maurie Markman, MD, Series Editor

Breast Cancer: *A Guide to Detection and Multidisciplinary Therapy,* edited by Michael H. Torosian, 2002

Colorectal Cancer: *Multimodality Management,* edited by Leonard Saltz, 2002

Melanoma: *Biologically Targeted Therapeutics,* edited by Ernest C. Borden, 2002

Treatment of Acute Leukemias: *New Directions for Clinical Research,* edited by Ching-Hon Pui, 2002

Allogenic Stem Cell Transplantation: *Clinical Research and Practice,* edited by Mary J. Laughlin and Hillard M. Lazarus, 2002

Chronic Leukemias and Lymphomas: *Clinical Management,* edited by Gary J. Schiller, 2003

Palliative Care of the Cancer Patient: *The Physician's Practical Guide,* edited by Kristine Nelson, 2003

Cancer of the Spine: *Handbook of Comprehensive Care,* edited by Robert F. McLain, Maurie Markman, Ronald M. Bukowski, Roger Macklis, and Edward Benzel, 2003

Cancer of the Lung: *From Molecular Biology to Treatment Guidelines,* edited by Alan B. Weitberg, 2001

Renal Cell Carcinoma: *Molecular Biology, Immunology, and Clinical Management,* edited by Ronald M. Bukowski and Andrew Novick, 2000

Current Controversies in Bone Marrow Transplantation, edited by Brian J. Bolwell, 2000

Regional Chemotherapy: *Clinical Research and Practice,* edited by Maurie Markman, 2000

Intraoperative Irradiation: *Techniques and Results,* edited by L. L. Gunderson, C. G. Willett, L. B. Harrison, and F. A. Calvo, 1999

BREAST CANCER

A GUIDE TO DETECTION AND MULTIDISCIPLINARY THERAPY

Edited by

MICHAEL H. TOROSIAN, MD

Department of Surgery, Fox Chase Cancer Center
Philadelphia, PA

Foreword by

ROBERT C. YOUNG, MD

President, Fox-Chase Cancer Center
President, American Cancer Society

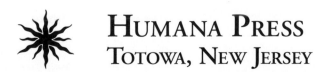

HUMANA PRESS
TOTOWA, NEW JERSEY

© 2002 Humana Press Inc.
999 Riverview Drive, Suite 208
Totowa, New Jersey 07512

www.humanapress.com

The content and opinions expressed in this book are the sole work of the authors and editors, who have warranted due diligence in the creation and issuance of their work. The publisher, editors, and authors are not responsible for errors or omissions or for any consequences arising from the information or opinions presented in this book and make no warranty, express or implied, with respect to its contents.

Due diligence has been taken by the publishers, editors, and authors of this book to assure the accuracy of the information published and to describe generally accepted practices. The contributors herein have carefully checked to ensure that the drug selections and dosages set forth in this text are accurate and in accord with the standards accepted at the time of publication. Notwithstanding, since new research, changes in government regulations, and knowledge from clinical experience relating to drug therapy and drug reactions constantly occur, the reader is advised to check the product information provided by the manufacturer of each drug for any change in dosages or for additional warnings and contraindications. This is of utmost importance when the recommended drug herein is a new or infrequently used drug. It is the responsibility of the treating physician to determine dosages and treatment strategies for individual patients. Further, it is the responsibility of the health care provider to ascertain the Food and Drug Administration status of each drug or device used in their clinical practice. The publishers, editors, and authors are not responsible for errors or omissions or for any consequences from the application of the information presented in this book and make no warranty, express or implied, with respect to the contents in this publication.

This publication is printed on acid-free paper. ∞

ANSI Z39.48-1984 (American National Standards Institute) Permanence of Paper for Printed Library Materials.

Cover design by Patricia F. Cleary.

Cover illustration: Round and oval masses are more often benign, and irregularly shaped masses or masses with spiculated margins are usually malignant. In this patient with a palpable lump in the left breast, an irregularly shaped mass was later found to represent carcinoma. (Fig. 11, Chapter 2; *see* full caption and discussion on p. 34.)

For additional copies, pricing for bulk purchases, and/or information about other Humana titles, contact Humana at the above address or at any of the following numbers: Tel: 973-256-1699; Fax: 973-256-8341; E-mail: humana@humanapr.com or visit our website at http://humanapress.com

Photocopy Authorization Policy:

Printed in the United States of America.   10 9 8 7 6 5 4 3 2 1

Library of Congress Cataloging-in-Publication Data

Breast cancer : a guide to detection and multidisciplinary therapy / edited by Michael H. Torosian.

 p. ; cm. -- (Current clinical oncology)
 Includes bibliographical references and index.
 ISBN 0-89603-839-4 (alk. paper)
 1. Breast--Cancer. I. Torosian, Michael, 1952 Apr. 23- II. Current clinical oncology (Totowa, N.J.)
 [DNLM: 1. Breast Neoplasms--therapy. WP 870 B82118 2002]
 RC280.B8 B665565 2002
 616.99'449--dc21

                       2001039599

Foreword

Breast cancer is responsible for one of every three cancers diagnosed in women. In 2001, approximately 192,200 new cases of invasive breast cancer were diagnosed along with 46,600 cases of *in situ* breast cancer. Approximately 40,200 women and 400 men will die of breast cancer this year. Excluding skin cancer, breast cancer is the commonest cancer occurring in women and certainly the most feared. Although the lifetime risk of developing breast cancer is one in eight (12.5%), this reflects the risk of a child just born developing breast cancer during her lifetime. Risks of developing breast cancer over the next ten years for women of any age are substantially lower (i.e., 2.5% for a 50-year-old woman).

The incidence of breast cancer rose progressively in the latter half of the 20th century, but appears to have stabilized since the 1990s. The rise in breast cancer mirrored the lifestyle changes in our country, with delayed pregnancies, fewer pregnancies, and the concomitant improved nutritional status of our society, influencing earlier menarche and later menopause. We have recently witnessed a national decline in breast cancer mortality associated with increasing use of mammography and improved breast cancer treatment. Between 1990 and 1997, breast cancer death rates decreased approximately 2% per year and are expected to continue in this pattern for some time to come.

The principal goal of the editor and authors of *Breast Cancer: A Guide to Detection and Multidisciplinary Therapy* is to produce a work that is both concise and clinically focused, but nevertheless provides the reader, regardless of level of expertise, with up-to-date information on the latest treatment standards and outcomes. Since breast cancer management is one of the most continually evolving areas of oncology practice, the authors have sought to address some of the current controversies, including breast conserving surgery without radiation therapy, sentinel node mapping, and bone marrow transplantation, among others. Their purpose here is not to resolve the controversial issues, but to provide the reader with the rationale for the treatment approaches as well as the robustness of the data supporting their use.

The great strength of the book is its multidisciplinary format. In virtually all aspects of cancer treatment, optimal cancer management is becoming a coordinated effort among multiple experts. *Breast Cancer: A Guide to Detection and Multidisciplinary Therapy* seeks to gather expertise from a wide array of oncology disciplines to provide the reader with a broad and balanced perspective on the optimal management of breast cancer.

One of the remarkable and somewhat unique aspects of breast cancer is the intense involvement of patients, survivors, and family members in the quest for progress. More has been written, discussed, and debated about breast cancer treatment than about any other single cancer. In this discussion, breast cancer patients have become educated, informed, and active in seeking optimal care. They come to physicians as the most broadly knowledgeable about the disease of any cancer patients. They ask important and penetrating questions. Many of the answers to their questions are found in this book.

Robert C. Young, MD
President, Fox-Chase Cancer Center
President, American Cancer Society

Preface

Breast Cancer: A Guide to Detection and Multidisciplinary Therapy offers comprehensive coverage of the multidisciplinary management of patients with breast cancer. Breast cancer is the most common noncutaneous malignancy of women. Fortunately, the incidence of breast cancer in the United States has begun to decline in the past few years and its diagnosis is being made at increasingly earlier stages. Nevertheless, this cancer causes especially devastating effects not only because of the typical burdens associated with cancer, but also because of its strong emotional, social, and family stresses. Multidisciplinary evaluation and treatment of those with breast cancer is essential to provide optimal management of these patients.

Breast Cancer: A Guide to Detection and Multidisciplinary Therapy is designed as a concise, clinically relevant state-of-the-art book composed by experts in the clinical, research, and epidemiologic aspects of breast cancer. Part I presents comprehensive diagnostic and management aspects of treating breast cancer patients from a multidisciplinary, clinical perspective. Epidemiologic and genetic development of breast cancer, diagnostic breast imaging, surgical biopsy, oncologic treatment options, radiation oncology rationale and techniques, and systemic therapies are clearly elucidated. In Part II, special clinical situations are addressed, including adjuvant chemotherapy, axillary adenopathy as initial presentation, breast cancer during pregnancy, local/regional recurrence, nipple discharge, and miscellaneous tumors of the breast. Finally, Part III provides a current review of controversies and areas of clinical research in breast cancer. Clinical issues such as breast-conserving surgery without radiation therapy, axillary lymph node management, the role of sentinel lymph node mapping and biopsy, management of internal mammary lymph nodes, transplantation, immunotherapy, and gene therapy are discussed, along with their potential implications to alter the management of breast cancer patients in the future.

The goal of *Breast Cancer: A Guide to Detection and Multidisciplinary Therapy* is to provide a comprehensive and clinically relevant paradigm for treating the breast cancer patient. The multidisciplinary approach evident throughout this book should appeal to surgeons, medical oncologists, radiation oncologists, gynecologists, primary care physicians, gerontologists, and all other physicians and health care personnel involved in the management of the breast cancer patient.

Michael H. Torosian, MD, FACS

Contents

Foreword, **Robert C. Young**, MD v

Preface vii

Contributors xi

I CLINICAL MANAGEMENT

1 Epidemiology and Clinical Risk Factors 3
   Mary B. Daly, MD, PhD

2 Breast Imaging 19
   Julia A. Birnbaum, MD, and Emily F. Conant, MD

3 Breast Biopsy Techniques 71
   Lisa A. Newman, MD, and Frederick C. Ames, MD

4 Clinical Classifications of Breast Cancer 81
   Michael H. Torosian, MD, FACS

5 Breast-Conserving Surgery:
   Lumpectomy With or Without Axillary Dissection 89
   Samuel W. Beenken, MD, and Kirby I. Bland, MD

6 Mastectomy 99
   David R. Brenin, MD, and David W. Kinne, MD

7 Breast Reconstruction 111
   Louis P. Bucky, MD, and Gary A. Tuma, MD

8 Radiation Therapy 129
   Barbara Fowble, MD, and Gary Freedman, MD

9 Chemotherapy in Breast Cancer 145
   Michael P. Russin, MD, and Lori J. Goldstein, MD

10 Hormonal Therapy of Breast Cancer 161
   Halle C. F. Moore, MD, and Kevin R. Fox, MD

11 The Role of Surgery for Metastatic Breast Cancer 175
   Lori Jardines, MD

12 Male Breast Cancer 183
   Mahmoud El-Tamer, MD, FACS, and Lucy J. Kim, MD

13 Oncogenes in the Development of Breast Cancer 193
   *Xiao Tan Qiao, MD, Kenneth L. van Golen, PhD,
   and Sofia D. Merajver, MD, PhD*

II SPECIAL CLINICAL SITUATIONS

14 Primary Chemotherapy 213
   Deborah L. Toppmeyer, MD

15   Axillary Adenopathy as the Initial Presentation of Breast Cancer 227
     Shirley Scott, MD, and Monica Morrow, MD

16   Breast Cancer During Pregnancy 235
     Mary L. Gemignani, MD, and Jeanne A. Petrek, MD

17   Local-Regional Recurrence in Breast Cancer 245
     Thomas J. Kearney, MD, FACS, and David A. August, MD, FACS

18   Nipple Discharge 255
     Marcia Boraas, MD

19   Sarcoma and Lymphoma of the Breast:
     Presentation, Diagnosis, and Treatment 263
     Helena Chang, MD, PhD, and Jane Kakkis, MD

III CURRENT CONTROVERSIES AND RESEARCH

20   Breast Conservation Without Radiation Therapy
     for Carcinoma of the Breast 273
     Gordon F. Schwartz, MD, MBA

21   Axillary Node Dissection in Breast Cancer 285
     James F. Pingpank, Jr., MD, and Elin R. Sigurdson, MD, PhD

22   Internal Mammary Lymph Nodes: *Management and Other Controversies* 295
     James C. Watson, MD, and John P. Hoffman, MD

23   High-Dose Chemotherapy and Autologous Stem Cell Transplantation
     for Breast Cancer 313
     Edward A. Stadtmauer, MD

24   Immunotherapy and Gene Therapy for Breast Cancer 325
     Daniela Santoli, PhD, and Sophie Visonneau, PhD

     Index 343

Contributors

FREDERICK C. AMES, MD, *Department of Surgical Oncology, University of Texas M.D. Anderson Cancer Center, Houston, TX*

DAVID A. AUGUST, MD, FACS, *Division of Surgical Oncology, UMDNJ-Robert Wood Johnson Medical School, The Cancer Institute of New Jersey, New Brunswick, NJ*

SAMUEL W. BEENKEN, MD, *Comprehensive Cancer Center, University of Alabama at Birmingham, Birmingham, AL*

JULIA A. BIRNBAUM, MD, *Hospital of The University of Pennsylvania, Philadelphia, PA*

KIRBY I. BLAND, MD, *Comprehensive Cancer Center, University of Alabama at Birmingham, Birmingham, AL*

MARCIA BORAAS, MD, *Department of Surgical Oncology, Fox Chase Cancer Center, Philadelphia, PA*

DAVID R. BRENIN, MD, *Department of Surgery, Columbia-Presbyterian Medical Center, New York, NY*

LOUIS P. BUCKY, MD, *Division of Plastic Surgery, University of Pennsylvania School of Medicine, Philadelphia, PA*

HELENA CHANG, MD, PhD, *Revlon/UCLA Breast Center, Los Angeles, CA*

EMILY F. CONANT, MD, *Hospital of The University of Pennsylvania, Philadelphia, PA*

MARY B. DALY, MD, PhD, *Fox Chase Cancer Center, Philadelphia, PA*

MAHMOUD EL-TAMER, MD, FACS, *Department of Surgery, Columbia-Presbyterian Medical Center, New York, NY*

BARBARA FOWBLE, MD, *Department of Radiation Oncology, Fox Chase Cancer Center, Philadelphia, PA*

KEVIN R. FOX, MD, *Division of Hematology-Oncology, University of Pennsylvania School of Medicine, Philadelphia, PA*

GARY FREEDMAN, MD, *Department of Radiation Oncology, Fox Chase Cancer Center, Philadelphia, PA*

MARY L. GEMIGNANI, MD, *Breast Service, Department of Surgery, Memorial Sloan-Kettering Cancer Center, New York, NY*

LORI J. GOLDSTEIN, MD, *Division of Population Science, Fox Chase Cancer Center, Philadelphia, PA*

JOHN P. HOFFMAN, MD, *Department of Surgical Oncology, Fox Chase Cancer Center, Philadelphia, PA*

LORI JARDINES, MD, *The Breast Center, Medical College of Pennsylvania Hospital, Philadelphia, PA*

JANE KAKKIS, MD, *UCLA School of Medicine, Los Angeles, CA*

THOMAS J. KEARNEY, MD, FACS, *Division of Surgical Oncology, UMDNJ-Robert Wood Johnson Medical School, The Cancer Institute of New Jersey, New Brunswick, NJ*

DAVID W. KINNE, MD, *Department of Surgery, College of Physicians & Surgeons, Columbia University, New York, NY*

LUCY J. KIM, MD, *Department of Surgery, Columbia-Presbyterian Medical Center, New York, NY*

SOFIA D. MERAJVER, MD, PhD, *Department of Internal Medicine, Comprehensive Cancer Center, University of Michigan Health Center, Ann Arbor, MI*

HALLE C. F. MOORE, MD, *Division of Hematology-Oncology, University of Pennsylvania School of Medicine, Philadelphia, PA*

MONICA MORROW, MD, *Department of Surgery, Northwestern University Medical School, Chicago, IL*

LISA A. NEWMAN, MD, *Department of Surgery, The University of Texas M.D. Anderson Cancer Center, Houston, TX*

JEANNE A. PETREK, MD, *Breast Service, Department of Surgery, Memorial Sloan-Kettering Cancer Center, New York, NY*

JAMES F. PINGPANK, JR., MD, *Fox Chase Cancer Center, Philadelphia, PA*

XIAO TAN QIAO, MD, *Department of Internal Medicine, Comprehensive Cancer Center, University of Michigan Health Center, Ann Arbor, MI*

MICHAEL P. RUSSIN, MD, *Fox Chase Cancer Center, Philadelphia, PA*

DANIELA SANTOLI, PhD, *The Wistar Institute, Philadelphia, PA*

GORDON F. SCHWARTZ, MD, MBA, *Department of Surgery, Jefferson Medical College, and the Breast Health Institute, Philadelphia, PA*

SHIRLEY SCOTT, MD, *Department of Surgery, Northwestern University Medical School, Chicago, IL*

ELIN R. SIGURDSON, MD, PhD, *Department of Surgery, Fox Chase Cancer Center, Philadelphia, PA*

EDWARD A. STADTMAUER, MD, *Bone Marrow and Stem Cell Transplant Program, University of Pennsylvania Cancer Center, Philadelphia, PA*

DEBORAH L. TOPPMEYER, MD, *The Cancer Institute of New Jersey, New Brunswick, NJ*

MICHAEL H. TOROSIAN, MD, FACS, *Department of Surgical Oncology, Fox Chase Cancer Center, Philadelphia, PA*

GARY A. TUMA, MD, *Division of Plastic Surgery, University of Pennsylvania School of Medicine, Philadelphia, PA*

KENNETH L. VAN GOLEN, PhD, *Department of Internal Medicine, Comprehensive Cancer Center, University of Michigan Health Center, Ann Arbor, MI*

SOPHIE VISONNEAU, PhD, *The Wistar Institute, Philadelphia, PA,*

JAMES C. WATSON, MD, *Department of Surgical Oncology, Fox Chase Cancer Center, Philadelphia, PA*

I

CLINICAL MANAGEMENT

1

Epidemiology and Clinical Risk Factors

Mary B. Daly, MD, PhD

CONTENTS

INTRODUCTION
GENERAL FEATURES
EPIDEMIOLOGIC RISK FACTORS
GENETIC RISK FACTORS
REFERENCES

1. INTRODUCTION

Breast cancer remains the most common cancer among women in the United States, and the second leading cause of death due to cancer, with approximately 43,300 deaths expected a year. After decades of increasing incidence rates, data from the Surveillance, Epidemiology, and End Results (SEER) program indicate a plateau in rates of new cases between 1990 and 1996 and a shift in stage from regional and distant stages to more localized disease *(1)*. Over the same period, breast cancer death rates have declined (on average) by 1.7% a year *(2)* (Fig. 1). Despite these recent promising trends, breast cancer represents a significant personal and societal burden that affects women in the prime of their lives and accounts for a large portion of the health care budget. A long history of classical epidemiologic studies, now coupled with the new information emerging from the field of molecular genetics, is beginning to elucidate the basic mechanisms of breast carcinogenesis and allow development of novel treatment and prevention strategies.

2. GENERAL FEATURES

2.1. Age

The risk of developing breast cancer increases throughout a woman's lifetime, and the disease is relatively rare in very young women. Rates begin to rise steeply at age 45 *(3)* (Fig. 2). Despite the lower rates for young, premenopausal women, those whose cancer is diagnosed before age 35 are more likely to be carriers of a breast cancer susceptibility gene and to present with higher grade tumors and more advanced stages, and to experience a more biologically aggressive form of the disease, which results in decreased disease-free and overall survival rates *(4,5)*. The overall association of breast cancer incidence with increasing age is consistent with a stochastic model of breast cancer, wherein a progressive series of genetic changes within the cell is necessary for the evolution of the molecular changes leading to cancer initiation. It is

From: *Current Clinical Oncology:*
Breast Cancer: A Guide to Detection and Multidisciplinary Therapy
Edited by: M. H. Torosian © Humana Press Inc., Totowa, NJ

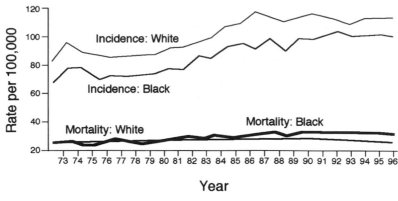

American Cancer Society, Surveillance Research, 1999
Data from SEER, 1999 and NCHS, 1999

Fig. 1. Incidence and mortality Surveillance, Epidemiology, and End Results (SEER) data indicating that during the period 1990–1996, breast cancer death rates declined by an average of 1.7% a year. (Data from refs. *1* and 2.)

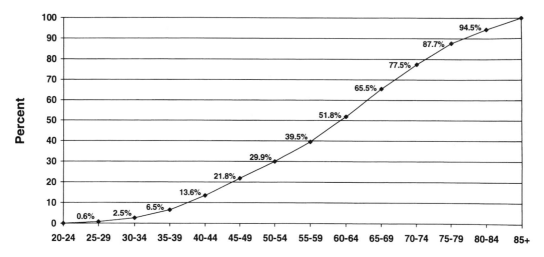

Fig. 2. Distribution of breast cancer diagnoses by age for the period 1987–1989 indicates that the rates begin to rise steeply at age 45. (From ref. *3.*)

becoming increasingly clear that these genetic changes are the result of a multitude of risk-related factors.

2.2. Race/Ethnicity

There are striking racial/ethnic differences in both the incidence and mortality rates for breast cancer. Overall, rates are highest for Caucasian women, lowest for Native American and Korean women, and intermediate for African-American, other Asian, and Hispanic women *(6)* (Fig. 3). An interesting crossover phenomenon occurs among African-American women, with rates for women under age 40 significantly higher than those seen in young Caucasian women, while the opposite is seen in women over age 40 *(7).* Temporal differences among groups also exist, the most notable being the dispropor-

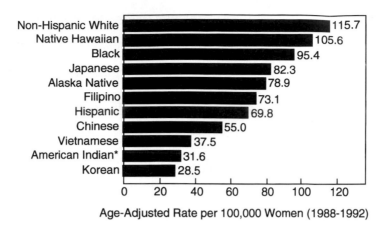

Fig. 3. Breast cancer incidence patterns by race and ethnicity in the United States. (From ref. 6.)

tionate increment in incidence rates seen among Hispanic women over the last 30 years *(8).* Epidemiologic studies have also consistently noted increased rates of breast cancer among Jewish women, an observation most likely explained by the recent identification of mutations in the *BRCA1/2* genes that are more prevalent among individuals of Ashkenazi Jewish descent.

2.3. Country of Origin

The general international pattern of breast cancer incidence reveals higher rates for Western, industrialized nations and lower rates for less industrialized and Asian countries *(9)* (Fig. 4). Furthermore, breast cancer incidence rates increase in migrants as they move from low-risk to high-risk countries *(10).* These significant differences are thought to be attributable to variations in important risk factors such as reproductive practices, diet, and perhaps genetic heterogeneity. Although the long-term trend in increasing mortality rates for breast cancer has begun to be reversed in some countries, the trend is not universal, and mortality rates continue to rise in Italy, Japan, and other less industrialized nations *(9).*

Even within the United States, there is significant geographic diversity in breast cancer rates, with mortality rates highest in the Northeast and lowest in the South *(11).* Most of this variation is thought to be caused by regional differences in breast cancer risk factors, although a number of ongoing studies are examining the possibility of environmental hazards in high-risk areas *(12).*

3. EPIDEMIOLOGIC RISK FACTORS

3.1. Hormonal Risk Factors

One of the most consistent epidemiologic observations is the association of reproductive factors with risk of breast cancer. The first observation noted was the increased risk for breast cancer documented among nulliparous women. Not only was it noted that parous women have a decreased risk for breast cancer, but it was also observed that the degree of protection afforded by pregnancy depends on the age at time of first live birth (FLB), with the greatest protection seen among women whose first full-term pregnancy occurred before age 20. In fact, when the FLB is delayed to age 35 or older, the risk for breast cancer equals or exceeds that of a nulliparous woman. The addition of subsequent pregnancies

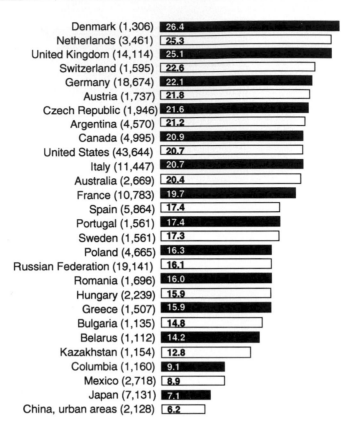

Denmark (1,306) 26.4
Netherlands (3,461) 25.3
United Kingdom (14,114) 25.1
Switzerland (1,595) 22.6
Germany (18,674) 22.1
Austria (1,737) 21.8
Czech Republic (1,946) 21.6
Argentina (4,570) 21.2
Canada (4,995) 20.9
United States (43,644) 20.7
Italy (11,447) 20.7
Australia (2,669) 20.4
France (10,783) 19.7
Spain (5,864) 17.4
Portugal (1,561) 17.4
Sweden (1,561) 17.3
Poland (4,665) 16.3
Russian Federation (19,141) 16.1
Romania (1,696) 16.0
Hungary (2,239) 15.9
Greece (1,507) 15.9
Bulgaria (1,135) 14.8
Belarus (1,112) 14.2
Kazakhstan (1,154) 12.8
Columbia (1,160) 9.1
Mexico (2,718) 8.9
Japan (7,131) 7.1
China, urban areas (2,128) 6.2

Fig. 4. Age-standardized (world) breast cancer mortality rates per 100,000 women (in bars) for 1995, 1994[a], or 1993[b] and number of deaths (in parentheses) in areas with more than 1,000 deaths annually (source: World Health Organization database). (From Mettlin C (1999) Global breast cancer mortality statistics. *CA* **49,** 138–144. With permission from Lippincott Williams & Wilkins.)

and/or lactation add little to the protection associated with the FLB. By causing breast epithelial cells to become fully differentiated and mature, and thus less likely to undergo further mitoses, an early full-term pregnancy is thought to protect the cells from subsequent genotoxic events that may initiate the carcinogenic process. An alternative hypothesis is that pregnancy modifies age-related changes in plasma estrogen levels.

The total length of menstruation during a woman's lifetime contributes to risk. Both early age at menarche and late age at menopause are associated with an increased risk (Table 1). On the other hand, risk for breast cancer is significantly decreased among women undergoing surgical oophorectomy, particularly if the surgery is performed before age 35 years *(13)*. The relevance of these findings is the importance of the length of ovarian activity and the duration of exposure to ovarian hormones in the promotion of breast cancer. This is further supported by the modest increase in risk associated with both postmenopausal estrogen replacement therapy, particularly when the duration of use exceeds 15 years *(14),* and exposure to diethylstilbestrol (DES) during pregnancy *(15)*. The risk associated with the use of oral contraceptives appears to be negligible, which suggests that the risk of exposure to exogenous estrogens may vary during different stages of life.

An association between premature termination of pregnancy and subsequent risk of breast cancer has been observed in some epidemiologic case-control studies *(16)*. There is some biologic plausibility to support this observation in that a pregnancy that is terminated early

Table 1
Breast Cancer Risks Associated
with Hormonal Factors

Risk factor	Relative risk
Age at menarche *(14)*	
≤12	3.7
>13	1.6
Age at menopause *(21)*	
≤45	1.0
≥55	2.0
Years of use of estrogen replacement therapy *(22)*	
0	1.0
<5	0.9
5–9	1.1
10–14	1.3
15–19	1.2
≥20	1.5

may leave the breast epithelial tissue in an indeterminant state of proliferation without reaching full maturation. These studies, however, are fraught with design flaws, particularly that of recall bias. A recent cohort study from Denmark showed no association between induced abortion and breast cancer risk *(17)*.

The approach of correlating serum, plasma, or urinary levels of endogenous sex hormones or sex hormone-binding globulins with cancer rates has produced conflicting results. However, the Nurses' Health Study has prospectively evaluated relationships between plasma sex steroid hormone levels and breast cancer risk and has found statistically significant positive associations for circulating levels of estradiol, estrone, estrone sulfate, prolactin, and dehydroepiandrosterone sulfate *(18,19)*. Other investigators are examining the intermediate metabolic pathways of endogenous hormones that may have more significance at the level of the end organ *(20)*.

Although the complex set of interactions that determine breast cancer risk are incompletely known, the significant body of data linking factors associated with reproductive hormones to breast cancer incidence has led to the proposal that endogenous sex hormones are major determinants of breast cancer risk and that the role of other factors, including genetic polymorphisms, environmental exposures and lifestyle events may be in the modulation or metabolism of estrogen, progesterone, and/or androgenic hormones *(21,22)*. Furthermore, the data suggest that there is differential susceptibility of breast tissue to the adverse effects of hormone exposure, with the highest vulnerability found among less differentiated cells during periods of rapid growth and the lowest vulnerability seen in cells that have undergone complete maturation during a full-term pregnancy. In this model, the initiation of cancer is seen as a multifactorial event, depending on the stage of development of the breast, the hormonal environment, the genetic susceptibility, and the presence or absence of modifying factors.

3.2. Diet

The weight of epidemiologic data from international comparisons, migration studies, and time trends supports an important role for dietary fat in the etiology of breast cancer.

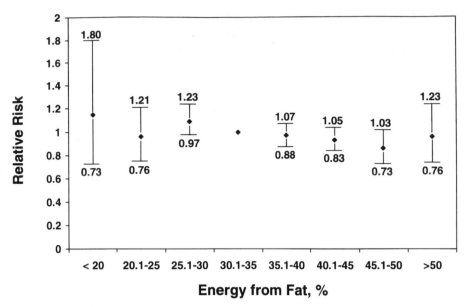

Fig. 5. Relative risk of breast cancer by percentage of energy derived from dietary fat. (Data from ref. *24.*)

International rates, for example, show a fivefold difference in breast cancer incidence between countries with the highest and lowest fat intake *(23)*. Animal studies have shown an association between mammary cancer and both dietary fat and total caloric intake *(14)*. Several case-control studies have also found a strong positive association between breast cancer risk and self-reported fat intake, particularly in postmenopausal women. Cohort studies, which have a stronger power to detect a causal association, however, have had mixed results. The Nurses' Health Study, for instance, found no association between total dietary fat intake and breast cancer incidence, after an 8-year follow-up *(24)* (Fig. 5). The data on fiber and micronutrients are even more contradictory. Recently, interest in the relationship between dietary components and breast cancer has shifted to the role of phytoestrogens, plant compounds that are structurally similar to endogenous estrogens with mixed estrogenic/antiestrogenic effects. Vegetarian and macrobiotic diets, more typical of diets in countries where breast cancer incidence is low, are thought to contain higher levels of phytoestrogens. It is postulated that isoflavones in phytoestrogens may act as antiestrogens and bind to estrogen receptors, thus reducing estrogen induction of breast cell proliferation.

What has also emerged from the dietary studies is a fairly consistent but weak association of breast cancer risk and moderate to heavy alcohol consumption. Data from the first National Health and Nutrition Examination Survey (NHANES I), for example, demonstrated a dose-response relationship between alcohol consumption and breast cancer risk, with relative risks ranging from 1.4 to 2.0 as intake level rises *(25)*. A number of confounding factors associated with the use of alcohol, however, may account for some of the association seen.

Another approach to the study of diet and cancer risk is to examine the association of body weight, or the prevalence of obesity, with cancer incidence. In general, body weight has been positively correlated with both breast cancer incidence and mortality, although the association is confined to postmenopausal women, among whom incidence rates increase with age more rapidly among overweight than among lean women. Proposed mechanisms include the increased availability of endogenous estrogens by conversion of adrostenedione, derived from the adrenal gland, to estrone in adipose tissue, and/or alterations in the distribution of steroid hormones in the plasma produced by dietary fat intake *(26)*. A recent metaanalysis of dietary fat intervention studies provides evidence for a significant reduction in estradiol levels among postmenopausal women whose fat intake was reduced to 10–12% *(27)*.

Finally, limited data support a protective role for physical activity (both during leisure time and at work), and breast cancer risk *(28)*. The effect is most pronounced among premenopausal and younger postmenopausal women. The known association of vigorous physical activity with decreased circulating levels of ovarian hormones may provide a plausible biologic mechanism to explain this finding, which could have significant public health implications.

3.3. Radiation Exposure

Observations of women exposed to the Hiroshima and Nagasaki atomic bombs have documented an association between radiation exposure and subsequent risk for breast cancer. These findings are substantiated by the increased risk experienced by women exposed to multiple fluoroscopies for the treatment of tuberculosis, to diagnostic X-rays for the evaluation of scoliosis, to X-ray treatment for postpartum mastitis, and to mantle radiation for Hodgkin's disease *(29–31)*. The risk is greatest among women exposed during puberty and occurs after a latent period of 10–20 years *(21)*. Even women irradiated in infancy for an enlarged thymus appear to have a significant, dose-dependent risk for breast cancer 30 years after exposure *(32)*. These cancers tend to be bilateral, with a high frequency of intraductal disease *(33)*. There does not, however, appear to be any risk associated with routine diagnostic imaging or to employment as a radiologic technologist *(34)*.

3.4. Benign Breast Disease

Fibrocystic breast disease has often been cited as a risk factor for subsequent breast cancer. However, careful evaluation of histologic patterns of benign disease have identified those groups in whom the risk is truly elevated. In the largest retrospective cohort study published, Dupont and Page *(35)* reevaluated more than 10,000 consecutive biopsies performed over almost two decades and correlated histologic pattern with subsequent incidence of breast cancer. Women undergoing breast biopsies whose tissue show no evidence of proliferation have no increase in the relative risk of breast cancer. Risk increases from 1.4 to 4.4 with the degree of proliferation and atypia seen in the biopsy specimen. There also appears to be an interaction between the presence of proliferative breast disease and family and reproductive history, with relative risk increasing to as high as 8.0 in the setting of a positive family history, nulliparity, or late age at first birth, suggesting that the proliferative process itself is affected by other risk factors *(35)*. Data from this series also identified sclerosing adenosis and fibroadenoma as independent risk factors for invasive disease, with relative risks in the 1.5–2.0 range *(36,37)*. Confirmatory evidence of these findings comes from the prospective Nurses' Health Study in which a prior diagnosis of atypical ductal hyperplasia or atypical lobular hyperplasia conferred odds ratios for subsequent breast cancer of 2.4 and 5.3, respectively *(38)*.

Lobular carcinoma *in situ* (LCIS) is the most common benign lesion to present as a multicentric and/or bilateral process and is often associated with sclerosing adenosis, stromal fibrosis, fat necrosis, duct ectasia, and fibroadenoma *(39)*. A diagnosis of LCIS increases the risk of subsequent breast cancer in either breast by a factor of four to nine times that of the general population and is thought to be a marker of proliferation rather than a premalignant

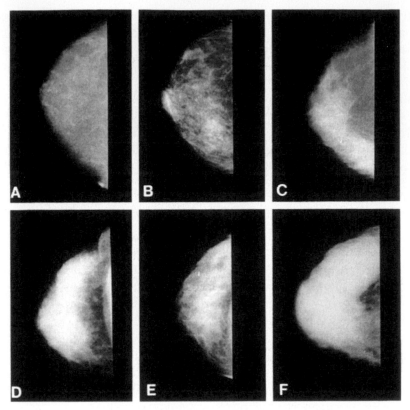

Fig. 6. Categories of breast density. **(A)** Density 0%. **(B)** Density < 10%. **(C)** Density 10% to < 25%. **(D)** Density 25% to < 50%. **(E)** Density 50% to < 75%. **(F)** Density ≥ 75%. (From ref. *44.*)

lesion itself *(21,40)*. The excess risk seen is highest for women who develop LCIS before the age of 40 years *(41)*.

3.5. Mammographic Density

A growing body of data suggests an association between the degree of mammographic density and risk for breast cancer, independent of other risk factors. In 1976, Wolfe *(42,43)* proposed a classification scheme of mammographic breast density with four categories, N1, P1, P2, and DY. In his initial studies, patterns P2 and DY, characterized by ductal and irregular densities, were associated with an increased risk of breast cancer. Since then several studies have explored the relationship between mammographic density and breast cancer risk, using a variety of classification schemes *(44)* (Figs. 6 and 7). The association of radiodensity with age, weight, reproductive factors, and ethnicity is unclear and may contribute to the contradictory findings. A nested case-control study from the Breast Cancer Detection Demonstration Project (BCDDP) data, however, found a linear association of increasing breast density and breast cancer risk, independent of other known risk factors *(45)*. Among participants in the Canadian National Breast Screening Study (NBSS), women with the most extensive densities on mammogram had a significantly increased risk of being diagnosed with atypical hyperplasia or carcinoma *in situ (46)*. Finally, segregation analysis in a cohort of women followed since 1944 indicates that the presence of at least one dominant gene may account for 29% of the variability of breast density seen in that population *(47)*. Preliminary

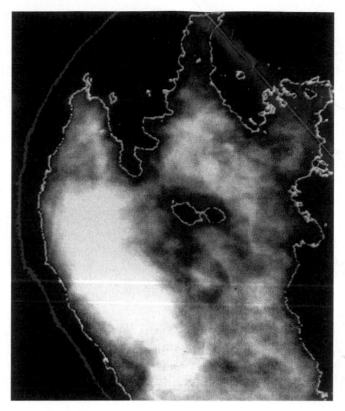

Fig. 7. Method used to measure mammographic features. Thick line, edge of breast; thin line, edge of dense tissue. (From ref. *44.*)

data from a randomized dietary intervention trial to reduce fat intake, conducted among women with extensive areas of radiographic density on mammogram, has shown a significant decrease in density associated with a reduction in total or saturated fat intake *(48)*. Further research in this area may offer new opportunities for risk reduction.

3.6. Occupation

The observation of increased risk of breast cancer among Catholic nuns, now known to be attributable to the confounding factor of nulliparity, was probably the first attempt to link risk of the disease to an occupation. Several studies that have subsequently sought to identify occupational risks for breast cancer have failed to detect specific and modifiable workplace exposures causally related to breast cancer. A number of significant associations between professional, managerial, and administrative positions and breast cancer have been found but are likely to be related to the association of occupational choices and other socioecomic, cultural, and lifestyle factors such as reproductive choices, diet, and physical activity *(49)*.

3.7. Environmental Factors

Concern about the excess of breast cancer in the industrialized and densely populated Northeastern portion of the country has led to a search for potential environmental hazards found in this geographic area. The organochlorine compounds used in pesticides have been a prime suspect because of their storage in adipose tissue, their estrogenic activity, and their conversion to highly reactive compounds *(50)*. An early series of small studies comparing serum levels of organochlorine compounds between cases and controls showed inconsistent results. More recent community-based studies with larger samples have failed to find increased serum or plasma levels of 1,1-dichloro-2,2-bis(p-chlorophenyl)ethylene (DDE) and polychlorinated biphenyls (PCBs) in women who subsequently developed breast cancer *(50–52)* or increased breast adipose tissue levels of hexachlorobenzene (HCB) and β-benzene hexachloride in newly diagnosed women *(53,54)*. Although additional studies are ongoing, there appears to be a growing consensus that exposure to pesticides does not account for the excess rates of breast cancer seen in certain geographic areas.

4. GENETIC RISK FACTORS

Even though most breast cancers are sporadic, no factor other than age alters the magnitude of risk more than a family history of the disease. Several epidemiologic studies have documented that a history of breast cancer in first-, second-, or third-degree relatives confers an increased risk of the disease of approximately two- to fourfold *(55)*. In a large population-based case-control study, the Cancer and Steroid Hormone (CASH) Study, the risk for breast cancer among women under the age of 45 was increased threefold if a mother or a sister had been diagnosed with breast cancer. The risk was particularly elevated among women with two or more affected first-degree relatives (odds ratio 21.68; 95% confidence interval 3.09–94.74) *(56)*. Prospective data from the Nurses' Health Study found that the relative risk of breast cancer was highest among women whose mother was diagnosed before the age of 40 *(57)*. Risk varies with age of onset of the affected relative and the number of affected relatives.

Although historically the contribution of the traditional reproductive risk factors (e.g., nulliparity) to the expression of hereditary breast cancer has been unclear, data from the Nurses' Health Study show little protection from late age at menarche, early age at first live birth, or multiparity among women with a family history of breast cancer *(58)*. Likewise, data from the Iowa Women's Health Study, a population-based longitudinal cohort study, suggested that the increased risk of breast cancer among sisters of postmenopausal breast cancer cases is independent of other risk factors *(59)*. The identification of a histologic pattern characterizing hereditary breast cancer has been elusive, although medullary carcinoma has been associated with younger age at onset. Claus et al. *(60)* and Rosen et al. *(61)* have noted an excess of medullary histology in multicase families. One consistent histologic finding has been the exponential increase in breast cancer risk in women diagnosed with atypical hyperplasia who also have a positive family history *(62)*. Clarification of these associations has recently been facilitated by the discovery of breast cancer susceptibility genes.

4.1. The BRCA1 and BRCA2 Genes

The clinical evidence of an autosomal dominant inherited predisposition to breast cancer has been supported by segregation analysis, a quantitative method to determine whether a particular trait is distributed in the population in a Mendelian manner of inheritance. Applied to the CASH data set, segregation analysis and goodness-of-fit tests of genetic models provided evidence for the existence of a rare autosomal dominant allele associated with increased susceptibility to breast cancer *(63)*. Approximately 5–10% of all breast cancer demonstrates an autosomal dominant pattern of inheritance. Hereditary breast cancer is characterized by early age at onset (5–15 years earlier than sporadic

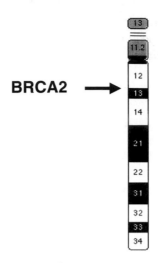

BRCA2 ⟶

Chromosome 13

Fig. 8. Location of *BRCA2* on chromosome 13.

cases), bilaterality, vertical transmission through both maternal and paternal lines, and association with tumors of other organs, particularly the ovary, colon, endometrium, and prostate gland *(64–66)*.

In 1990, a susceptibility gene for breast cancer was mapped by genetic linkage to the long arm of chromosome 17, in the interval 17q12–21 *(67)*. The linkage between breast cancer and genetic markers on chromosome 17q was soon confirmed by others, and evidence for the coincident transmission of both breast and ovarian cancer susceptibility in linked families was observed *(64)*. The *BRCA1* gene was subsequently identified by positional cloning methods and has been found to encode a protein of 1863 amino acids. This susceptibility gene appears to be responsible for disease in 45% of families with multiple cases of breast cancer only, and up to 90% of families with both breast and ovarian cancer *(68)*. A second breast cancer susceptibility gene, *BRCA2,* was localized through linkage studies of 15 families with multiple cases of breast cancer to the long arm of chromosome 13 (Fig. 8). Germline mutations in *BRCA2* are thought to account for approximately 35% of multiple case breast cancer families and are also associated with male breast cancer, ovarian cancer, prostate cancer, and pancreatic cancer *(69,70)*. The risk for breast cancer in female *BRCA2* mutation carriers appears similar to that for *BRCA1* carriers, but the age of onset is shifted to an older age distribution *(71)*.

Of the several hundred mutations described in these genes, most lead to a frameshift resulting in missing or nonfunctional proteins *(72)*. In addition, tumors from individuals with *BRCA1/2* mutations show deletion of the wild-type allele, supporting speculation that these genes play a role in tumor suppression. Both *BRCA1* and *BRCA2* are also involved in the control of meiotic and mitotic recombination and in the maintenance of genomic stability, suggesting an additional role in the DNA repair process *(73–75)*. In vitro models of *BRCA2*-deficient cell lines have demonstrated hypersensitivity to both radiation and chemotherapeutic agents that induce DNA breaks *(76,77)*. The growing body of data elucidating the functions of these genes suggests a gatekeeper role, characterized by interactions with other genes in the regulation of the cell cycle and DNA repair and may provide novel opportunities to develop genotype-based therapeutic approaches to treatment and prevention.

The frequency of mutations in *BRCA1* in the general population has been estimated to be 0.0006, which corresponds to a carrier frequency of 1 in 800. Carrier rates are not distributed evenly, however, and tend to concentrate in families with multiple cases of breast and/or breast/ovarian cancer. *BRCA1* and *BRCA2* also share differential prevalence rates in certain ethnic groups. Most notably, three specific mutations, the 185delAG mutation and the 5382insC mutation on *BRCA1* and the 6174delT mutation on *BRCA2,* have been found to be common in Ashkenazi Jews. The frequency of these three mutations approximates 1 in 40 in this population and accounts for up to 25% of early-onset breast cancer and up to 90% of families with both breast and ovarian cancer *(78).* Additional "founder effects" have been described in the Netherlands and in Iceland *(79,80).*

The actual expression of disease in gene mutation carriers, known as penetrance, is estimated to range from 36 to 85% for breast cancer and from 16 to 60% for ovarian cancer. Among female *BRCA1* carriers who have already developed a primary breast cancer, estimates for a second contralateral breast cancer are as high as 64% by age 70, and for ovarian cancer as high as 44% by age 70 *(81).* It is not known whether specific mutations confer differential rates of penetrance, or what other genetic and/or environmental/lifestyle factors may interact with the presence of a mutation to determine expressivity. Ongoing studies are addressing the role of reproductive factors, endogenous and exogenous hormone exposure, diet, and lifestyle factors in the modulation of risk among carriers.

The phenotypic expression of *BRCA1/2* breast cancer indicates distinctive pathologic features. Historically, medullary, tubular, and lobular histologies and improved survival have been associated with familial breast cancer *(82).* The Breast Cancer Linkage Consortium examined histopathologic features of breast cancer in women with *BRCA1/2* mutations and (compared with controls) showed an excess of high-grade tumors in *BRCA1* carriers and a relative lack of *in situ* components adjacent to invasive lesions *(83).* High mitotic and total grades, as well as higher rates of aneuploidy and high proliferative fractions, were also reported for *BRCA1* carriers in kindreds followed by Henry Lynch's group, who also noted higher rates of medullary histology *(84).* The phenotype for *BRCA2*-related tumors appears to be more heterogeneous and may include an excess of lobular histology *(85).* In accordance with the poor prognostic features noted histologically for *BRCA1*-related breast cancer, two European studies recently reported survival rates that were similar to or worse than sporadic cases, with a significantly increased risk of contralateral breast cancer *(86,87).*

4.2. Li-Fraumeni Syndrome

Breast cancer is also a component of the rare Li-Fraumeni syndrome in which germline mutations of the p53 gene on chromosome 17p have been documented *(88).* First reported by Bottomley and Condit *(89),* this syndrome is characterized by premenopausal breast cancer in combination with childhood sarcoma, brain tumors, leukemia and lymphoma, lung cancer, and adrenocortical carcinoma. A germline mutation in the p53 gene has been identified in over 50% of families exhibiting this syndrome, and inheritance is autosomal dominant with a penetrance of at least 50% by age 50. Although highly penetrant, the Li-Fraumeni gene is thought to account for less than 1% of breast cancer cases *(90).*

4.3. Other Factors

One of the more than 50 cancer-related genodermatoses, Cowden's syndrome, is characterized by an excess of breast cancer, gastrointestinal malignancies, and thyroid disease, both benign and malignant *(91)*. Skin manifestations include multiple trichilemmomas, oral fibromas and papillomas, and acral, palmar, and plantar keratoses. Germline mutations in PTEN, a protein tyrosine phosphatase with homology to tensin located on chromosome 10q23, are responsible for this syndrome. Loss of heterozygosity observed in a high proportion of related cancers suggests that PTEN functions as a tumor suppressor gene. Its defined enzymatic function indicates a role in maintenance of the control of cell proliferation *(92)*. Disruption of PTEN appears to occur late in tumorigenesis and may act as a regulatory molecule of cytoskeletal function. Although it accounts for a small fraction of hereditary breast cancer, the characterization of PTEN function will provide valuable insights into signal pathways and maintenance of normal cell physiology *(93)*.

Ataxia telangiectasia is an autosomal recessive disorder characterized by neurologic deterioration, telangiectasias, immunodeficiency states, and hypersensitivity to ionizing radiation. It is estimated that approximately 1% of the general population may be heterozygote carriers of the gene, which has been localized to chromosome 11q22–23 *(94)*. Ataxia telangiectasia cells are sensitive to ionizing radiation and radiomimetic drugs and lack cell cycle regulatory properties after exposure to radiation *(95)*. Several epidemiologic studies have suggested a statistically increased risk of breast cancer among female heterozygote carriers, with an estimated relative risk of 3.9 *(96)*. Given the high heterozygote carrier rate in the population, this association could account for a significant proportion of hereditary breast cancer and poses a potential risk related to diagnostic radiation exposure in these individuals.

The identification and location of these breast cancer genes will now permit further investigation of the precise role they play in cancer progression and will allow us to determine the percentage of total breast cancer caused by the inheritance of mutant genes. This in turn will ultimately enrich our understanding of all breast cancer, sporadic as well as hereditary, and will facilitate the identification of high-risk individuals.

REFERENCES

1. Chu KC, Tarone RE, Kessler LG, et al. (1996) Recent trends in U.S. breast cancer incidence, survival, and mortality rates. *J. Natl. Cancer Inst.* **88**, 1571–1579.
2. Wingo P, Ries L, Giovino G, et al. (1999) Annual report to the nation on the status of cancer, 1973–1996, with a special section on lung cancer and tobacco smoking. *J. Natl. Cancer Inst.* **91**, 675–690.
3. Hankey BF, Miller B, Curtis R, Kosary C (1994) Trends in breast cancer in younger women in contrast to older women. *Monogr. Natl. Cancer Inst.* **16**, 7–14.
4. Winchester D, Osteen R, Menck H (1996) The national cancer data base report on breast carcinoma characteristics and outcome in relation to age. *Cancer* **78**, 1838–1843.
5. De La Rochefordiere A, Asselain B, Campana F, et al. (1993) Age as prognostic factor in premenopausal breast carcinoma. *Lancet* **341**, 1039–1043.
6. Stat Bite (1996) Breast cancer incidence by race/ethnicity. *J. Natl. Cancer Inst.* **88**, 577.
7. Krieger N (1990) Social class and the black/white crossover in the age-specific incidence of breast cancer: a study linking census-derived data to population-based registry records. *Am. J. Epidemiol.* **131**, 804–814.
8. Eidson M, Becker T, Wiggins C, Key C, Samet J (1994) Breast cancer among Hispanics, American Indians and Non-Hispanic whites in New Mexico. *Int. J. Epidemiol.* **23**, 231–237.
9. Mettlin C (1999) Global breast cancer mortality statistics. *CA* **49**, 138–144.
10. Berg J (1984) Clinical implications of risk factors for breast cancer. *Cancer* **53**, 589–591.
11. National Cancer Institute (1999) *Atlas of Cancer Mortality in the United States, 1950–94*. NIH Publication No. 99–4564. NIH, Bethesda, MD, pp. 211–212.
12. Sturgeon S, Schairer C, Gail M, McAdams M, Brinton L, Hoover R (1995) Geographic variation in mortality from breast cancer among white women in the United States. *J. Natl. Cancer Inst.* **87**, 1846–1853.
13. MacMahon B, Cole P, Brown J (1973) Etiology of human breast cancer: a review. *J. Natl. Cancer Inst.* **50**, 21–42.
14. Henderson IC (1993) Risk factors for breast cancer development. *Cancer* (Suppl.) **71**, 2127–2140.

15. Colton T, Greenberg R, Noller K, et al. (1993) Breast cancer in mothers prescribed diethylstilbestrol in pregnancy. *JAMA* **269,** 2096–2100.
16. Rookus M, van Leeuwen F (1996) Induced abortion and risk for breast cancer: reporting (recall) bias in a Dutch case-control study. *J. Natl. Cancer Inst.* **88,** 1759–1764.
17. Melbye M, Wohlfahrt J, Olsen J, et al. (1997) Induced abortion and the risk of breast cancer. *N. Engl. J. Med.* **336,** 81–85.
18. Hankinson S, Willett W, Manson J, et al. (1998) Plasma sex steroid hormone levels and risk of breast cancer in postmenopausal women. *J. Natl. Cancer Inst.* **90,** 1292–1299.
19. Hankinson S, Willett W, Michaud D, et al. (1999) Plasma prolactin levels and subsequent risk of breast cancer in postmenopausal women. *J. Natl. Cancer Inst.* **91,** 629–634.
20. Michnovicz J, Bradlow H (1990) Induction of estradiol metabolism by dietary indole-3-carbinol in humans. *J. Natl. Cancer Inst.* **82,** 947–949.
21. Henderson IC (1990) What can a woman do about her risk of dying of breast cancer? *Curr. Probl. Cancer* **14,** 165–229.
22. Kelsey J, Berkowitz G (1988) Breast cancer epidemiology. *Cancer Res.* **48,** 5615–5623.
23. Greenwald P, Kramer B, Weed D (1993) Expanding horizons in breast and prostate cancer prevention and early detection. *J. Cancer Educ.* **8,** 91–107.
24. Holmes MD, Hunter DJ, Colditz GA, et al. (1999) Association of dietary intake of fat and fatty acids with risk of breast cancer. *JAMA* **281,** 914–920.
25. Schatzkin A, Jones Y, Hoover R, et al. (1987) Alcohol consumption and breast cancer in the epidemiologic follow-up study of the first National Health and Nutrition Examination Survey. *N. Engl. J. Med.* **316,** 1169–1173.
26. Reed MJ, Beranek PA, Cheng RW, McNeill JM, James VH (1987) Peripheral oestrogen metabolism in postmenopausal women with or without breast cancer: the role of dietary lipids and growth factors. *J. Steroid Biochem.* **27,** 985–989.
27. Wu A, Pike M, Stram D (1999) Meta-analysis: dietary fat intake, serum estrogen levels, and the risk of breast cancer. *J. Natl. Cancer Inst.* **91,** 529–534.
28. Thune I, Brenn T, Lund E, Gaard M (1997) Physical activity and the risk of breast cancer. *N. Engl. J. Med.* **336,** 1269–1275.
29. Aisenberg A, Finkelstein D, Doppke K, Koerner F, Boivin J, Willett C (1997) High risk of breast carcinoma after irradiation of young women with Hodgkin's disease. *Cancer* **79,** 1203–1210.
30. Miller A, Howe G, Sherman G, et al. (1989) Mortality from breast cancer after irradiation during fluoroscopic examinations in patients being treated for tuberculosis. *N. Engl. J. Med.* **321,** 1285–1289.
31. Hoffman D, Lonstein J, Morin M, Visscher W, Harris B, Boice J (1989) Breast cancer in women with scoliosis exposed to multiple diagnostic X rays. *J. Natl. Cancer Inst.* **81,** 1307–1312.
32. Hildreth N, Shore R, Dvoretsky P (1989) The risk of breast cancer after irradiation of the thymus in infancy. *N. Engl. J. Med.* **321,** 1281–1284.
33. Anderson N, Lokich J (1990) Bilateral breast cancer after cured Hodgkin's disease. *Cancer* **65,** 221–223.
34. Boice J, Mandel J, Doody M (1995) Breast cancer among radiologic technologists. *JAMA* **274,** 394–401.
35. Dupont W, Page D (1987) Breast cancer risk associated with proliferative disease, age at first birth, and a family history of breast cancer. *Am. J. Epidemiol.* **125,** 769–779.
36. Jensen R, Page D, Dupont W, Rogers L (1989) Invasive breast cancer risk in women with sclerosing adenosis. *Cancer* **64,** 1977–1983.
37. Dupont W, Page D, Parl F, et al. (1994) Long-term risk of breast cancer in women with fibroadenoma. *N. Engl. J. Med.* **331,** 10–15.
38. Marshall L, Hunter D, Connolly J, et al. (1997) Risk of breast cancer associated with atypical hyperplasia of lobular and ductal types. *Cancer Epidemiol. Biomarkers Prev.* **6,** 297–301.
39. Osborne M, Hoda S (1994) Current management of lobular carcinoma in situ of the breast. *Oncology* **8,** 45–49.
40. Hutter R (1982) Lobular carcinoma in situ. *CA* **32,** 231–2.
41. Bodian C, Perzin K, Lattes R (1996) Lobular neoplasia, long term risk of breast cancer and relation to other factors. *Cancer* **78,** 1024–1034.
42. Wolfe J (1976) Risk for breast cancer development determined by mammographic parenchymal pattern. *Cancer* **37,** 2486–2492.
43. Wolfe J (1976) Breast patterns as an index of risk for developing breast cancer. *AJR* **126,** 1130–1139.
44. Boyd N, Lockwood G, Byng J, Trichtler D, Yaffe M (1998) Mammographic densities and breast cancer risk. *Cancer Epidemiol. Biomarkers Prev.* **7,** 1133–1144.
45. Byrne C, Schairer C, Wolfe J, et al. (1995) Mammographic features and breast cancer risk: effects with time, age, and menopause status. *J. Natl. Cancer Inst.* **87,** 1622–1629.

46. Boyd N, Jensen H, Cooke G, Han H (1992) Relationship between mammographic and histological risk factors for breast cancer. *J. Nalt. Cancer Inst.* **84,** 1170–1179.
47. Pankow J, Vachon C, Kuni C, et al. (1997) Genetic analysis of mammographic breast density in adult women: evidence of a gene effect. *J. Natl. Cancer Inst.* **89,** 549–556.
48. Knight J, Martin L, Greenberg C, et al. (1999) Macronutrient intake and change in mammographic density at menopause: results from a randomized trial. *Cancer Epidemiol. Biomarkers Prev.* **8,** 123–128.
49. Zheng W, Shu X, McLaughlin J, Chow W, Gao Y, Blot W (1993) Occupational physical activity and the incidence of cancer of the breast, corpus uteri, and ovary in Shanghai. *Cancer* **71,** 3620–3624.
50. Helzlsouer K, Alberg A, Huang H, et al. (1999) Serum concentrations of organochlorine compounds and the subsequent development of breast cancer. *Cancer Epidemiol. Biomarkers Prev.* **8,** 525–532.
51. Krieger N, Wolff M, Hiatt R, Rivera M, Vogelman J, Orentreich N (1994) Breast cancer and serum organochlorines: a prospective study among white, black and Asian women. *J. Natl. Canser Inst.* **86,** 589–599.
52. Hunter D, Hankinson S, Laden F, et al. (1997) Plasma organochlorine levels and the risk of breast cancer. *N. Engl. J. Med.* **337,** 1253–1258.
53. Zheng T, Holford T, Mayne S, et al. (1999) Environmental exposure to hexachlorobenzene (HCB) and risk of female breast cancer in Connecticut. *Cancer Epidemiol. Biomarkers Prev.* **8,** 407–411.
54. Zheng T, Holford T, Mayne S, et al. (1999) β-Benzene hexachloride in breast adipose tissue and risk of breast carcinoma. *Cancer* **85,** 2212–2218.
55. Horn–Ross PL (1993) Multiple primary cancers involving the breast. *Epidemiol. Rev.* **15,** 169–176.
56. Thompson WD (1994) Genetic epidemiology of breast cancer. *Cancer* **74,** 279–287.
57. Colditz GA, Willett WC, Hunter DJ, et al. (1993) Family history, age, and risk of breast cancer. *JAMA* **270,** 338–343.
58. Colditz GA, Rosner BA, Speizer FE for the Nurses' Health Study Research Group (1996) Risk factors for breast cancer according to family history of breast cancer. *J. Natl. Cancer Inst.* **88,** 365–371.
59. Chen P-L, Sellers TA, Rich SS, Potter JD, Folsom AR (1994) Examination of the effect of nongenetic risk factors on the familial risk of breast cancer among relatives of postmenopausal breast cancer patients. *Cancer Epidemiol. Biomarkers Prev.* **3,** 549–555.
60. Claus EB, Risch N, Thompson WD, Carter D (1993) Relationship between breast histopathology and family history of breast cancer. *Cancer* **71,** 147–153.
61. Rosen PP, Lesser ML, Senie RT, Kinne DW (1982) Epidemiology of breast carcinoma III: relationship of family history to tumor type. *Cancer* **50,** 171–179.
62. DuPont W, Page D (1985) Risk factors for breast cancer in women with proliferative breast disease. *N. Engl. J. Med.* **312,** 146.
63. Claus EB, Risch N, Thompson WD (1991) Genetic analysis of breast cancer in the cancer and steroid hormone study. *Am. J. Hum. Genet.* **48,** 232–242.
64. Narod S, Feunteun J, Lynch H, et al. (1991) Familial breast-ovarian locus on chromosome 17q12–23. *Lancet* **338,** 82.
65. Phipps RF, Perry PM (1988) Familial breast cancer. *Postgrad. Med. J.* **64,** 847–849.
66. Sellers TA, Potter JD, Rich SS, et al. (1994) Familial clustering of breast and prostate cancers and risk of postmenopausal breast cancer. *J. Natl. Cancer Inst.* **86,** 1860–1865.
67. Hall J, Lee M, Newman B, et al. (1990) Linkage of early onset familial breast cancer to chromosome 17q21. *Science* **250,** 1684–1689.
68. Easton DF, Bishop DT, Ford D, Crockford GP, the Breast Cancer Linkage Consortium (1993) Genetic linkage analysis in familial breast and ovarian cancer: results from 214 families. *Am. J. Hum. Genet.* **52,** 678–701.
69. Wooster R, Neuhausen SL, Mangion J, et al. (1994) Localization of a breast cancer susceptibility gene, *BRCA2,* to chromosome 13q12–13. *Science* **265,** 2088–2090.
70. Gayther SA, Mangion J, Russell P, et al. (1997) Variation of risks of breast and ovarian cancer associated with different germline mutations of the *BRCA2* gene. *Nat. Genet.* **15,** 103–105.
71. Schubert EL, Lee MK, Mefford HC, et al. (1997) *BRCA2* in American families with four or more cases of breast or ovarian cancer: recurrent and novel mutations, variable expression, penetrance, and the possibility of families whose cancer is not attributable to *BRCA1* or *BRCA2. Am. J. Hum. Genet.* **60,** 1031–1040.
72. Miki Y, Swensen J, Shattuck-Eidens D, et al. (1994) A strong candidate for the breast and ovarian cancer susceptibility gene *BRCA1. Science* **266,** 66–71.
73. Scully R, Chen J, Plug A (1997) Association of *BRCA1* with Rad51 in mitotic and meiotic cells. *Cell* **88,** 265–275.
74. Sharan SK, Morimatsu M, Albrecht U, et al. (1997) Embryonic lethality and radiation hypersensitivity mediated by Rad51 in mice lacking *BRCA2. Nature* **386,** 804–810.

75. Blackwood A, Weber B (1998) *BRCA1* and *BRCA2*. From molecular genetics to clinical medicine. *J. Clin. Oncol.* **16**, 1969–1977.
76. Abbot D, Freeman M, Holt J (1998) Double-strand break repair deficiency and radiation sensitivity in *BRCA2* mutant cancer cells. *J. Natl. Cancer Inst.* **90**, 978–985.
77. Biggs P, Bradley A (1998) A step toward genotype-based therapeutic regimens for breast cancer in patients with *BRCA2* mutations? *J. Natl. Cancer Inst.* **90**, 951–953.
78. Neuhausen S, Gilewski T, Norton L, et al. (1998) Recurrent *BRCA2* 6174delT mutations in Ashkenazi Jewish women affected by breast cancer. *Nat. Genet.* **13**, 126–128.
79. Peelen T, van Vliet M, Petrij-Bosch A, et al. (1997) A high proportion of novel mutations in *BRCA1* with strong founder effects among Dutch and Belgian hereditary breast and ovarian cancer families. *Am. J. Hum. Genet.* **60**, 1041–1049.
80. Thorlacius S, Olafsdottir G, Kryggvadottir L, et al. (1996) A single *BRCA2* mutation in male and female breast cancer families from Iceland with varied cancer phenotypes. *Nat. Genet.* **13**, 117–119.
81. Greene MH (1997) Genetics of breast cancer. *May. Clin. Proc.* **72**, 54–65.
82. Malone KE, Daling JR, Weiss NS, McKnight B, White E, Voigt LF (1996) Family history and survival of young women with invasive breast carcinoma. *Cancer* **78**, 1417–1425.
83. Breast Cancer Linkage Consortium (1997) Pathology of familial breast cancer: differences between breast cancers in carriers of *BRCA1* and *BRCA2* mutations and sporadic cases. *Lancet* **349**, 1505–1510.
84. Marcus JN, Page DL, Watson P, Narod SA, Lenoir GM, Lynch HT (1997) *BRCA1* and *BRCA2* hereditary breast carcinoma phenotypes. *Cancer* **80**, 543–556.
85. Marcus JN, Watson P, Page DL, et al. (1996) Hereditary breast cancer—pathobiology, prognosis, and *BRCA1* and *BRCA2* gene linkage. *Cancer* **77**, 697–709.
86. Verhoog LC, Brekelmans CTM, Seynaeve C, et al. (1998) Survival and tumour characteristics of breast-cancer patients with germline mutations of BRCA1. *Lancet* **351**, 316–321.
87. Johannsson OT, Ranstam J, Borg A, Olsson H (1998) Survival of BRCA1 breast and ovarian cancer patients: a population-based study from southern Sweden. *J. Clin. Oncol.* **16**, 397–404.
88. Garber JE, Goldstein AM, Kantor, AF, Dreyfus MG, Fraumeni JF Jr, Li FP (1991) Follow-up study of twenty-four families with Li-Fraumeni syndrome. *Cancer Res.* **51**, 6094–6097.
89. Bottomley R, Condit P (1968) Cancer families. *Cancer Bull.* **20**, 22.
90. Ford D, Easton DF (1995) The genetics of breast and ovarian cancer. *Br. J. Cancer* **72**, 805–812.
91. Tsou HC, Teng DHF, Ping XL, et al. (1997) The role of MMAC1 mutations in early-onset breast cancer: causative in association with Cowden syndrome and excluded in *BRCA1*-negative cases. *Am. J. Hum. Genet.* **61**, 1036–1043.
92. Lynch ED, Ostermeyer EA, Lee MK, et al. (1997) Inherited mutations in PTEN that are associated with breast cancer, Cowden disease, and juvenile polyposis. *Am. J. Hum. Genet.* **61**, 1254–1260.
93. Myers MP, Tonks NK (1997) Invited Editorial—PTEN: sometimes taking it off can be better than putting it on. *Am. J. Hum. Genet.* **61**, 1234–1238.
94. Savitsky K, Bar-Shira A, Gilad S, et al. (1995) A single ataxia telangiectasia gene with a product similar to PI-3 kinase. *Science* **268**, 1749–1753.
95. Gilad S, Chessa L, Khosravi R, et al. (1998) Genotype-phenotype relationships in ataxia-telangiectasia and variants. *Am. J. Hum. Genet.* **62**, 551–561.
96. Easton DF (1994) Cancer risks in A-T heterozygotes. *Int. J. Radiat. Biol.* **66(suppl. 6)**, S177–182.

2

Breast Imaging

Julia A. Birnbaum, MD
and Emily F. Conant, MD

CONTENTS

INTRODUCTION
MAMMOGRAPHY
OTHER BREAST IMAGING MODALITIES
CONCLUSIONS
BIBLIOGRAPHY

1. INTRODUCTION

The combination of high-quality breast imaging and improved compliance with screening mammography guidelines has begun to alter the course of breast cancer and its mortality rates in the United States. Although film-screen mammography remains the foundation of breast imaging, other modalities such as ultrasound, magnetic resonance imaging (MRI), nuclear medicine, and digital mammography are now included in the radiologist's armementarium to allow earlier detection and diagnosis of this all too common disease.

2. MAMMOGRAPHY

Mammographic imaging can be divided into two approaches for two different patient populations: *screening mammography* and *diagnostic mammography.*

2.1. Screening Mammography

Screening mammography is used to detect breast cancer in the asymptomatic patient, based on the rationale that early diagnosis of breast cancer improves morbidity and mortality. Beginning in the 1960s, several randomized trials have documented a statistically significant decrease in mortality (approximately 30%) from breast cancer with annual screening mammography for women at least 50 years of age. Whether or not annual screening mammography is equally beneficial to women aged 40–49 years has been a subject of much debate.

To date, eight randomized trials have included women between the ages of 40 and 49 years. These studies, using different methodologies (i.e., annual versus biennial screening intervals, single versus two views per breast), have demonstrated disparate results. Because no single trial *by itself* has included a sufficient number of younger women to

From: *Current Clinical Oncology:*
Breast Cancer: A Guide to Detection and Multidisciplinary Therapy
Edited by: M. H. Torosian © Humana Press Inc., Totowa, NJ

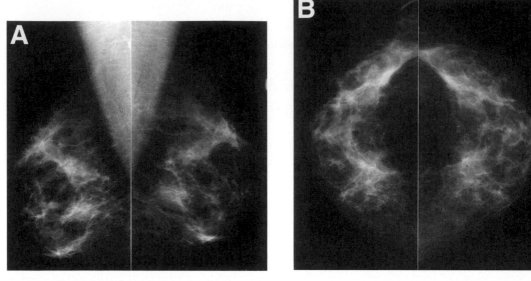

Fig. 1. Routine mediolateral oblique (**A**) and craniocaudal (**B**) views in a 49-year-old asymptomatic woman with scattered fibroglandular densities.

ensure statistical adequacy or has involved an adequate follow-up period, several investigators have performed meta-analyses on pooled data. Depending on which studies are included in the meta-analysis, a significant decrease in mortality (up to 40%) can be shown for younger women.

Conflicting results from the numerous randomized trials have led to confusion among patients and physicians. However, as of 1997, the National Cancer Institute, the American Cancer Society, and the American College of Radiology have all recommended that annual screening mammography begin at the age of 40.

To be cost-effective, screening mammography must be performed at high volume and low cost. Most breast imaging centers use several strategies to decrease the cost and increase the volume. Commonly, the radiologic technologist takes routine views of each breast; these films are evaluated for technical adequacy and the patient is discharged. Multiple examinations can then be batch-read by the interpreting radiologist at a later time. The batch reading of screening cases allows for optimization of viewing and processing conditions as well as double reading of studies in some practices. Double reading of screening cases has been shown to increase the cancer detection rate by up to 15%. If an abnormality is detected on a screening mammography study, the patient is recalled for a diagnostic evaluation, which may include additional mammographic views and/or a breast ultrasound.

2.1.1. STANDARD MAMMOGRAPHIC VIEWS

A routine screening mammogram includes *craniocaudal (CC)* and *mediolateral oblique (MLO) views* of each breast; the combination of these two views should image almost the entire volume of the breast tissue (Fig. 1).

To obtain the CC view, the technologist compresses the breast in a horizontal plane. The lateralmost portion of glandular tissue, including the axillary tail, may not be visualized on a routine CC view owing to the curvature of the chest wall.

The MLO view is used for routine imaging in order to include the extension of breast tissue into the axillary tail. The exact degree of obliquity varies from patient to patient, as optimal positioning is with the plane of compression parallel to the fibers of the pectoralis major muscle.

Compression during breast imaging is necessary for many reasons. Compression holds the breast still, thereby limiting motion artifact. It decreases overlap of superimposed breast structures, which increases the likelihood that an abnormality will be visualized rather than obscured by overlying breast tissue. Decreasing the thickness of the breast reduces X-ray beam scatter, which may cause blurring. Reducing breast thickness and scatter also decreases radiation dose by decreasing exposure time; the same decrease in exposure time also reduces the likelihood of motion.

2.2. Diagnostic Mammography

Diagnostic mammography is used to evaluate the patient with clinical signs and/or symptoms of breast cancer (i.e., palpable lump, pain, nipple discharge) and to characterize and localize further abnormalities detected on screening mammography. The diagnostic evaluation, which is tailored to each individual patient, may involve routine as well as special mammographic views and is often supplemented by breast sonography. Other indications for diagnostic mammography include a history of breast cancer and prior benign breast biopsy. The radiologist evaluates the images on-line and generally discusses the results with the patient in person after completion of the diagnostic study.

2.2.1. Additional Mammographic Views

A diagnostic evaluation may be indicated to characterize further and/or localize a lesion detected on a screening mammogram or to determine whether an abnormality is real or is the result of summation artifact (superimposition of normal glandular tissue) or other artifact.

There are several mammographic views that aid in better imaging of certain areas of breast tissue. The *exaggerated craniocaudal lateral (XCCL) view* is also known as the *internally rotated CC view* because the breast is internally (medially) rotated in relation to the compression plate and film. This projection places the far lateral breast tissue, which is usually included only on the MLO view, within the imaging field for a CC view (Fig. 2). Far medial lesions may be imaged utilizing an *externally rotated CC view* or a *cleavage (valley) view*. In the latter view, the medial portion of both breasts is imaged. The *axillary tail view* is performed at an angle between the CC and MLO views and is used to visualize deeper into the axilla, an area that is not entirely included on the routine CC view.

The *90-degree lateral view* (usually a *mediolateral [ML] view* but may also be performed as a *lateromedial [LM] view*) has many additional uses. The lateral view is used with one or both of the routine mammographic views (CC and MLO) to triangulate the exact location of a lesion in the breast and can help determine whether or not a possible lesion is indeed real or the result of superimposition of breast tissue (Fig. 3). However, since the 90-degree lateral view may not include as much of the axillary tail and high central breast tissue as the MLO view, some lesions deep in the lateral and deep superior breast may not be visible on the 90-degree lateral view.

Other views may be used to visualize specific areas of breast tissue better. *Rolled views* displace superimposed structures. Thus, a lesion previously obscured may become apparent on a rolled view. Similarly, pseudolesions produced by summation artifact may be clearly elucidated as such by rolled views.

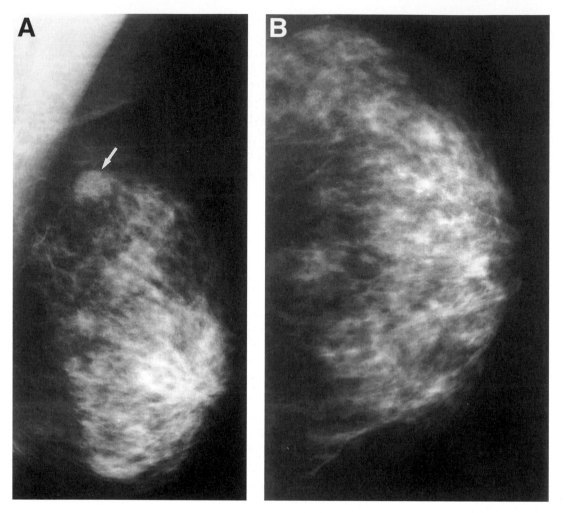

Fig. 2. The exaggerated craniocaudal lateral view (XCCL). Screening mediolateral oblique view **(A)** demonstrates an irregularly shaped density in the superior breast (long arrow). However, no corresponding abnormality is seen on the routine craniocaudal view **(B).** *(Figure continues)*

Tangential views can be used to evaluate palpable abnormalities obscured by overlying breast tissue. Additionally, they are used to verify the dermal location of suspected skin calcifications (Fig. 4).

Spot compression, which can be performed in any projection, is used to evaluate further equivocal or obscured findings on a screening mammogram (Fig. 5). The smaller compression device allows for greater compression of a focal area of interest. Not only does this view displace overlapping breast tissue and thus decrease summation artifact, but by decreasing breast thickness, it decreases scatter and therefore improves contrast. Spot compression is often combined with *magnification* for further evaluation of indeterminate or suspicious calcifications and margin characteristics of a density or mass (Fig. 6). Using varying focal spot sizes, the area of interest can be magnified between 1.5 and 2.0 times.

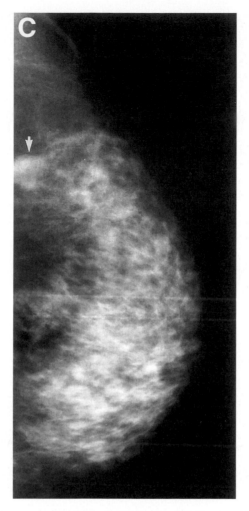

Fig. 2. *(Continued).* The patient was rotated internally for the XCCL view **(C),** which places more of the lateral breast tissue within the field of view. The mass is visualized at the edge of the film in the deep lateral breast (short arrow). This mass proved to be a fibroadenoma upon biopsy.

2.3. Mammography Reporting and BI-RADS

In 1992, the FDA Food and Drug Administration passed the Mammography Quality Standards Act (MQSA) in an attempt to ensure high-quality mammography. One of the components of MQSA is clear and concise communication of the results of mammographic interpretation. Recognizing the importance of accurate communication in mammography reporting, the Breast Task Force of the American College of Radiology appointed a committee of experts to develop standardized mammography terminology and an organized reporting system. The result is known as BI-RADS: Breast Imaging Reporting and Data System.

BI-RADS includes five major sections:

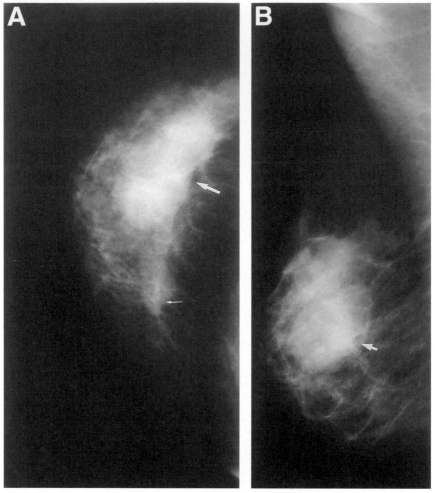

Fig. 3. Use of the mediolateral (ML) view. **(A)** The left craniocaudal view demonstrates a large lobulated mass occupying the central and lateral breast (thick arrow), as well as an irregular density with the suggestion of distortion in the medial breast (thin arrow). However, on the left mediolateral oblique view **(B),** only the large mass is seen (short arrow). Is the second lesion not real, or is it obscured by the larger mass? *(Figure continues)*

1. A breast imaging lexicon
2. A reporting system
3. A report coding system
4. A pathology coding system
5. A description of follow-up and outcome monitoring.

The last three sections offer recommendations for data collection for those interpreting mammograms and will not be further discussed here. However, as breast imagers nationwide are now required to use BI-RADS, an understanding of the lexicon and reporting system used in mammography reports is imperative for all clinicians who refer patients for routine screening as well as diagnostic breast imaging.

The reporting system divides the organization of the mammography report into four sections:

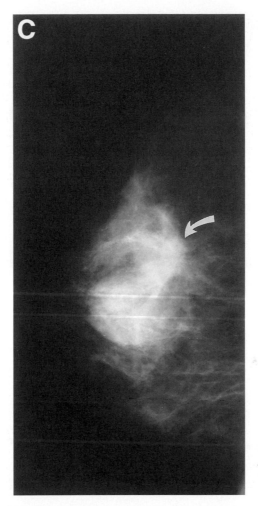

Fig. 3. *(Continued).* **(C)** The ML view not only confirms the presence of a second abnormality but also localizes it to the superior breast (curved arrow). Further examination with ultrasound (not shown) demonstrated several large cysts in the central and lateral breast and a suspicious solid mass in the inner upper quadrant, later proved to represent an invasive carcinoma.

1. A mention of comparison with prior studies
2. A brief description of the type of breast tissue
3. A description of significant findings
4. A final assessment category.

2.3.1. TYPE OF BREAST TISSUE

Because breast tissue has the same X-ray attenuation as, and thus may obscure, focal masses, the sensitivity of mammography decreases with increasing glandularity of the breast. By briefly describing the type of breast tissue, the mammographer provides the referring clinician with an estimated sensitivity of the mammogram for each patient and also offers a description of the parenchymal pattern, which may be correlated with the physical examination of the breast by the clinician.

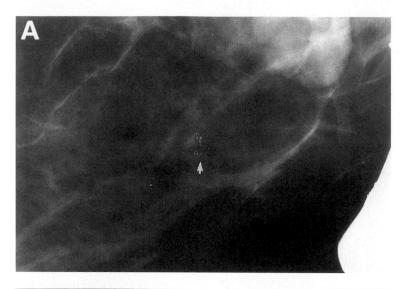

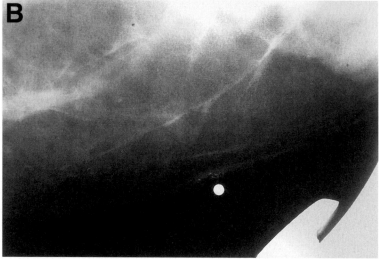

Fig. 4. Skin calcifications. **(A)** A spot magnification in the craniocaudal projection demonstrates pleomorphic calcifications in the inner right breast (arrow). A dermal location was suspected since the calcifications appeared peripherally near the inferior skin surface on the mediolateral oblique view (not shown). **(B)** A tangential film reveals that the calcifications are located in the skin layer next to the metallic BB skin marker.

The four general breast tissue types as described by the BI-RADS lexicon are as follows (Fig. 7):

1. Almost entirely fat
2. Scattered fibroglandular densities
3. Heterogeneously dense
4. Extremely dense.

2.3.2. DESCRIPTION OF SIGNIFICANT FINDINGS

The BI-RADS lexicon is a dictionary of terms used in the description of mammographic findings. The categories and recommended descriptors in these categories are as follows:

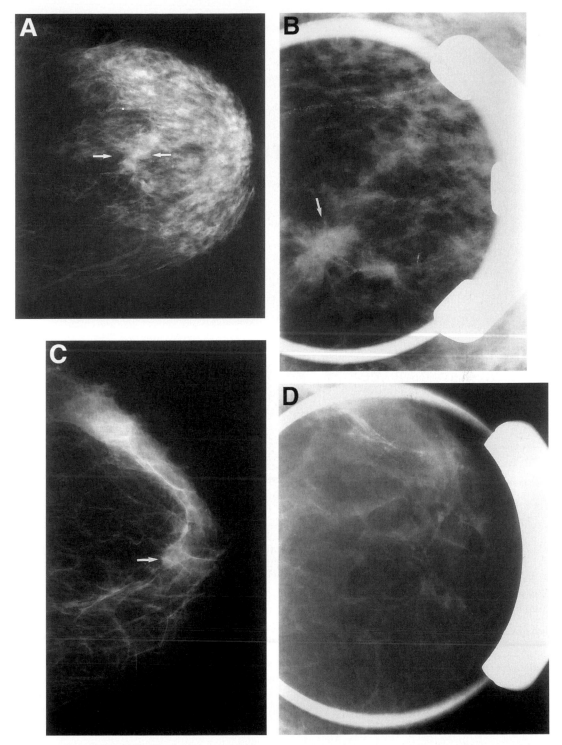

Fig. 5. Use of spot compression views. (**A** and **B**) Spot compression can confirm the presence of an abnormality by reducing the superimposition of overlying structures. In (**A**), there is the suggestion of distortion in the central breast at a middle depth on a routine craniocaudal view (arrows). Spot compression (**B**) of this area demonstrates a spiculated mass (arrow). (**C** and **D**) Spot compression may also resolve an equivocal finding. On a routine craniocaudal view (**C**), there is a subareolar focal asymmetric density (arrow). The density does not persist on the spot compression view (**D**).

27

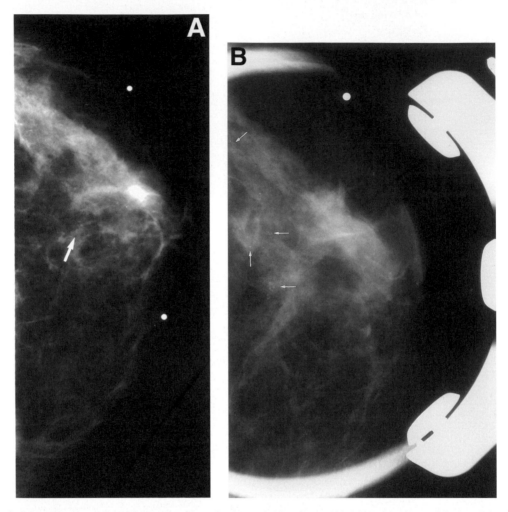

Fig. 6. Magnification views for evaluation of microcalcifications. **(A)** Right craniocaudal view identifies calcifications in the central breast (thick arrow). **(B)** The number and morphology of the calcifications are better evaluated with magnification, which also demonstrates that the calcifications are more extensive than appreciated on the routine view (thin arrows). The metallic markers were placed on a cutaneous scar from a prior biopsy.

Masses: described in terms of their shape, margin, and density relative to the surrounding breast tissue.

Calcifications: described in terms of their morphology, or shape of the individual particles, and distribution within the breast.

Architectural distortion: identified in association with other findings or as an isolated finding (Fig. 8).

Associated findings: the secondary signs of breast cancer (such as skin retraction or thickening, nipple retraction, trabecular thickening, architectural distortion, and axillary adenopathy) (Figs. 9 and 10).

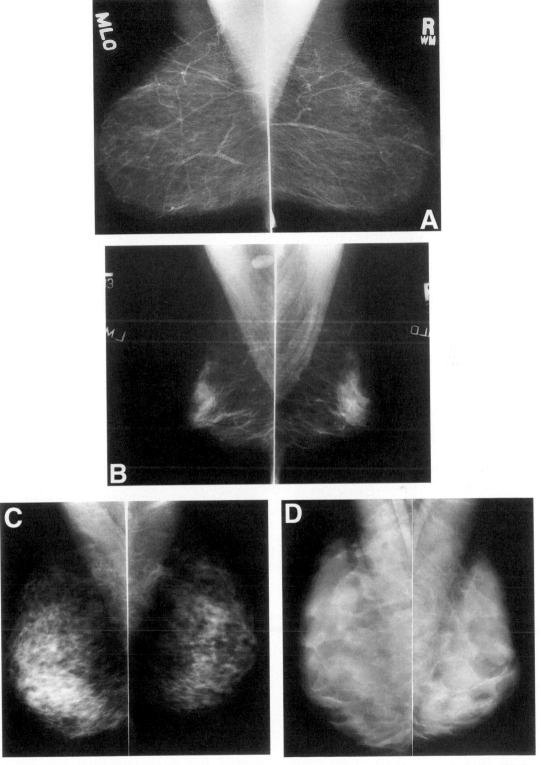

Fig. 7. Normal mediolateral oblique views with varying breast density. (**A**) Almost entirely fat. (**B**) Scattered fibroglandular densities. (**C**) Heterogeneously dense. (**D**) Extremely dense.

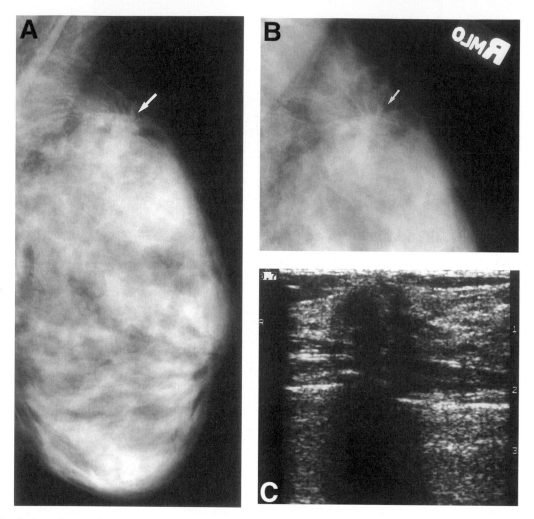

Fig. 8. Invasive carcinoma presenting as architectural distortion. Routine mediolateral oblique (MLO) view (**A**) and close-up of the superior breast also in the MLO view (**B**) demonstrate distortion in the superior breast (arrows). (**C**) Ultrasound confirms a highly suspicious hypoechoic mass with ill-defined margins and posterior acoustic shadowing.

Special cases: mammographic findings that do not readily fit into the above categories include focal asymmetric densities (which may or may not be indicative of a true lesion), solitary dilated ducts, and intramammary lymph nodes.

2.3.3. ASSESSMENT CATEGORIES

One of the most important parts of a clear, concise radiology report is the conclusion, or recommendations based on the imaging findings. According to BI-RADS guidelines, the reporting radiologist should offer an overall impression of the significance of the findings described in the body of the report. There are five assessment categories in BI-RADS, as follows:

Category 1: Normal
Category 2: Benign
Category 3: Probably benign

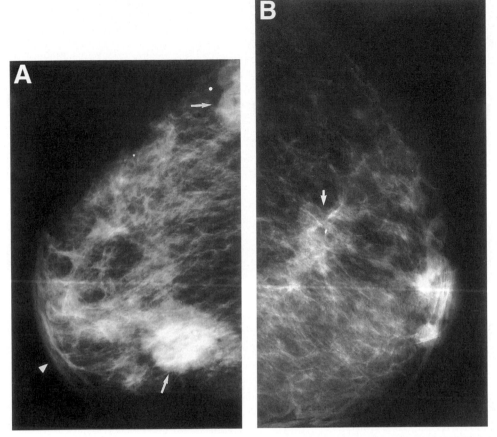

Fig. 9. Associated findings of breast cancer. Bilateral mediolateral (**A** and **B**) and bilateral craniocaudal (CC) (**C** and **D**; p. 32) views. This 82-year-old patient presented with two palpable masses in the left breast, indicated by the metallic skin markers. Note two suspicious masses in the left breast (thick arrows); the lateral mass in the left breast is not visualized on the left CC view (**C**) owing to its far lateral location. Also note trabecular thickening (thin arrow), which appears as many crisscrossing white lines, and skin thickening, which is best seen in the periareolar breast (arrowhead). There is also an irregularly shaped suspicious mass in the right breast (short arrows). The periareolar right breast mass was confirmed as a cyst on ultrasound.

Category 4: Suspicious
Category 5: Highly suggestive of malignancy.

Implicit in each of these categories is a likelihood of malignancy and a recommendation for follow-up or further action. For categories 1 and 2, in which the breast shows either no abnormality or a definitely benign finding, the likelihood of malignancy is thought to be 0%, and routine yearly follow-up is recommended. For category 3, the likelihood of malignancy is less than 2%; a short-interval follow-up is recommended, usually at 6 months. Tissue diagnosis is recommended for category 4 and 5 examinations; the likelihood of malignancy is between 2 and 90% for category 4 and more than 90% for category 5 lesions.

Category 0 is utilized when the evaluation is incomplete. This most often occurs with screening mammograms when additional evaluation is necessary to characterize a possible abnormality and may include comparison with prior films, additional mammographic views, and/or breast ultrasound.

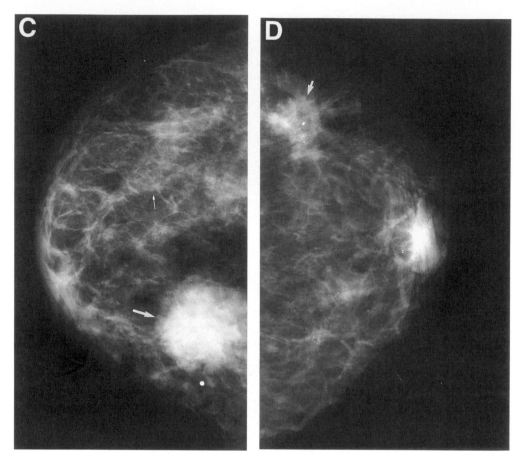

Fig. 9. *(continued).*

3.4. The Normal Breast

There is a wide spectrum of appearance of the normal breast. As mentioned above, BI-RADS describes four types of breast composition: fatty, scattered fibroglandular densities, heterogeneously dense, and extremely dense. In general, younger women tend to have more glandularity and thus a denser mammographic appearance. With age (and without stimulation from exogenous hormones), the glandular tissue atrophies, resulting in an increasingly fatty mammographic appearance. However, the mammographic appearance also reflects body habitus and history of lactation, since increased body fat and lactation are both associated with increased breast fat relative to glandular tissue.

Other normal structures that can be visualized on mammography include skin, arteries and veins, lactiferous ducts, and Cooper's ligaments. Normal skin is usually 0.8–2 mm thick, although skin in the inframammary fold area can often be more than 3 mm. With current mammographic technique, a bright light is often necessary to visualize the skin. Because malignant as well as benign processes can affect the skin, evaluation of the skin should be a routine aspect of mammographic interpretation.

Blood vessels, both arteries and veins, can also be seen on mammographic views. Because early arterial calcifications and tortuous, superimposed vessels can sometimes mimic the suspicious appearance of malignant calcifications and masses, respectively, an

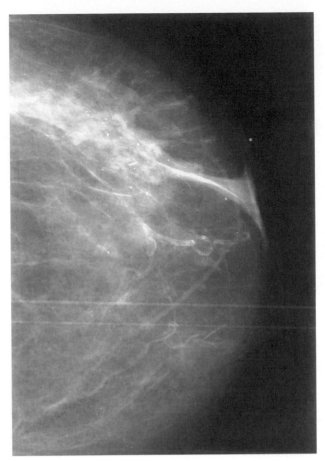

Fig. 10. Associated findings of breast cancer. Right craniocaudal view demonstrates a palpable lateral breast mass with associated pleomorphic calcifications. Note extension to the nipple, causing thickening and retraction of the nipple.

appreciation of the tubular nature of the finding (sometimes requiring spot compression with or without magnification) may help avoid unnecessary biopsy.

Lactiferous ducts, especially if dilated, may be visualized in a subareolar location. If imaged in cross-section, the appearance may simulate a subareolar nodule. Spot compression views may help clarify the true tubular nature of the structure.

Cooper's ligaments, fibrous bands that help support the breast, are seen as a thin trabeculations extending from the glandular parenchyma to their insertion in the skin. Trabecular thickening, which often accompanies skin thickening, can be seen in malignant (i.e., inflammatory carcinoma) as well as benign processes (i.e., inflammation, infection, and venous/lymphatic obstruction) and manifests mammographically as prominent crisscrossing lines (Fig. 9C).

3.5. *The Abnormal Breast*

3.5.1. MASSES

3.5.1.1. Shape. In general, round and oval masses are usually benign; the more irregular the shape, the higher the likelihood of malignancy (Fig. 11). However, there is a large amount of overlap between benign and malignant masses. For example, a benign process such as sclerosing adenosis or fat necrosis may have an irregular shape, whereas certain can-

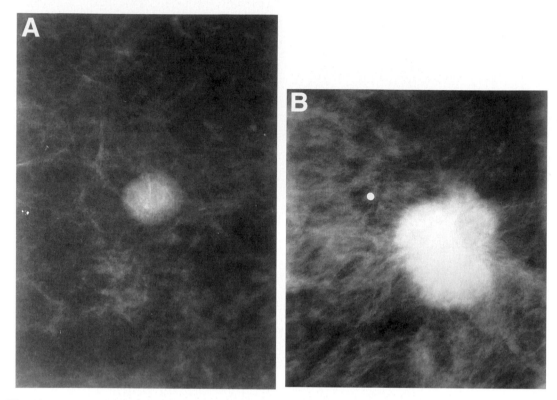

Fig. 11. Round and oval masses are more often benign, and irregularly shaped masses or masses with spiculated margins are usually malignant. **(A)** This round, circumscribed mass was shown to be a simple cyst on ultrasound. **(B)** In another patient with a palpable lump in the left breast, an irregularly shaped mass was later found to represent carcinoma. Note also spiculated margins and high density relative to the surrounding breast parenchyma.

cers (i.e., mucinous and medullary carcinomas) may infrequently present as round or oval masses. Ultrasound is necessary to determine whether masses are cystic or solid; with solid masses, ultrasound may provide some insight into the etiology of the mass.

3.5.1.2. Margin. Most circumscribed masses, those with an abrupt transition between the mass and the surrounding tissue, are benign. The likelihood of malignancy increases as margins become more irregular. However, as with the shape of a mass, there is overlap between benign and malignant masses. The classic breast carcinoma is indistinct or spiculated, and the classic cyst and fibroadenoma are circumscribed (Fig. 11). However, a benign mass process can have indistinct or even spiculated margins, and some cancers may be circumscribed. Some margins may appear circumscribed at low resolution but appear less well-defined with magnification views.

3.5.1.3. Density. Low-density (fat-containing) masses are benign. Examples include hamartomas, lymph nodes, oil cysts, and galactoceles. Malignant processes tend to be of high density relative to breast tissue, but benign processes can be of high or equal density (Fig. 12).

3.5.2. Benign Masses

Most *cysts* are round or oval, whereas *fibroadenomas* tend to be oval or macrolobulated (Fig. 13; see also Fig. 11). Both usually have circumscribed margins. Overlying breast tissue

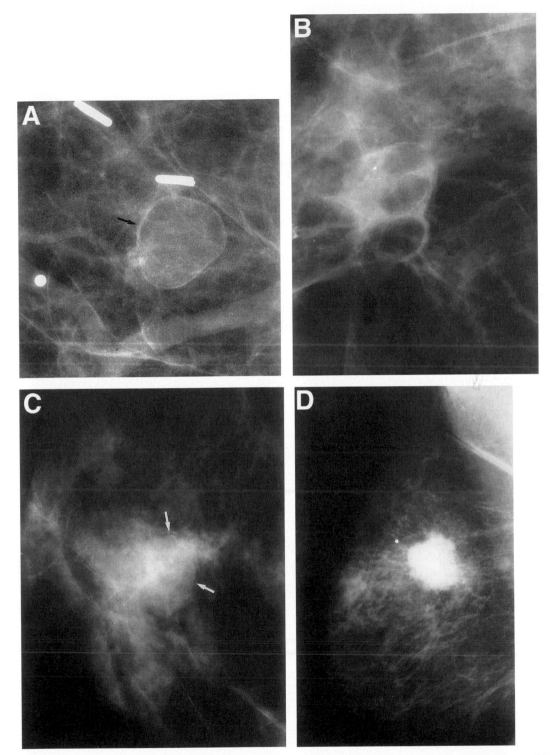

Fig. 12. Density of masses. (**A** and **B**). Fat-containing masses are benign. (**A**) A palpable lipid cyst (black arrow), a benign circumscribed mass with the internal density of fat. (**B**) In a different patient, several findings of fat necrosis included an irregularly shaped density, irregular coarse calcifications, and three lipid cysts. The presence of the lipid cysts confirms a benign process. (**C**) This partially obscured fibroadenoma (white arrows) is isodense to the surrounding glandular tissue. (**D**) An extremely dense carcinoma is very obvious when surrounded by lower density breast tissue. This is the same patient as in Figure 11.

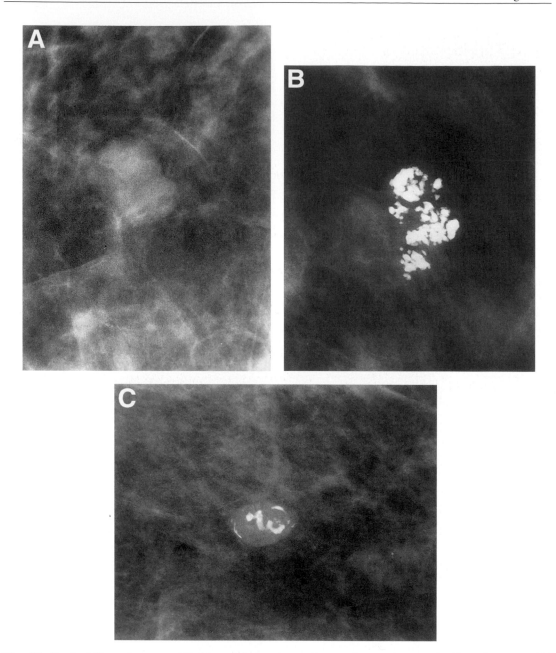

Fig. 13. Typical fibroadenomas. **(A)** Macrolobulated margins are frequently seen in fibroadenomas. **(B)** Diffuse coarse calcifications are throughout this fibroadenoma. The associated mass is just barely visible. **(C)** Coarse curvilinear calcifications with a peripheral distribution are associated with this circumscribed fibroadenoma.

may cause obscuration of the margins, and spot compression views may be necessary to characterize them. Inflammatory change in a cyst can create an ill-defined margin. Cysts and fibroadenomas cannot be differentiated mammographically, unless degeneration of a fibroadenoma has led to formation of typical coarse calcifications (Fig. 13). The density of cysts and fibroadenomas can be equal to or greater than the surrounding breast parenchyma.

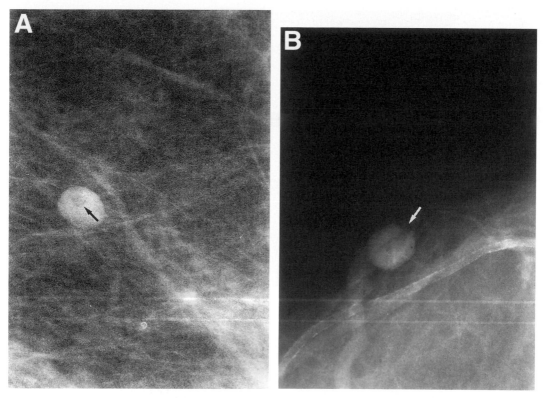

Fig. 14. Intramammary lymph nodes. The mammographic appearance depends on the orientation of the node relative to the X-ray beam. **(A)** Viewed *en face* with the hilum superimposed on cortex, the hilum is seen as a central lucency (black arrow). **(B)** If the hilum is viewed in tangent, it presents as a lucent notch (white arrow).

Intramammary lymph nodes are often present in the upper outer quadrant of the breast at the surface of the parenchymal tissue near the subcutaneous fat. They are usually oval or slightly lobulated (reniform) in shape, with a circumscribed or obscured margin. The presence of a fatty hilum is diagnostic. Viewed *en face,* the hilum manifests as a central lucency; viewed in tangent, a fatty hilum presents as a lucent notch. Spot compression, possibly with magnification, may help visualize the fatty hilum and thus confirm the diagnosis on mammography alone; otherwise, ultrasound may be helpful (Fig. 14).

The characteristic mammographic appearance of a *hamartoma* is an oval, round, or lobulated circumscribed mass containing both fat and soft tissue elements, reflecting its composition of fat, glandular, and fibrous tissue (Fig. 15). The appearance has been likened to a cut sausage. Hamartomas containing little or no fat are difficult, if not impossible, to differentiate from a cyst or noncalcified fibroadenoma.

3.5.3. MALIGNANT MASSES

Most *invasive breast carcinomas* appear mammographically as a mass, classically a dense, irregularly shaped spiculated mass with or without associated microcalcification (Fig. 16). Unfortunately, breast cancer does not always demonstrate these classic findings and can mimic a benign lesion with a lobulated or oval shape, or with indistinct, microlobulated, or even circumscribed margins. Certain histologic subtypes of breast carcinoma, such

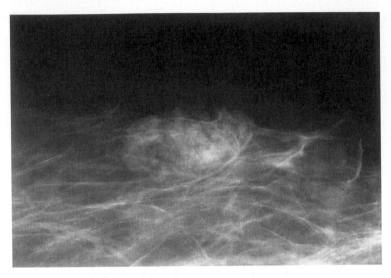

Fig. 15. A hamartoma is generally circumscribed and has an internal matrix of fat and soft tissue density.

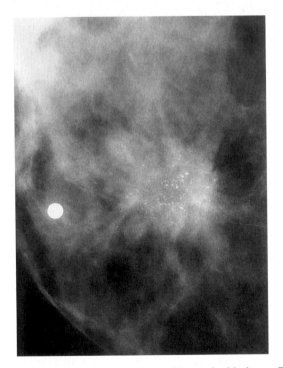

Fig. 16. Left craniocaudal view of a 42-year-old woman with a palpable lump. This carcinoma is irregular in shape, has spiculated margins, and contains pleomorphic calcifications.

as medullary, mucinous, and intracystic cancers, are more likely to present a benign mammographic appearance with round or oval shapes and often partially well-defined margins (Fig. 17). In other cases, especially with invasive lobular carcinoma, the mammographic finding may be of a rather poorly defined density or simply of an asymmetric density with or without clinical findings. Invasive lobular carcinoma may also be an elusive mammographic

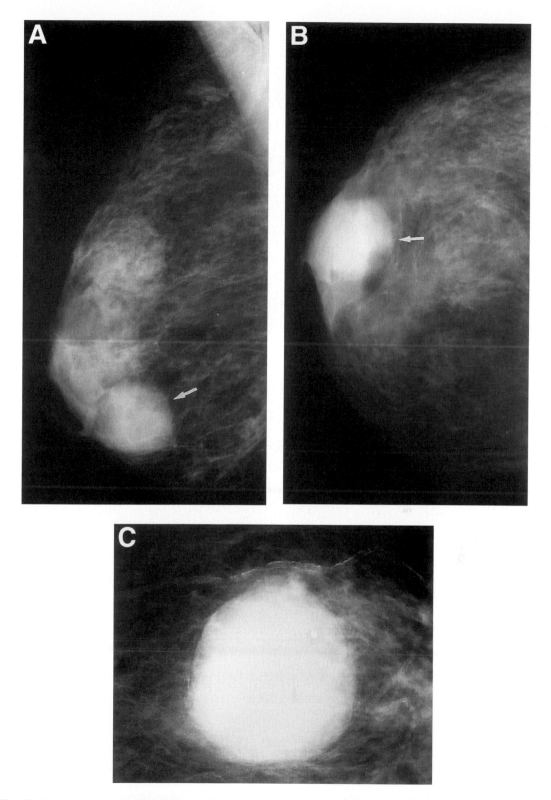

Fig. 17. Benign-appearing breast cancer. (**A** and **B**) Invasive ductal carcinoma presenting as a round, partially circumscribed mass in the periareolar left breast (arrows). (**C**) In a different patient, medullary carcinoma presents as a large rounded mass, but the margins are poorly defined, raising the suspicion of malignancy.

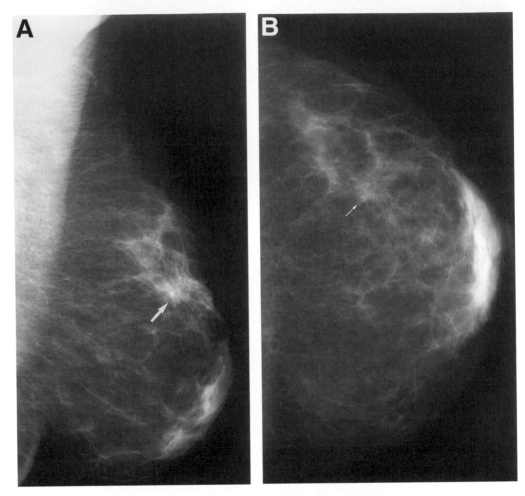

Fig. 18. Invasive lobular carcinoma with subtle mammographic findings. (**A**) mediolateral oblique view of the right breast (**A** and **B**) demonstrates an ill-defined density with associated distortion (thick arrow). However, the findings on the craniocaudal view (**B**) are much less pronounced (thin arrow). *(Figure continues)*

lesion that is well visualized on only one of the routine mammographic views (Fig. 18). The difficulty in diagnosing invasive lobular carcinoma on mammography is thought to be because of the planar, cellular growth of the tumor.

Although *ductal carcinoma in situ* usually presents with microcalcifications, it may infrequently manifest as a noncalcified mass (Fig. 19).

Malignant breast masses other than primary breast carcinoma are extremely rare. Primary or secondary *lymphoma* can appear as a solitary mass or as multiple masses that may be circumscribed, indistinct, or a combination of both. Metastatic lesions (most commonly from melanoma) are usually round masses with indistinct margins and occur multiply in both breasts.

3.5.4. CALCIFICATIONS

3.5.4.1. Morphology. Morphology refers to the shape of each individual particle of calcification and also to the homogeneity or heterogeneity of shapes among those calcifications identified. In general, the likelihood of malignancy increases with the irregularity of the indi-

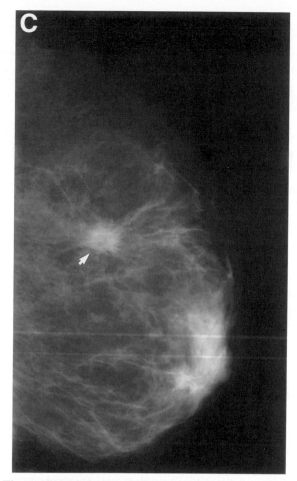

Fig. 18. *(Continued).* **(C)** The mediolateral view confirms a spiculated mass with architectural distortion (short arrow). Pathologic evaluation revealed invasive lobular carcinoma.

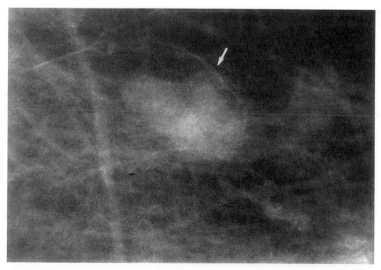

Fig. 19. This irregularly shaped mass with indistinct margins (arrow) underwent core biopsy. Histologically, the mass was solid and cribriform ductal carcinoma *in situ* without evidence of microinvasion.

vidual shapes and with increasingly heterogeneous populations. Adequate assessment of morphology often requires the use of magnification views as well as a magnifying glass.

Typically benign morphologies include skin, vascular, coarse, popcorn-like, large rod-like, round, punctate, lucent-centered, rim (eggshell), milk of calcium, and sutural calcifications. Indeterminate calcifications include amorphous and indistinct calcifications. Fine linear and/or branching calcifications and those that are pleomorphic (heterogeneous) in their morphology are associated with a high probability of malignancy.

3.5.4.2. Distribution. Calcifications are also characterized by their distribution in breast tissue. A cluster is defined as a group of five or more calcifications in 1 cm^3. Both benign and malignant processes can produce focal clusters of calcifications. Segmental calcifications involve a ductal system; this is a suspicious pattern because many breast carcinomas begin as ductal processes. Regional calcifications are present within a larger volume of breast tissue that may not conform to an anatomic structure or division. Like clustered calcifications, regional calcifications may be benign or malignant. Diffuse and scattered calcifications are widely distributed throughout the breast and are usually (but not always!) benign.

Comparison with prior mammograms is crucial in the evaluation of calcifications. Coarsening of individual particles (growth in size of a particle as opposed to an increase in number of particles) generally indicates a benign etiology; this is commonly appreciated with degenerating fibroadenomas and calcifications of fat necrosis. Without comparison mammograms, indeterminate calcifications may require tissue diagnosis; however, confirmation of long-term stability (i.e., several years) often supports a benign diagnosis, favoring continued follow-up rather than intervention. However, low-grade intraductal carcinoma may remain stable for several years; thus, visualization of pleomorphic calcifications or linear/branching forms should prompt tissue diagnosis even if there has been no interval change.

Improvement in imaging technique and resolution in the past several years has unquestionably improved the diagnostic capabilities of film/screen mammography. The improved quality has also created an occasional diagnostic dilemma. When calcifications appear more prominent on current mammograms, is it because they are new, increasing in number, or merely better visualized? Careful analysis or morphology should help select those calcifications that are suspicious and therefore should be biopsied regardless of the presence or absence of interval change in recent years. Possibly stable calcifications of indeterminate morphology may warrant a short-interval follow-up with magnification views, to assess true interval stability.

3.5.5. BENIGN CALCIFICATIONS

Typical *skin calcifications* are round or polygonal with lucent centers and are seen in the medial, inferior, periareolar, and axillary portions of the breast. They may be scattered but can also form tight clusters or rosettes (Fig. 20). They usually appear peripheral on at least one routine mammographic view; however, because the breast is curved, dermal calcifications may possibly project over the breast parenchyma on both views. If confirmation of the dermal origin is necessary, a tangential view should be obtained.

Advanced *vascular calcifications* do not present a diagnostic dilemma: they are linear and parallel, and the associated vessel is often identified (Fig. 21). However, early vascular calcifications may be mistaken for malignant calcifications. Spot magnification views may reveal additional parallel calcifications and may also delineate an associated blood vessel.

Milk of calcium refers to precipitated calcium in microcysts, which are actually cystically dilated lobules. Because calcium pools in the dependent portion of microcysts, the mammographic appearance depends on the direction of the X-ray beam. On the craniocaudal view, the

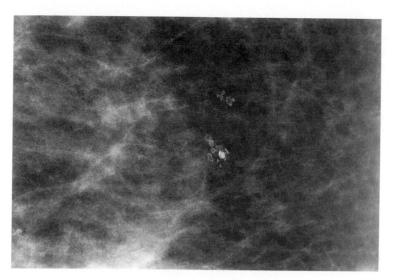

Fig. 20. Dermal calcifications. Note the round and oval lucent-centered calcifications seen in small rosettes. This appearance makes the diagnosis of skin calcifications obvious.

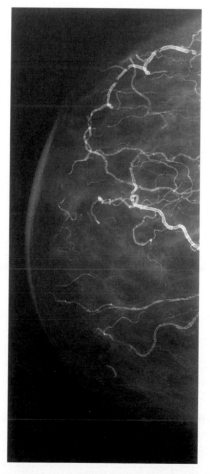

Fig. 21. Extensive vascular calcifications are seen in this elderly patient

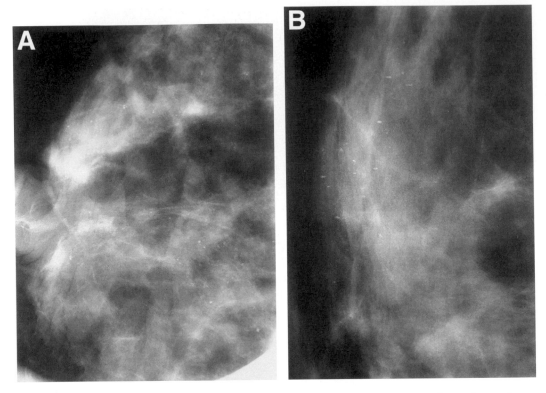

Fig. 22. Milk of calcium. The calcifications appear round, with indistinct or "smudgy" margins on the cran-iocaudal view (**A**). On the mediolateral view (**B**), the calcifications appear linear or curvilinear. The hori-zontal X-ray beam identifies the calcifications layering in the dependent portion of tiny microcysts.

calcifications appear round but with "smudgy" edges. However, with the 90-degree lateral view, the calcifications appear as tiny horizontal lines or crescents with the concave surface superior, as the horizontal beam identifies them layering in the bottom of microcysts (Fig. 22).

Fat necrosis produces a varied mammographic appearance, including calcifications, lipid cysts, neodensities, and spiculated masses. The wall of an oil cyst may calcify; such cysts may be seen as curvilinear or plaque-like calcifications surrounding a lucent or mixed-den-sity mass (Fig. 23). The morphology of each individual particle may create suspicion; how-ever, additional views, including magnification views, often reveal that the calcifications are peripheral and associated with a lucent mass.

Adenosic calcifications form in the acini. Consequently, each particle is typically punctate or round. Because each lobule contains several acini, these calcifications are often grouped together in rosettes (Fig. 24). The process is usually diffuse and bilateral.

Calcification of intraductal secretions produces the characteristic appearance of *secre-tory calcifications*. These are usually larger than malignant calcifications (>1 mm versus <0.5 mm), have a smooth contour, gently taper, and are often bilateral in a predominantly subareolar distribution (Fig. 25). Although they are less likely than malignant calcifica-tions to branch, the presence of a linear, branching calcification does not always imply carcinoma. The presence of a lucent center within a linear, rod-shaped calcification con-firms a benign etiology, as this represents calcification of periductal stroma that does not occur in intraductal carcinoma.

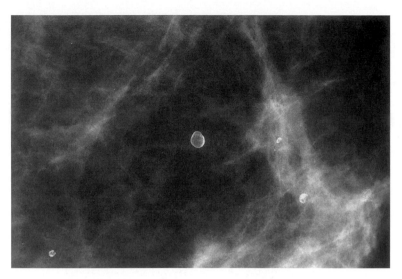

Fig. 23. Peripherally calcified lipid cyst. Like dermal calcifications, a calcified lipid cyst contains a lucent center. However, the calcified lipid cyst is usually larger and is not often seen in small groups or rosettes.

3.5.6. MALIGNANT CALCIFICATIONS

Malignant calcifications may be present with or without a mammographically detectable mass. Most cases of ductal carcinoma *in situ* manifest mammographically as calcifications, 75% as calcifications alone and 10% as calcifications with a mass.

Classic malignant calcifications are clustered fine, linear, and branching pleomorphic microcalcifications often distributed in a linear fashion (Fig. 26). This appearance reflects the underlying process, which is calcification of intraductal necrotic debris, or comedonecrosis; the calcifications are actually casts of the ducts. Noncomedo malignant calcifications tend to be smaller than calcifications associated with comedonecrosis and are often granular, irregular, or amorphous in morphology.

Calcifications associated with an invasive malignancy may be present in the area of the soft tissue mass or in the surrounding tissue. The morphology of the calcifications in invasive malignancies is similar to that of intraductal carcinoma.

3.6. Evaluation of the Patient with Breast Cancer

Imaging plays an important role in the diagnosis, staging, surgical planning, and long-term follow-up of the patient with breast cancer. Mammography is integral in determining the extent of disease and the possibility of multifocal or multicentric carcinoma. Following primary excision, mammography is used to evaluate residual disease, especially if the carcinoma presented as malignant calcifications. Finally, routine imaging evaluation of the conservatively treated breast may allow early detection of recurrent disease. Ultrasound and MR imaging may be used as adjunct modalities for these purposes in certain circumstances.

3.6.1. PRIOR TO TREATMENT

Optimal treatment planning requires accurate assessment of extent of disease, which includes not only the size of the primary lesion but whether or not there is multifocal, multicentric, and/or bilateral disease. Traditionally, mammography has performed these roles.

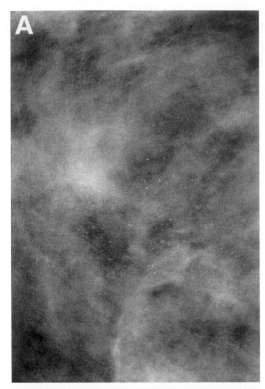

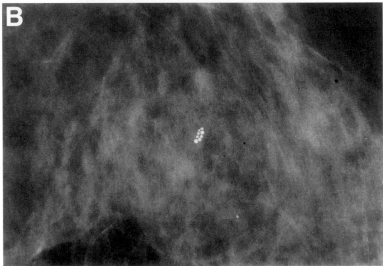

Fig. 24. Punctate and round calcifications. **(A)** These tiny calcifications are referred to as punctate, like small grains of sand. They most likely formed in the lobules of the breast acini. **(B)** Although slightly differing in size, these calcifications are round and very smooth in contour, supporting a benign etiology.

However, in a dense breast, or with a characteristically subtle lesion such as invasive lobular carcinoma, mammographic evaluation may not be able to determine the true extent of disease and may not visualize multicentric and multifocal disease. Ultrasound has been shown to be useful in detecting mammographically occult masses associated with malignant calcifications, suggesting an invasive component to what was thought to be intraductal disease

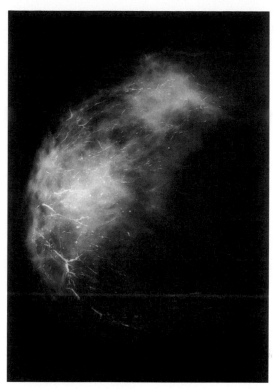

Fig. 25. Secretory calcifications. These extensive linear calcifications have smooth contours with tapered or blunt ends and are characteristic of secretory calcifications.

(Fig. 27). Recent studies have shown that MRI demonstrates one or more additional foci of disease in one-third of patients and upstages patients with invasive lobular carcinoma; both of these findings would thus affect patient management (Fig. 28).

3.6.2. POSTBIOPSY EVALUATION

For patients electing breast conservation, complete excision of disease is an important goal prior to the onset of radiation therapy. If the preoperative mammogram demonstrates suspicious calcifications (and pathologic evaluation confirms that these calcifications are involved with the malignant process), postsurgical mammographic evaluation is indicated to evaluate for residual calcifications (Fig. 29). Because the presence of residual suspicious calcifications correlates with the pathologic finding of residual disease, suspicious calcifications detected on the postexcision mammogram should undergo needle localization for removal at the time of reexcision.

3.6.3. MAMMOGRAPHIC EVALUATION FOLLOWING BREAST CONSERVATION

Interpretation of the mammographic images of the conservatively treated breast requires a knowledge of benign posttreatment changes and the ability to differentiate them from recurrent disease.

The most common changes in the breast following lumpectomy include architectural distortion, skin thickening and retraction, fluid collections presenting as masses, increased parenchymal density without mass or distortion (i.e., scar), lipid cysts, and calcifications. Although these changes also occur following surgery for benign disease, they are more

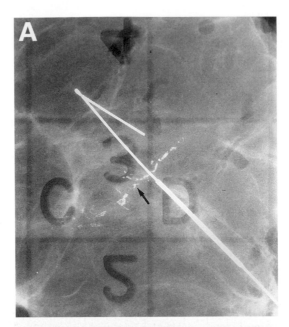

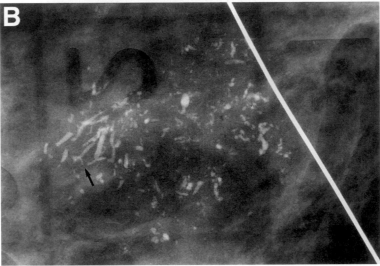

Fig. 26. Ductal carcinoma *in situ* (DCIS) with comedonecrosis. **(A)** Specimen radiograph following needle localization. These calcifications exhibit several suspicious features: they are heterogeneous in size and shape; several are linear in shape with a few branching forms (arrow); and many of the calcifications are linearly distributed. **(B)** Although not in a linear distribution, these calcifications of DCIS are extremely pleomorphic. Note the irregular and angular shapes, as well as branching forms (arrow).

prominent in patients with malignancy owing to more extensive resection. Additionally, they are accentuated in scope and prolonged in duration because of radiation therapy, which itself may induce mammographic changes.

Postsurgical changes such as stromal edema, distortion, and fluid collections usually peak by 6 months. Subsequent mammographic evaluation should then demonstrate gradual resolution of these findings. In most cases, the appearance stabilizes after 2 years. A subsequent increase in density and/or architectural distortion in the lumpectomy bed may indicate recur-

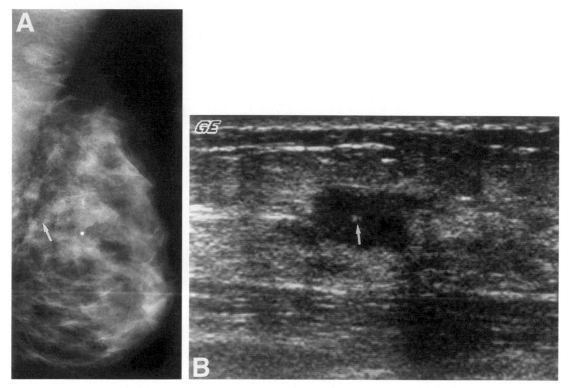

Fig. 27. Calcifications associated with a mass not clearly seen mammographically. (**A**) The right mediolateral oblique view in this 41-year-old woman with a new palpable lump (metallic BB) demonstrates a tiny cluster of plemorphic calcifications (arrow) suspicious for ductal carcinoma *in situ*. (**B**) On sonographic evaluation, a small solid mass is also identified, suggesting an invasive component. The two tiny echogenic foci within the mass (arrow) correspond to microcalcifications. Pathology from core biopsy demonstrated both intraductal and invasive components.

rent disease and should prompt further evaluation with additional mammographic views and possibly ultrasound.

Postoperative fat necrosis may present mammographically as a spiculated mass or density, with or without calcifications and lipid (oil) cysts. Without other findings, the density may be difficult to differentiate from malignancy, and biopsy may be necessary. Over time, the zone of fat necrosis becomes increasingly lucent as debris and hemorrhage are replaced by fat. The fat necrosis may calcify, producing typically curvilinear peripheral, plaque-like, or egg-shell calcifications (Fig. 30). Fat necrosis may also produce pleomorphic microcalcifications that are not associated with oil cysts and are thus indistinguishable from malignant calcifications based on imaging alone.

Radiation therapy results in diffuse parenchymal and skin edema. The mammographic manifestations of these changes are increased overall density, trabecular thickening, and skin thickening. Unlike postsurgical changes, skin thickening may take several years to stabilize.

Mammography is less sensitive for detecting local recurrence compared with detecting the initial cancer, probably because of postsurgical and postradiation changes. The reported sensitivity for recurrence in the lumpectomy bed is approximately 43%, whereas 90% of primary cancers are detected mammographically.

Recent studies have investigated the potential use of MRI in patients following breast conservation with suspicious mammographic and/or clinical findings. With intravenous con-

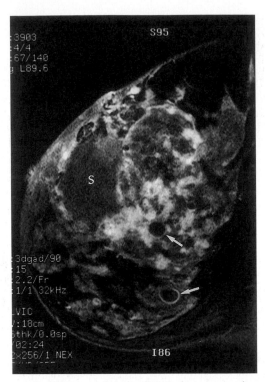

Fig. 28. Mammographically occult diffuse carcinoma detected on magnetic resonance (MR). This patient presented with a palpable mass. Following a negative mammogram, excisional biopsy of the palpable abnormality was performed, demonstrating invasive lobular carcinoma. Contrast-enhanced breast MR demonstrates the postoperative seroma (S), as well as diffuse patchy abnormal enhancement suggesting malignancy. Mastectomy confirmed diffuse carcinoma. Also noted on the MR are scattered cysts (arrows).

trast, recurrent disease but not benign postsurgical scarring has demonstrated enhancement (Fig. 31). Further investigation is necessary to define the role of MRI further in the follow-up of patients with breast cancer.

3.6.4. MAMMOGRAPHIC EVALUATION FOLLOWING MASTECTOMY

Imaging of the mastectomy bed is not routinely performed. However, if the patient develops a palpable lump, sonographic evaluation may help differentiate between postoperative scar and other findings such as lymph nodes or chest wall recurrence (Fig. 32). In certain patients, there is enough residual tissue to permit mammographic evaluation of a region of palpable concern, if sonography has been noncontributory.

4. OTHER BREAST IMAGING MODALITIES

Because of mammography's limited sensitivity and specificity, alternative methods of breast cancer detection and diagnosis have been proposed. These include ultrasound, MRI nuclear medicine, and digital mammography.

4.1. Breast Ultrasound

Breast ultrasound has become an indispensable imaging adjunct to mammography in the diagnosis of breast diseases. Thus far, no other modality has increased the specificity of mammography while simultaneously offering versatility and cost effectiveness.

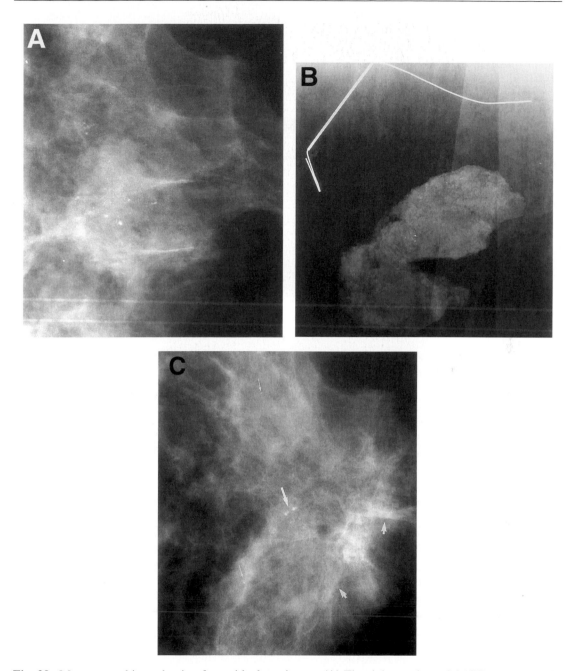

Fig. 29. Mammographic evaluation for residual carcinoma. (**A**) The right craniocaudal (CC) spot magnification view demonstrates loosely grouped heterogeneous calcifications in the subareolar breast. (**B**) Multiple calcifications were excised during primary excision (following needle localization), as shown in this specimen radiograph. (**C**) The postexcision right CC spot magnification view demonstrates a cluster of calcifications (thick arrow) and a few scattered calcifications (thin arrows) remaining in the subareolar region, as well as postsurgical architectural distortion (short arrows).

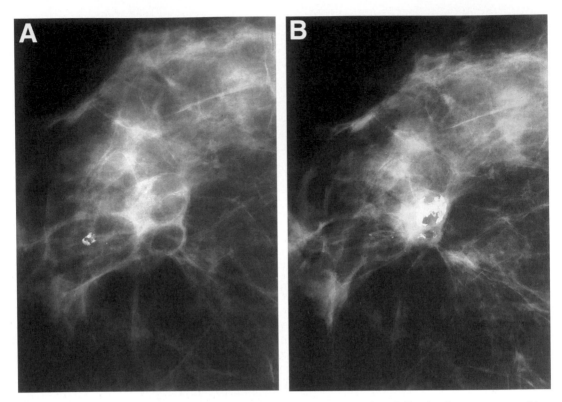

Fig. 30. Left craniocaudal views from 1995 (**A**) and 1998 (**B**) in a patient following lumpectomy and irradiation for carcinoma. Note marked increase in peripheral calcifications around three lipid cysts.

4.1.1. INDICATIONS

The indications for breast sonography are well-established:

1. To characterize palpable or nonpalpable breast masses as either cystic or solid
2. To provide an initial triage of palpable abnormalities in young (usually under age 30) or pregnant women
3. To evaluate a mammographic abnormality further
4. To localize or confirm a subtle or questionable mammographic finding
5. To provide real-time guidance for interventional breast procedures.

4.1.2. EQUIPMENT AND TECHNIQUE

State-of-the-art sonographic imaging requires a high-frequency, high-resolution hand-held transducer. Optimal imaging is acquired with a linear 10–13-MHz transducer.

Scanning is usually performed with the patient in the supine or supine-oblique position so that the quadrant of the breast to be examined is compressed against the chest wall rather than in a pendulous and mobile position. Various other positions (sitting-up, reverse oblique, and so on) may be necessary to tailor the breast exam to the patient and area of concern. The radial and antiradial scanning technique (Fig. 33) optimizes skin contact and, in comparison with transverse and longitudinal imaging, allows visualization of the breast structures (ducts, stromal tissue, and so on) in an anatomic plane in the breast as they course toward the nipple.

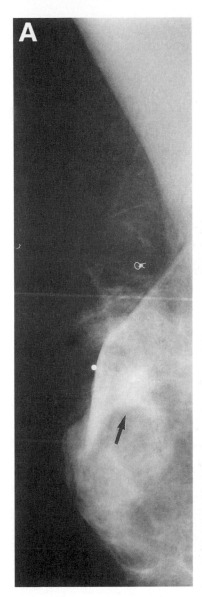

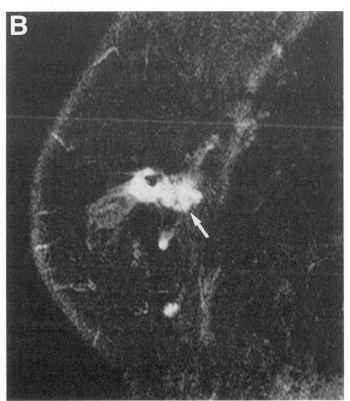

Fig. 31. Breast magnetic resonance image following breast conservation. This patient developed a palpable mass in the region of prior lumpectomy. Left mediolateral oblique view **(A)** demonstrates postsurgical distortion and a focal region of increased density (black arrow), which could represent postsurgical change or a mass. **(B)** Contrast-enhanced MR image reveals an enhancing mass (white arrow) suggesting recurrence. Carcinoma was confirmed on biopsy.

4.1.3. Normal Anatomy

Although the anatomic structures of the breast and surrounding tissue have recognizable sonographic characteristics, the normal features of the breast can be highly variable among patients. Just as some breasts are mammographically "dense" owing to a large amount of glandular and stromal tissue and others are "fatty" owing to very little glandular tissue, breasts have different recognizable parenchymal patterns on ultrasound related to the relative amounts of glandular and fatty tissues (Fig. 34).

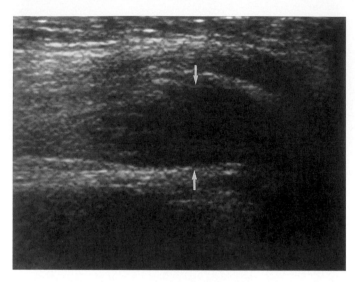

Fig. 32. Ultrasound of the mastectomy bed. In the region of a palpable lump, sonography revealed abnormal hypoechogenicity and expansion of the fibers of the pectoralis major muscle (arrows). Fine needle aspiration revealed adenocarcinoma.

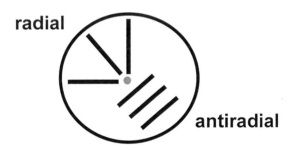

Fig. 33. Radial and antiradial scanning planes. The radial plane extends from the nipple like the spokes of a wheel. The antiradial plane is perpendicular to the radial plane.

The skin is composed of two thin echogenic lines separated by an inner hypoechoic line representing the dermis. The entire skin complex may measure up to 2 mm; skin thickening can be easily seen and measured.

Beneath the skin is a hypoechoic fatty layer that surrounds the entirety of the glandular parenchyma. Breast fat, unlike fat elsewhere in the body, appears relatively more hypoechoic than the surrounding fibroglandular and ligamentous tissue owing to the numerous attenuating and scattering surfaces that interlace throughout the glandular regions.

Though its distribution and quantity may vary, glandular tissue usually appears relatively more echogenic than the hypoechoic fatty lobules. Cooper's ligaments, the thin hyperechoic linear connective tissue structures, can be seen as scalloping striations between fat lobules usually just below the superficial fatty layer (Fig. 35).

Ductal structures are seen as hypoechoic or anechoic tubular structures that may often be followed toward the nipple-areola complex. Ducts may vary greatly in size from imperceptible to almost 8 mm in diameter. Ductal enlargement, owing to thick tenacious secretions or intraductal masses, may sometimes be demonstrated sonographically.

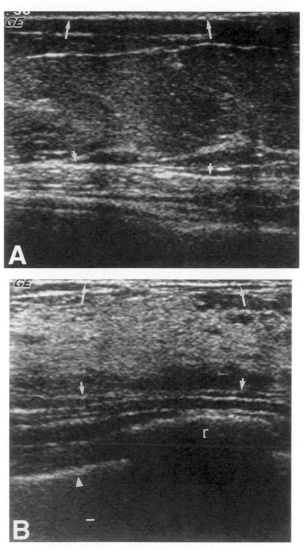

Fig. 34. The sonographic appearance of the normal breast is dependent on the amount of glandular tissue. A normal fatty breast is shown in **(A),** with normal fat relatively hypoechoic. The skin layer is extremely thin (long arrows). Deep to breast fat, the parallel fibers of the pectoralis muscle are visualized (short arrows). A normal dense breast is shown in **(B).** Most of the breast tissue between the skin (long arrows) and the pectoralis muscle (short arrows) is composed of extremely echogenic glandular tissue. A shadowing rib (r) can be seen just deep to the pectoralis muscle. The thin echogenic line of the pleura is also visualized (arrowhead).

Deep to the stromal and glandular tissue is a layer of retromammary fat. The retromammary fascia, a thin layer of connective tissue, is rarely seen sonographically. The pectoralis muscles are seen deep to the glandular and fatty tissues as striated planes; frequently, two layers may be visualized. Behind the musculature, the ribs are identifiable as oval structures in the sagittal plane, often with a hyperechoic central nidus owing to the core of fatty marrow.

4.1.4. LESION ANALYSIS

Breast ultrasound has an accuracy of almost 100% in differentiating a simple cyst from a solid mass. To achieve this high accuracy, strict sonographic criteria for a simple cyst must be met (Fig. 36):

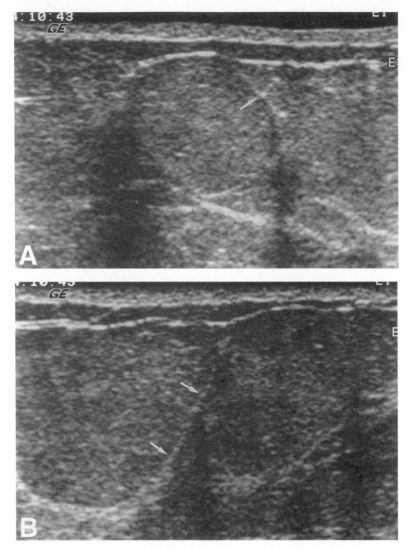

Fig. 35. Cooper's ligaments. (**A** and **B**) Thin echogenic Cooper's ligaments (arrows) are seen coursing toward the skin layer. Although they are extremely small, they can cause prominent posterior acoustic shadowing.

1. Anechoic contents
2. Well-circumscribed margin
3. Thin, imperceptible wall
4. Enhanced through transmission.

However, with the advent of high-frequency ultrasound transducers, the internal contents of a cyst are now more easily visualized. Complex cysts usually are a variant of benign cystic or benign epithelial proliferative changes of the breast and are extremely common. The internal echoes seen inside these complex cysts are caused by cellular debris or other proteinaceous material (Fig. 37). Often, with a change in patient position, the material may be seen to shift position to the dependent portion of the cyst. The presence of thin septations in an otherwise simple cyst should not be considered worrisome. Often, with careful scanning,

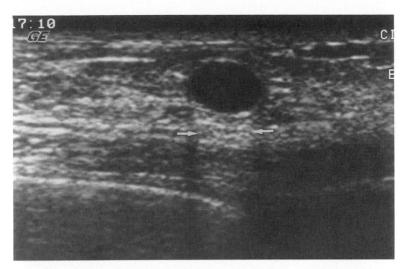

Fig. 36. Simple cyst. This sonographic lesion meets all the criteria for a simple cyst. It has a thin, imperceptible wall, a circumscribed margin, anechoic contents, and posterior acoustic enhancement (arrows). The few echoes seen within the cyst are the result of reverberation artifact.

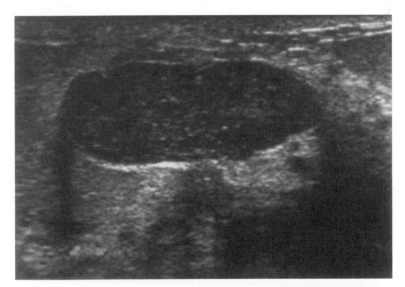

Fig. 37. Complex cyst. Although this sonographic lesion demonstrates a thin wall, circumscribed margin, and posterior acoustic enhancement, the internal contents are hypoechoic. Ultrasound-guided aspiration was performed, resulting in complete resolution of the complex cyst.

these apparent septations may even be identified as walls between contiguous cysts rather than intracystic septations.

Simple cysts have no chance of harboring a malignancy and do not need to be aspirated or have short-term follow-up. Mildly complicated cysts with layering debris or thin septations are likewise benign. If sonography cannot differentiate between a cyst and a solid lesion, ultrasound-guided aspiration may be necessary. If mural nodules, thick internal septations, or wall irregularities are present, evaluation with pulsed Doppler or color Doppler may demonstrate internal vascularity, suggesting the possibility of a papilloma or an intracystic papillary carcinoma (Fig. 38). Excisional rather than core biopsy is recommended for tissue diagnosis of these lesions.

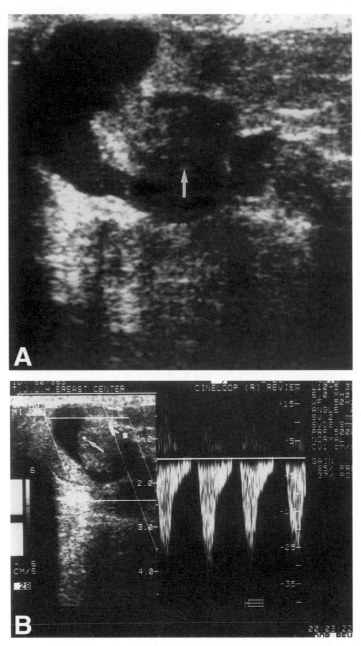

Fig. 38. Intracystic mass. Sonographic evaluation was performed in a 72-year-old woman with a palpable lump. **(A)** Hypoechoic soft tissue (arrow) is present within a cystic lesion. The differential diagnosis includes debris, hemorrhage, and intracystic mass. **(B)** Color Doppler evaluation demonstrates internal vascularity (arrow) within the soft tissue, confirming an intracystic mass. Pulsed Doppler interrogation identifies an arterial waveform.

Recent reports (Stavros et al., 1995), have suggested that if strict criteria for the sonographic analysis of solid masses are followed, the specificity for differentiating malignant from benign masses can reach over 90%. It is well-recognized that no single sonographic feature characterizes breast lesions and the tissue morphology. A battery of image parameters based on echogenicity, echotexture, and lesion shape is used. The key features used to characterize breast carcinomas are hypoechogenicity relative to the surrounding fibroglandular tissue; inhomogeneous echotexture; an echogenic rim representing desmoplasia; posterior acoustic shadowing; margin and border characteristics such as spiculation, microlobulation, and angulation; borders with diffuse lesion-to-tissue transition; and duct extensions and branching pattern (Fig. 39).

In contrast, a fibroadenoma, the most common benign solid mass of the breast, is most often seen as a circumscribed mass with homogeneous internal echoes, usually with posterior acoustic enhancement. The fibroadenoma's benign growth pattern frequently results in a lesion that is oblong in shape, differentiating it from the aggressive, vertical growth pattern and shape of an infiltrating carcinoma (Fig. 40). Fibroadenomas frequently have a thin echogenic pseudocapsule and up to two or three macrolobulations, rather than the angular or irregular margins of an infiltrative breast carcinoma. Thin, echogenic septations may also be visualized within the fibroadenoma.

Taken together, the qualitative descriptors of ultrasound have been successful in improving the specificity of clinical and mammographic findings of breast lesions.

4.1.5. VASCULAR IMAGING OF BREAST LESIONS

Several research groups have explored the possibility of using color or power Doppler imaging to differentiate between benign and malignant lesions, taking advantage of increased vascularity owing to neoangiogenesis in malignant lesions. However, there appears to be a significant overlap in vascularity of benign and malignant masses. Further investigation, especially into the quantitative evaluation of blood flow, may provide an additional tool in the differentiation of benign from malignant tumors.

4.1.6. CONCLUSION

Breast sonography has greatly increased the specificity of breast imaging while offering versatility and cost effectiveness. The advances in high-resolution transducers allow detailed characterization of breast lesions; with the adherence to strict criteria, close follow-up of many solid lesions may be possible, thus decreasing the false-positive rate of breast biopsies. Investigations into lesion characterization, especially using lesion vascularity, are ongoing and will hopefully provide further means for differentiation. If tissue sampling is necessary, ultrasound provides an excellent means of real-time guidance.

4.2. Magnetic Resonance Imaging

An accepted indication for breast MRI is to evaluate the integrity of breast implants. Many studies have investigated the utility of breast MRI in the detection and diagnosis of breast cancer. Potential applications of breast MRI include lesion characterization (i.e., benign versus malignant); further evaluation of equivocal mammographic and sonographic findings; evaluation of palpable abnormalities with negative mammographic and sonographic assessment; and evaluation of nipple discharge. In patients diagnosed with carcinoma, breast MRI may prove useful in staging of breast carcinoma; detection of mammographically occult multifocal and/or multicentric disease; evaluation of patients with axillary node involvement from an unknown primary; detection of recurrence in patients treated with breast conservation; and screening of high-risk patients (*BRCA1* and *-2* carriers; contralateral breast cancer).

In most centers, breast MRI remains an investigational tool. Both false-positive and false-negative results do occur (Figs. 41 and 42). Additionally, its relatively high cost will prohibit its use in all women with signs/symptoms or a new diagnosis of breast cancer. Further work

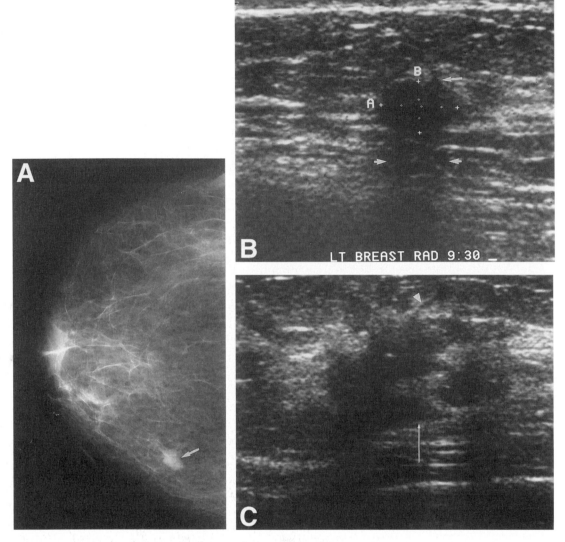

Fig. 39. Typical sonographic findings of malignancy. (**A** and **B**) Corresponding mammographic and sonographic findings in a 56-year-old asymptomatic woman. The left craniocaudal view (**A**) demonstrates a spiculated mass in the medial breast (arrow). Sonographic evaluation of the left medial breast (**B**) identified an irregularly shaped hypoechoic mass with extremely indistinct margins. Additional suspicious sonographic features of this mass include angularity (long arrow) and posterior acoustic shadowing (short arrows). (**C**) This 37-year-old patient presented with a palpable lump in the left breast. Sonographic evaluation demonstrates another typical malignancy with marked angularity (long thin arrow) and spiculations extending toward the skin (arrowhead).

is necessary to define those situations in which breast MRI will be most useful. Additionally, the caveat for its use in clinical situations is that there must be a way to localize and/or biopsy mammographically and clinically occult lesions. Some centers do have the capability to perform MRI-guided needle localizations and core biopsies (Fig. 43). If MRI localization or biopsy is not an option, the utility of breast MRI in the management of breast masses will be limited.

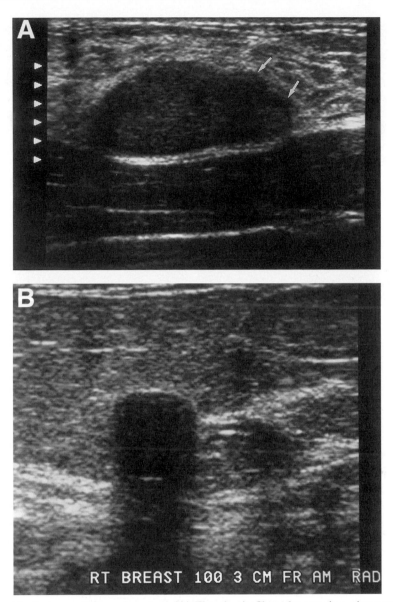

Fig. 40. Sonographic features of fibroadenomas. **(A)** The classic fibroadenoma is a circumscribed hypoechoic mass with two to three macrolobulations (arrows). Posterior acoustic enhancement can often be seen, as in this case, due to a homogeneous internal consistency. **(B)** Some fibroadenomas, although circumscribed and homogeneous, may cause posterior acoustic shadowing, as in this patient. Histologic diagnosis using ultrasound-guided core biopsy demonstrated a sclerotic fibroadenoma. Fibrosis is a common cause of posterior acoustic shadowing.

4.3. Nuclear Medicine in Breast Imaging

Imaging with radionuclides has been used for sestamibi studies and for sentinel node mapping, which is discussed in Chapters 5, 21, and 22.

4.3.1. SESTAMIBI BREAST IMAGING

Nuclear medicine recently made front page news with announcements that the use of scintimammography could prevent unnecessary biopsies in women suspected of having

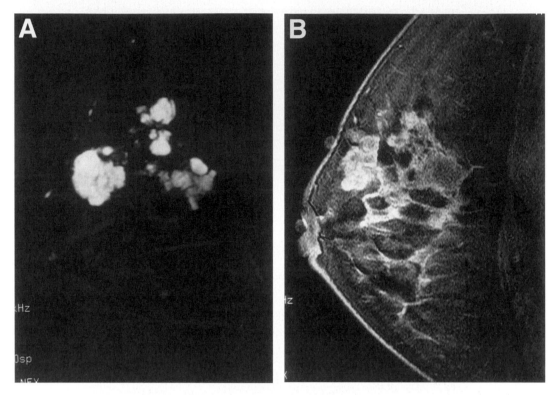

Fig. 41. False-negative breast magnetic resonance (MR) image. T2-weighted image **(A)** demonstrates multiple high-intensity masses that have a thin rim of enhancement following gadolinium injection **(B).** The MR findings were thought to represent multiple breast cysts. On pathology, colloid carcinoma was found.

breast cancer. The most frequently used tracer for scintimammography has been Tc-99m-sestamibi. A few recent studies have reported a high positive predictive value, sensitivity, and specificity for the diagnosis of breast cancer, but the efficacy has largely been limited to the diagnosis of large, often palpable, cancers. Tumors smaller than 1 cm or medial lesions are poorly imaged with the technology. Khalkhali et al. (1997) evaluated 153 suspicious lesions in 147 patients. Cancer was correctly identified in 90% of cases, with a 7% false-positive rate and a 3% false-negative rate. Although these are encouraging numbers, the study population was drawn from patients with mammographic or clinical abnormalities, rather than from a true screening population; therefore, the false-positive rate based on an asymptomatic population is unknown. In another study (Palmedo et al., 1996), the reported sensitivities have ranged from 97% (for cancers >2 cm) to 26% (for those <0.5 cm). In addition, false-positive results have been reported in benign conditions such as fibroadenomas and regions of normal glandular tissue.

As with breast MRI, a limitation in the utility of sestamibi is the difficulty in localizing mammographically and/or clinically occult lesions.

4.4. Digital Mammography

Digital mammography has many potential advantages over film-screen techniques. Since digital systems acquire, display, and store the images independently, each of these functions can be individually optimized.

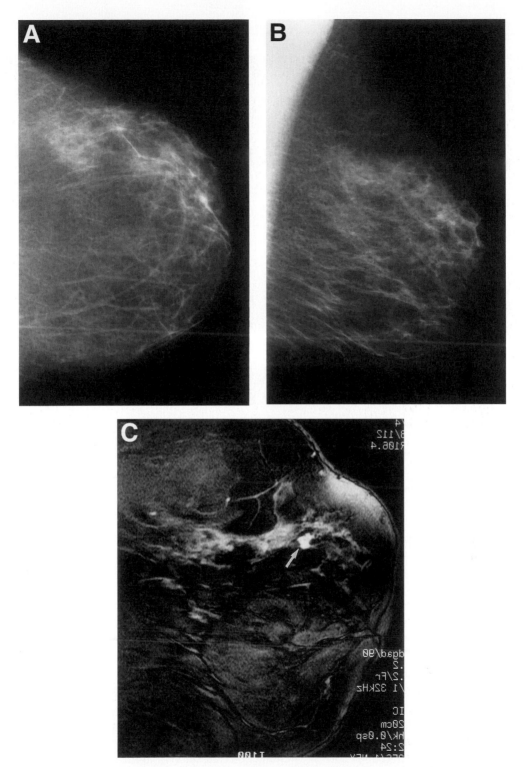

Fig. 42. False-positive breast magnetic resonance imaging (MRI). This 56-year-old patient presented with a palpable mass in the right breast. (**A** and **B**) No mammographic abnormality was identified on craniocaudal and mediolateral views of the right breast. (**C**) A small enhancing mass (arrow) was identified on MRI, which was considered suspicious for carcinoma. Excisional biopsy demonstrated benign breast tissue with fibrocystic changes.

63

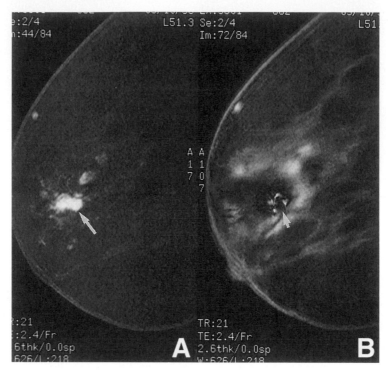

Fig. 43. Magnetic resonance-guided needle localization. (**A**) Contrast-enhanced image demonstrates a small enhancing mass (long arrow), which was not seen mammographically. (**B**) Wire placement within the mass causes a signal void (short arrow), obscuring visualization of the mass.

The success of the film-screen technique is related to the high spatial resolution and the ability to image tissues with inherently low contrast. This technique, however, is limited in the range of exposures over which clinically significant contrast can be displayed. In a single film-screen image, the range of densities in the breast that can be optimally presented are limited by the limited range of exposures that yield clinically significant contrast detail.

The ability to detect malignancies or the *sensitivity* of mammography is dependent on the conspicuity of lesions in a wide range of breast types. Unfortunately, up to 10% of clinically evident breast cancers are not detected mammographically, and the sensitivity of mammography is known to decrease as the glandularity of the breasts increases. The dense glandular tissue may obscure underlying pathology. In other words, if two breast lesions are located in two very different types of breast tissue, dense glandular tissue versus a very radiolucent fatty area, both the lesions may not be detected on the same film using a standard technique. This may lead to lack of detection of one of the lesions or the need for multiple films to evaluate fully the areas of differing densities.

Another major concern in screening with conventional mammography is the lack of *specificity* and the high rate of false-positive interpretations. Of all nonpalpable lesions detected by film-screen mammography and considered suspicious enough to warrant biopsy, only approximately 30% prove to be malignant histologically. The false-positive cases are physically as well as psychologically traumatic.

Digital mammography has the potential to be both more sensitive and specific than film-screen mammography. The sensitivity may be improved by the wide dynamic range of the digital detector, which may allow improved detection of lesions in both dense and fatty areas. The specificity may be improved by the ability to manipulate the images to optimize detection in all breast types. Since digital systems acquire, display, and store the image data independently, each of these functions can be optimized individually. The contrast, brightness, and magnification can be controlled at the display monitor or prior to printing a hard copy digital image to allow complete evaluation of all portions of the breast. To understand the limitations of film-screen or analog systems and to appreciate the potential advantages of direct digital imaging, we must first review the basic principles of image quality.

4.4.1. SPATIAL RESOLUTION

Mammography presents a unique challenge in imaging by requiring a very high spatial resolution (50–100 µm) over a large area (up to 24×30 cm). Under optimal conditions, film-screen systems have a limiting resolution of 20 lp/mm. To provide similar resolution, digital systems must have each imaging unit or pixel spaced no further apart than 0.025 mm. For large receptors such as a full field detector, this would require a pixel matrix on the order of $9600 \times 12,000$ pixels—a technologic feat! Digital systems presently provide a spatial resolution of 8–10 lp/mm, significantly less than film-screen systems.

4.4.2. CONTRAST RESOLUTION

Digital systems may have a spatial resolution less than that of film screen systems, but digital receptors provide markedly improved contrast resolution. Unlike a conventional film-screen system whose exposure response curve is nonlinear, the detectors used in digital systems have linear responses; therefore the digital imaging system provides good imaging efficiency over a wide range of exposures, allowing lesion detection even at the very outside ranges of exposures. Image processing (such as windowing and leveling) also allows the display of selected exposure ranges at high contrast.

It is possible for a system to have excellent spatial resolution but poor visibility of detail because of insufficient contrast resolution. Advances in mammography have always considered the balance of spatial and contrast resolution and the need to maintain a low dose. The exact spatial resolution requirements of digital systems are yet to be determined. Currently full-field digital systems have 50–100-µm resolution, but the superior contrast resolution compensates for the poor spatial resolution.

4.4.3. ADVANTAGES OF DIGITAL IMAGING

4.4.3.1. Separation of Acquisition and Display. One of the many advantages of digital imaging is the ability to optimize image acquisition by separating it from the image display. In film-screen images, the exposure technique dictates the optical density range that is visualized. The exposure technique is optimized so that with one image the range of densities within a breast are captured. In digital imaging, it is the desired signal-to-noise ratio that dictates the exposure (low dose, of course), and the resulting range of pixel intensities is then spread over the full range of the display. By separating image acquisition from the display function, the image information may be presented for interpretation in a multitude of formats.

The information is then available for storage, display, and manipulation. The image is displayed as a collection of discrete information samples, or pixels. The display matrix describes the pixel distribution or how many square units the image will be divided into for viewing. The matrix size directly affects the possible spatial resolution of the image, and the monitors necessary to display the digital data must be of a high enough resolution to allow

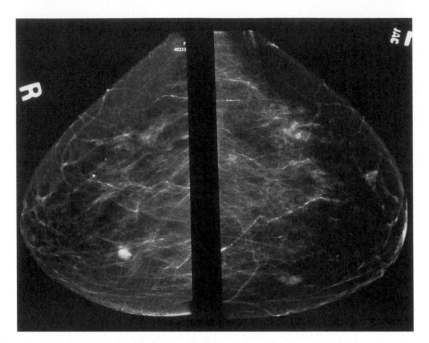

Fig. 44. Full-field digital mammography images. One technique for displaying the digital mammographic images includes a "thickness compensation" algorithm that reduces the number of gray levels without decreasing the diagnostic content of the displayed image. Note the detail in the very superficial subcutaneous zone. With the thickness compensation algorithm applied, all the tissue may be visualized at a high contrast level.

detection of lesions at the 50–100-µm size. These monitors are costly and, if not of adequate resolution, may limit the sensitivity in detecting small lesions.

4.4.3.2. Postacquisition Image Processing. The quality of the monitor for viewing direct digital images may be a limiting factor in image analysis. The matrix size, range of brightness, sharpness, and noise in the displayed image will vary with the quality of the monitor. The ability to manipulate the image with contrast and brightness controls allows the operator to alter the image to enhance image information. This allows tailoring of image presentations to individual breast types or reader preference (Fig. 44). The workstation also provides the capability to invert the displayed image so that densities are seen as black and areas of high penetration such as fat are seen as bright. Magnification or the zoom mode is helpful for visualizing faint objects such as microcalcifications or even the spicules in area of subtle architectural distortion (Fig. 45).

4.4.3.3. Other Advantages of Digital Systems. Cassettes are no longer necessary, and the images obtained may be quickly displayed on a nearby acquisition workstation. The postacquisition manipulation of images has been shown to reduce the number of retakes (improving specificity) and also decrease the exposure.

Computer-aided detection (CAD) has possible benefit as a second reader that is tireless, consistent, and undistracted. A second read by the computer may draw attention to overlooked areas by the first radiologist. CAD may also provide a statistical probability of malignancy based on lesion type and therefore ultimately decrease the number of biopsy recommendations.

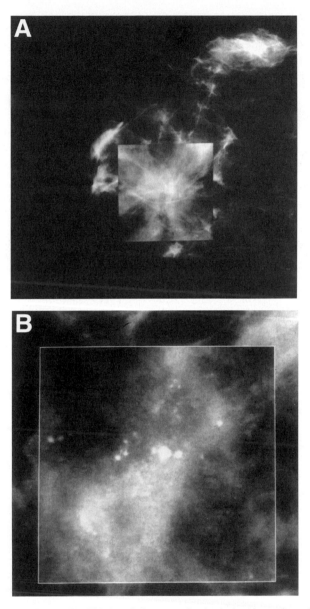

Fig. 45. Magnification or zoom mode. **(A)** A subtle area of spiculation in an invasive ductal carcinoma is made more evident by using the magnification tool available on the digital workstation. **(B)** Magnification as well as manipulation of the contrast helps resolve the morphology of these punctate calcifications, in this case of benign adenosis.

The archiving process provides copies of digital studies that should be as good as the "original." There should be no repeated exams owing to lost films. Storage is provided on an optical disk.

With the development of telemammography offsite expert mammography consultants may be made available to remote and underserved areas. Potentially, the ability to transmit images digitally will allow second opinions from geographically distant readers or teleconferencing of cases for teaching purposes.

5. CONCLUSIONS

Skillfully practiced, the art of multimodality breast imaging will provide the greatest hope for detecting the smallest, most treatable, and curable breast cancers. New modalities and new algorithms for breast cancer screening and for the evaluation of breast symptoms will continue to emerge; however, diligent, high-quality imaging remains the most significant factor in altering the course of breast cancer and reducing the mortality rate of this tragic disease.

BIBLIOGRAPHY

Mammography

ACR Standard for the Performance of Breast Ultrasound Examination (1999) American College of Radiology, Reston, VA, pp. 339–342.

ACR Standard for the Performance of Diagnostic Mammography (1999) American College of Radiology, Reston, VA, pp. 43–46.

ACR Standard for the Performance of Screening Mammography (1999) American College of Radiology, Reston, VA, pp. 35–42.

Bassett LW (1995) Clinical image evelution. *Radiol. Clin. North. Am.* **33,** 1027–1039.

Cardenosa G, Eklund GW (1995) Screening mammography in women 40–49 years old. *AJR* **164,** 1104–1106.

Conant EF, Maidment ADA (1996) Breast cancer imaging. *Sci. Am. Sci. Med.* **3,** 22–31.

Dershaw DD (1995) Mammography in patients with breast cancer treated by breast conservation (lumpectomy with or without radiation). *AJR* **164,** 309–316.

D'Orsi CJ, Bassett LW, Feig SA (1998) *Illustrated Breast Imaging Reporting and Data System (BI-RADS™),* 3rd ed. American College of Radiology, Reston, VA.

Evans WP (1995) Breast masses: appropriate evaluation. *Radiol. Clin. North Am.* **33,** 1085–1108.

Feig SA (1988) Importance of supplementary mammographic views to diagnostic accuracy. *AJR* **151,** 40–41.

Hogge JP, Robinson RE, Magnant CM, Zuurbier RA (1995) The mammographic spectrum of fat necrosis of the breast. *Radiographics* **15,** 1347–1356.

Kopans DB (1998) *Breast Imaging,* 2nd ed. Lippincott-Raven, Philadelphia.

Krecke KN, Gisvold JJ (1993) Invasive lobular carcinoma of the breast: mammographic findings and extent of disease at diagnosis in 184 patients. *AJR* **161,** 957–960.

Mendelson EB (1992) Evaluation of the postoperative breast. *Radiol. Clin. or North Am.* **30,** 107–138.

RSNA Categorical Course in Breast Imaging Syllabus (1995). Radiological Society of North America, Oak Brook, IL.

Sickles EA (1989) Breast masses: mammographic evaluation. *Radiology* **173,** 297–303.

Sickles EA (1995) Management of probably benign breast lesions. *Radiol Clin North Am* **33,** 1123–1130.

Stavros AT, Thickman D, Rapp CL, Dennis MA, Parker SH, Sisney GA (1995) Solid breast nodules: use of ultrasonography to distinguish between benign and malignant lesions. *Radiology* **96,** 123–134.

Magnetic Resonance Imaging

Hochman MG, Orel SG, Powell CM, Schnall MD, Reynolds CA, White LN (1997) Fibroadenomas: MR imaging appearances with radiologic-histopathologic correlation. *Radiology* **204,** 123–129.

Nunes LW, Schnall MD, Orel SG, et al. (1997) Breast MR imaging: interpretation model. *Radiology* **202,** 833–841.

Orel SG (1998) High-resolution MR imaging for the detection, diagnosis, and staging of breast cancer. *Radiographics* **18,** 903–912.

Orel SG, Hochman MG, Schnall MD, Reynolds CA, Sullivan DC (1996) High-resolution MR imaging of the breast: clinical context. *Radiographics* **16,** 1385–1401.

Orel SO, Schnall MD, Powell CM, et al. (1995) Staging of suspected breast cancer: effect of MR imaging and MR-guided biopsy. *Radiology* **96,** 115–122.

Nuclear Medicine

Khalkhali I, Iraniha S, Diggles LE, Cutrone JA, Mishkin FS (1997) Scintimammography: the new role of technetium-99m sestamibi imaging for the diagnosis of breast carcinoma. *Q. J. Nucl. Med.* **41,** 231–238.

Klaus AJ, Klingensmith WC 3rd, Parker SH, Stavros AT, Sutherland JD, Aldrete KD (2000) Comparative value of 99m Tc-sestamibi scintimammography and sonography in the diagnostic workup of breast masses. *AJR* **174,** 1779–1783.

Palmedo H, Schomburg A, Grunwald F, Mallmann P, Krebs D, Biersack HJ (1996) Technetium-99m-MIBI scinti-mammography for suspicious breast lesions. *J. Nucl. Med.* **37,** 626–630.

Tolmos J, Cutrone JA, Wang B, et al. (1998) Scintimammographic analysis of nonpalpable breast lesions previously identified by conventional mammography. *J. Natl. Cancer Inst.* **90,** 846–849.

Digital Mammography

Nawano S, Murakami K, Moriyama N, Kobatake H, Takeo H, Shimura K (1999) Computer-aided diagnosis in full digital mammography. *Invest. Radiol.* **34,** 310–316.

Pisano ED (2000) Current status of full-field digital mammography. *Radiology* **214,** 26–28.

3

Breast Biopsy Techniques

Lisa A. Newman, MD,
and Frederick C. Ames, MD

CONTENTS

INTRODUCTION
PERCUTANEOUS BREAST BIOPSY
OPEN SURGICAL BREAST BIOPSY
BIBLIOGRAPHY

1. INTRODUCTION

The past two decades have seen sweeping changes and expansion in the armamentarium of available approaches to detect and manage abnormal breast masses. In the past, all women requiring breast biopsies underwent single-stage procedures under general anesthesia, and the decision to proceed with definitive cancer therapy (which was always a mastectomy) was made intraoperatively, based on frozen section evaluation of the excised palpable mass.

Currently, however, patients have a variety of surgical treatment options for breast cancer (breast conservation therapy, mastectomy with or without immediate reconstruction), and every effort should be made to obtain a histologic diagnosis via needle biopsy (core or aspiration) of palpable masses as well as mammographically detected lesions. With this approach, management alternatives can be reviewed by the clinician and the patient before any incision on the breast is made. This shift in diagnostic strategy has several advantages:

1. The likelihood of obtaining negative margins with a single surgical procedure is greater if the diagnosis of malignancy has already been established at the time of definitive lumpectomy.
2. There are now broadened applications for induction chemotherapy, including tumor downstaging to improve rates of breast conservation therapy. It is preferable to have a histologic diagnosis via needle biopsy in this setting so that measurable disease is preserved for assessment of tumor response.
3. Improved breast cancer surveillance with screening mammography has resulted in increased numbers of indeterminate lesions detected; the ability to evaluate these lesions via needle biopsy will result in the avoidance of surgery for those patients whose lesions are actually benign.

With this background, the purpose of this chapter is to review the various forms of currently available needle as well as open surgical biopsy techniques and to discuss some of the common practice guidelines utilized on the Breast Service at the University of Texas M.D. Anderson Cancer Center.

From: *Current Clinical Oncology:*
Breast Cancer: A Guide to Detection and Multidisciplinary Therapy
Edited by: M. H. Torosian © Humana Press Inc., Totowa, NJ

2. PERCUTANEOUS BREAST BIOPSY

2.1. Palpable Masses

For palpable breast masses, a direct, freehand biopsy may be the most rapid means of establishing a cancer diagnosis, and this may be an appropriate initial maneuver for those patients who cannot (or will not) comply with the return visits necessary for thorough bilateral breast imaging. Otherwise, it is preferable to obtain a bilateral mammogram and possibly breast ultrasound as well, prior to performing an invasive procedure. The mammogram will provide valuable information regarding evidence of multicentric or contralateral lesions and may facilitate the distinction between a lobular, well-defined lesion, likely to represent a simple cyst, and an irregular, stellate lesion more consistent with a cancer. The addition of breast ultrasound to characterize the lesion further, and perhaps guide the percutaneous biopsy, also offers significant advantages. Some cystic lesions of the breast may be surrounded by a surprisingly thick quantity of dense breast tissue, which can mislead the clinician in identifying the cyst contents for aspiration. An ultrasound-guided aspiration should obviate this potential pitfall. If a needle biopsy has been attempted prior to ultrasound breast imaging, hemorrhage into the cyst cavity can distort the appearance of the lesion, and the resulting heterogeneity may falsely heighten concern regarding malignancy.

2.2. Fine Needle Aspiration versus Core Needle Biopsy

The second basic consideration regarding percutaneous breast biopsies is the choice between performing a fine needle aspiration biopsy (FNAB) for cytology or a core needle biopsy (CNB) to obtain tissue for pathologic assessment. The primary advantage of FNAB is its simplicity: 21-, 22-, or 23-gage needles, attached to a 5- or 10-mL syringe (readily available in most offices or clinics), may be utilized for the procedure; it is relatively atraumatic for the patient; and it is ideally suited for the aspiration of a simple cyst. However, it is optimal to have an experienced cytopathologist available for immediate evaluation of the sample adequacy. Sensitivity of FNAB varies with the experience of the clinician and the cytopathologist, ranging from 73 to 99% in published reports. Sample inadequacy rates range from 5 to 36%. The major limitation of FNAB is the inability of cytology to distinguish invasive cancer from *in situ* disease. A word of caution is warranted when considering FNAB to evaluate a breast mass in a pregnant patient; the proliferative changes of pregnancy can alter mammary tissue such that the cytologic appearance will be misinterpreted as atypia.

CNB is typically performed utilizing an automated biopsy gun attached to a 14-, 18-, or 20-gage cutting needle. Tissue cores can be processed for complete pathologic assessment and are generally adequate to determine level of invasion. Sensitivity rates are generally higher for CNB compared with FNAB, approaching 100% in many studies. The major disadvantage, however is the greater trauma for the patient.

The optimal way to integrate FNAB and CNB into clinical practice is to utilize both modalities sequentially. At the M.D. Anderson Cancer Center, the typical approach is to perform FNAB first. This specimen would be characterized as 1) benign, 2) atypical/indeterminate, 3) suspicious for carcinoma, 4) malignant, or 5) insufficient sample for diagnosis. If the overall clinical picture (mammographic, sonographic, and physical findings) is compatible with a benign lesion, then no further immediate intervention is necessary. All other categories may require subsequent CNB either to improve diagnostic accuracy or to distinguish *in situ* from invasive disease.

It is important to emphasize that concordance of the needle biopsy result and the clinical impression is crucial; proceeding with an open biopsy is always indicated if the needle biopsy appears benign in the face of a clinically or radiographically suspicious lesion. Similarly, if atypia (lobular or ductal) is detected based on the needle biopsy result, an adjacent focus of either carcinoma *in situ* or invasive cancer must be ruled out with an open biopsy. Atypia is found in 3.6–9.5% of needle biopsies (FNAB or CNB) and is ultimately found to be associated with cancer on open biopsy in 30–60% of cases.

2.3. Nonpalpable Lesions

The third consideration in the discussion of percutaneous needle biopsy regards the management of a nonpalpable lesion detected by either mammographic or sonographic breast imaging. The selection of mammography versus ultrasound to guide the biopsy should follow the simple guideline of utilizing whichever modality best visualizes the lesion in question. In general, lesions that are suspicious based on pattern of microcalcifications will be best evaluated by mammographically guided biopsy, and at the M.D. Anderson Cancer Center we are likely to biopsy most of the remaining lesions with ultrasound guidance. Breast ultrasound has the added benefit of being able to image the axillary and supraclavicular nodal basins. FNAB of a suspicious lymph node under ultrasound guidance that confirms metastatic cancer will obviate the need for CNB following FNAB of the primary tumor in the breast.

Widespread adoption of routine mammography screening guidelines has contributed to reductions in breast cancer mortality rates; however, the detection of indeterminate lesions, which then require open surgical biopsy, has generated excessive costs and unnecessary surgery for many thousands of patients whose lesions ultimately proved to be benign. The development of the stereotactic needle biopsy technique resulted from the quest for an accurate diagnostic procedure that would reliably ascertain the nature of suspicious lesions without subjecting the patient to an open surgical procedure.

Stereotaxis is a method of triangulation resulting in paired images that can then be localized to a three-dimensional site with the assistance of a computer. A variety of stereotactic devices are available, including a relatively less expensive add-on device that can be attached to the standard, dedicated mammogram unit, and the patient can undergo the procedure in the upright position with this equipment. Vasovagal reactions may complicate this approach, and it may be more difficult for the patient to remain motionless while sitting in the upright position. The prone biopsy tables are more expensive and require more space than standard screening mammography equipment. Patients are less likely to experience vasovagal reactions in the prone position, but they must be able to lie fairly motionless for 40–60 minutes. This may not be possible for patients with neck or back problems.

The stereotactic biopsy equipment may incorporate FNAB or CNB techniques. The relative advantages of each were summarized in the preceding discussion; the previously mentioned considerations regarding concordance of biopsy results with the clinical impression and follow-up for needle biopsies revealing atypia apply to this setting as well. In addition, 11- or 14-gage vacuum-assisted biopsy units are available (Mammotome; Biopsys Medical, Irvine, CA) that result in the retrieval of a larger quantity of tissue through the same size tract. A major advantage of stereotactically guided CNB for microcalcifications is the ability to obtain specimen radiographs of the tissue cores to confirm sample adequacy (Fig. 1). Experienced mammography centers have reported sensitivity rates of 85–100% for stereotactic CNB series over the past 5 years. Most centers recommend 5 needle passes for solid masses and at least 10 passes for microcalcifications. Although long-term follow-up is cru-

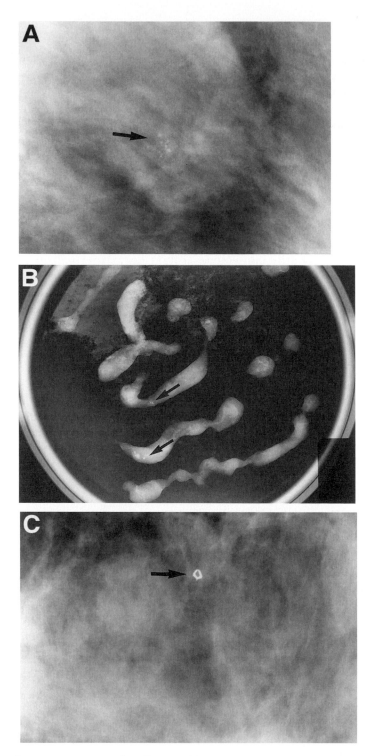

Fig. 1. (A) Screening mammogram of a 59-year-old woman reveals small area (arrow) of suspicious-appearing microcalcifications in the right upper inner quadrant. **(B)** Specimen radiograph of cores obtained following stereotactic breast biopsy with 11-gage needle showing suspicious calcifications (arrows) successfully sampled. **(C)** Postbiopsy mammogram showing metallic marker (arrow) placed at the time of stereotactic biopsy.

cial for those patients whose stereotactic needle biopsy reveals a benign finding, it has unfortunately been lacking in most published series. The actual false-negative rate of this procedure therefore remains questionable.

Some patients will be unable to undergo stereotactic biopsy because of technical considerations. Some of these considerations include body habitus too heavy for the stereotactic table; inability to remain relatively motionless for the duration of the procedure; very small breasts, for which the span of the biopsy needle may exceed the breast thickness; very superficial lesions; and vague, asymmetric densities or diffuse microcalcifications that will not be localized well on the stereotactic imaging system.

Very small lesions should be approached with caution when stereotactic or ultrasound-guided core biopsies are planned; complete evacuation of the lesion may make subsequent localization more difficult if wide local excision proves to be necessary. When this situation is anticipated, insertion of radiopaque clips at the time of percutaneous biopsy should be considered (Fig. 1C).

Another special circumstance deserves special mention. Mammographically detected lesions that appear compatible with a radial scar are generally approached more efficaciously with open surgical biopsy. It can be predicted in advance that a benign needle biopsy finding will be discordant with the very suspicious radiographic appearance of these lesions, and some investigators have reported coexistent carcinoma in 20% of the cases.

2.4. Advanced Breast Biopsy Instrumentation

Although the technique of stereotactic needle biopsy represents a major advance in the field of diagnostic maneuvers for nonpalpable breast lesions, it shares the same major limitation as other forms of needle biopsy: it is essentially a sampling procedure and cannot be relied on to completely remove the area of concern in most cases.

The Advanced Breast Biopsy Instrumentation (ABBI®) system (United States Surgical, Norwalk, CT) is the latest effort to increase the volume of breast tissue excised utilizing a percutaneous approach. The ABBI system utilizes the prone stereotactic biopsy table and localizing equipment; however, the cylindrical ABBI biopsy "guns" range from 5 to 20 mm in diameter, and an appropriately sized skin incision is made on the breast to accommodate the biopsy instrument. Since a larger volume of tissue is removed from the breast, this system can potentially completely excise a small breast neoplasm with negative margins (Fig. 2). However, data confirming the adequacy of margin control when this system is applied to mammographically detected cancers are lacking. In one of the largest reported series, final pathology review found positive margins in over 90% of ABBI-guided breast tissue extractions in which the margins appeared negative by specimen mammography. Although the percutaneous nature of the procedure would raise concerns regarding trauma to the breast, reported rates of hematoma complications have been less than 5%.

The appropriate indications for this procedure have not yet been defined. As mentioned above, the system has not been shown to be effective in excising small tumors with adequate margin control, and it should be noted that the ABBI equipment is not approved by the Food and Drug Administration for breast cancer therapy at this time. As a diagnostic modality, no improvement in accuracy over the more standard stereotactic core biopsy has been demonstrated, and the ABBI system, which does require a breast incision, is certainly a more invasive and traumatic procedure for the patient. One possible scenario that might be suitable for an ABBI-guided resection would be the patient with an early-stage breast cancer who wishes breast conservation therapy but who has an indeterminant, small lesion in another quadrant of the involved breast. In this setting, an ABBI resection could potentially excise the sec-

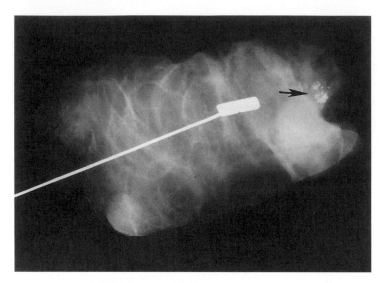

Fig. 2. Specimen radiograph of breast biopsy obtained with 2-cm Advanced Breast Biopsy Instrument (ABBI). Final pathology revealed focus of ductal carcinoma *in situ*, margins negative.

ondary lesion completely, so that it is no longer a concern on follow-up mammograms, while minimizing the volume of tissue excised and maximizing cosmesis.

3. OPEN SURGICAL BREAST BIOPSY

3.1. Incisional Biopsy

In an era of multiple forms of percutaneous needle biopsies, there are few remaining indications for an open surgical biopsy to incise a portion of a suspicious breast mass. However, occasionally the clinician is faced with the scenario of a palpable breast mass that is suspicious for a locally advanced breast cancer but a core needle biopsy is unavailable, or it reveals ductal carcinoma *in situ* (DCIS) only. In this circumstance an incisional biopsy would be warranted to rule out the presence of a large palpable form of DCIS versus an advanced cancer. Final pathology review would mandate a mastectomy as treatment for the former or induction chemotherapy for the latter. Cases that are clinically suspicious for inflammatory breast cancers may also be suitable for incisional biopsy, if core biopsy is not diagnostic.

3.2. Excisional Biopsy

Any breast lesion that requires definitive histopathologic evaluation is a candidate for excisional biopsy. Excisional biopsy may be performed with or without breast imaging guidance, depending on the confidence of the surgeon in his or her ability to palpate the full extent of the lesion. Image-directed guidance involves the use of mammography or ultrasound to insert localizing wires.

As mentioned previously, it is the practice of the M.D. Anderson Cancer Center and many other cancer centers to make every effort to obtain a histologic diagnosis for any suspicious breast lesion utilizing one of the needle biopsy techniques. If this is not possible, because of either technical considerations, concern that the lesion represents a radial scar, or the finding of atypia on needle biopsy, then an open diagnostic biopsy would be indicated.

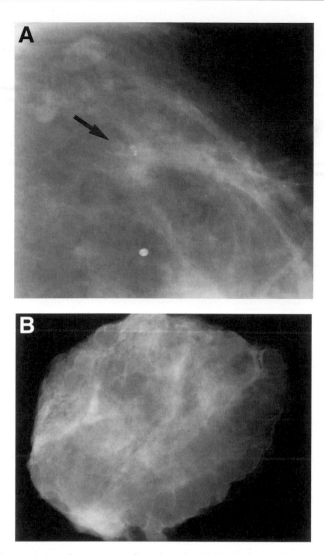

Fig. 3. A 65-year-old asymptomatic woman referred to the M.D. Anderson Cancer Center following excisional biopsy with needle localization of an abnormal mammographically detected lesion. **(A)** Preoperative magnification view revealing mass lesion and associated suspicious-appearing microcalcifications (arrow). **(B)** Specimen radiograph fails to reveal either mass or microcalcifications. *(Figure continues)*

Before proceeding with an open biopsy of a palpable mass in a patient with an abnormal mammogram, the operating surgeon is obligated to ensure that the palpable abnormality correlates with the mammographic lesion. When this is unclear, a breast ultrasound may be obtained to clarify the situation, or mammographic guidance for wire localization should be utilized.

For nonpalpable lesions requiring mammographic guidance to insert the localizing wires, a useful technique is to have the radiologist insert bracketing wires when the lesion involves a broad expanse of calcifications or asymmetric densities. It is crucial that a specimen mammogram be performed to confirm that the suspicious lesion was in fact excised (Fig. 3), and for lesions found to be cancerous a post-lumpectomy mammogram is necessary to rule out residual calcifications prior to institution of radiation therapy.

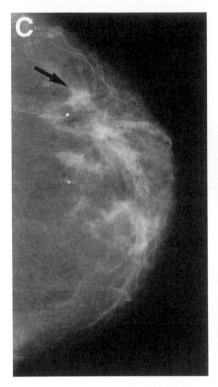

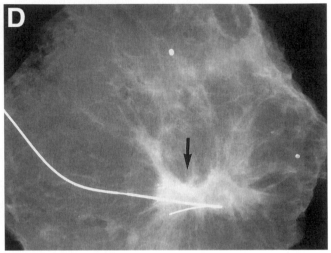

Fig. 3. *(Continued).* **(C)** Follow-up mammogram reveals persistent mass and calcifications (arrow). **(D)** Specimen radiograph following second needle localization biopsy confirming inclusion of the suspicious lesion (arrow) within the excised specimen.

The skin incision site should in general directly overlie the suspicious lesion, so that there is minimal risk of exposing extensive uninvolved breast tissue to the cancerous mass. The use of tunneling is also apt to make subsequent reexcision (when necessary for margin control) more difficult and may compromise the aesthetic result. When the lesion has been localized by mammographic guidance, the skin incision should be selected based on the location of the lesion, not the skin insertion site of the localizing needle.

A circumareolar approach is the most aesthetically acceptable incision site, and where possible this should be the attempted location. Additionally, for patients who ultimately require mastectomy, the circumareolar incision can easily be incorporated into the skin-sparing technique.

For excisional biopsies of known cancers, or lesions highly suspicious for harboring cancer, adequate margin control can be facilitated by several intraoperative maneuvers. Grossly, an attempt should be made to excise an approx 1-cm thickness of normal-appearing tissue surrounding the index lesion. The specimen should be oriented by the surgeon in three planes for the pathologist, and multiply colored inks should be used to define the margins. Mammography of the entire specimen, and of the specimen sections, can guide the surgeon to areas of suboptimal margin control, and efforts at excising more tissue in those areas or obtaining frozen section analysis can be focused on those sites. Metallic clips should then be left at the margins of the biopsy cavity to guide the radiation therapists if breast conservation therapy is contemplated.

Occasional patients will require surgical biopsy to evaluate bloody nipple discharge. At the M.D. Anderson Cancer Center we find it very helpful to perform galactography to localize the abnormal ductal structures. This is particularly useful in women with large, pendulous breasts, because in this setting the pathologic ductal lesion may be located more peripheral to the nipple areolar region than expected, and a "blind" terminal duct excision may miss the lesion.

Closure of biopsy wounds is generally performed in two layers, with use of absorbable suture for the subcutaneous tissue, and a subcuticular closure for the skin. No effort is made to approximate the deeper layers of the cavity, as this will usually result in greater skin retraction and distortion of the breast. Usually, seroma formation within the biopsy cavity will result in maintenance of the natural breast contour. However, if the volume of breast tissue resected does leave the patient with a significant deformity, then sterile saline can be injected into the cavity to facilitate cosmesis. Use of a support brassiere by the patient throughout the day may also be useful, to minimize tension and retraction of the breast against the suture line.

In summary, close communication among the surgeon, the radiologist, and the pathologist is crucial. This conversation regarding every patient should begin preoperatively, with biopsy planning, and should continue intraoperatively, with lesion confirmation via specimen imaging and margin assessment, and postoperatively, with evaluation of remaining breast tissue and final pathologic review to confirm concordance between initial impression and microscopic findings.

BIBLIOGRAPHY

Bassett L, Winchester DP, Caplan RB, et al. (1997) Stereotactic core-needle biopsy of the breast: a report of the Joint Task Force of the College of Radiology, American College of Surgeons, and College of American Pathologists. *CA Cancer J. Clin.* **47,** 171–191.

Bloomston M, D'Angelo P, Galliano D, Butler J, Dean R, Rosemurgy AS (1999) One hundred consecutive advanced breast biopsy instrumentation procedures: complications, costs, and outcome. *Ann. Surg. Oncol.* **6,** 195–199.

Brenner RJ, Fajardo L, Fisher PR, et al. (1996) Percutaneous core biopsy of the breast: effect of operator experience and number of samples on diagnostic accuracy. *AJR* **166,** 341–346.

Dowlatshahi K, Yaremko ML, Kluskens LF, et al. (1991) Nonpalpable breast lesions: findings of stereotactic needle-core biopsy and fine-needle aspiration cytology. *Radiology* **181,** 745–750.

Doyle AJ, Murray KA, Nelson EW, et al. (1995) Selective use of the image-guided large-core-needle biopsy of the breast: accuracy and cost-effectiveness. *AJR* **165,** 281–284.

Dronkers DJ (1992) Stereotaxic core biopsy of breast lesions. *Radiology* **183,** 631–634.

Elvecrog EL, Lechner MC, Nelson MJ (1993) Nonpalpable breast lesions: correlation of stereotaxic large-core-needle biopsy and surgical biopsy results. *Radiology* **188,** 453–455.

Ferzli GS, Puza T, Van Vorst-Bilotti S, Waters R (1999) Breast biopsies with ABBI®: experience with 183 attempted biopsies. *Breast J.* **5,** 26–28.

Gisvold JJ, Goellner JR, Grant CS, et al. (1994) Breast biopsy: a comparative study of stereotaxically guided core and excisional techniques. *AJR* **162,** 815–820.

Israel PZ, Fine RE (1995) Stereotactic needle biopsy for occult breast lesions: a minimally invasive alternative. *Am. Surg.* **61,** 87–91.

Jackman RJ, Nowels KW, Shepard MJ, et al. (1994) Stereotaxic large-core-needle biopsy of 450 nonpalpable breast lesions with surgical correlations in lesions with cancer or atypical hyperplasia. *Radiology* **193,** 91–95.

Janes RH, Bouton MS (1994) Initial 300 consecutive stereotactic core-needle-breast biopsies by a surgical group. *Am. J. Surg.* **168,** 533–536.

Liberman L, Dershaw DD, Rosen PP, et al. (1994) Stereotaxic 14-gauge breast biopsy: how many core biopsy specimens are needed? *Radiology* **192,** 793–795.

Liberman L, Evans WP, Dershaw DD, et al. (1994) Radiography of microcalcifications in stereotaxic mammary core biopsy specimens. *Radiology* **190,** 223–225.

Meyer JE, Christian RL, Lester SC, et al. (1996) Evaluation of nonpalpable solid breast masses with stereotaxic large-needle core biopsy using a dedicated unit. *AJR* **167,** 179–182.

Mikhail RA, Nathan RC, Weiss M, et al. (1994) Stereotactic core-needle biopsy of mammographic breast lesions as a viable alternative to surgical biopsy. *Ann. Surg. Oncol.* **1,** 363–367.

Parker SH, Burbank F, Jackman RJ, et al. (1994) Percutaneous large-core breast biopsy: a multi-institutional study. *Radiology* **193,** 359–364.

Parker SH, Lovin JD, Jobe WE, et al. (1991) Nonpalpable breast lesions: stereotactic automated large-core biopsies. *Radiology* **180,** 403–407.

Pisano ED, Fajardo LL, Tsimikas J, et al. (1998) Rate of insufficient samples for fine-needle aspiration for nonpalpable breast lesions in a multicenter clinical trial. *Cancer* **82,** 679–688.

Sneige N (1997) A comparison of fine needle aspiration, core biopsy, and needle localization biopsy techniques in mammographically detectable nonpalpable breast lesions. *Pathol. Case Rev.* **1,** 6–11.

Sneige N (1993) Fine-needle aspiration of the breast: a review of 1,995 cases with emphasis on diagnostic pitfalls. *Diagn. Cytopathol.* **9,** 106–112.

4

Clinical Classifications of Breast Cancer

Michael H. Torosian, MD, FACS

CONTENTS

INTRODUCTION
INVASIVE/INFILTRATING CARCINOMA
DUCTAL CARCINOMA *IN SITU*
MICROINVASIVE CARCINOMA
PAGET'S DISEASE
INFLAMMATORY CARCINOMA
LOBULAR CARCINOMA *IN SITU*
CONCLUSIONS
BIBLIOGRAPHY

1. INTRODUCTION

Epidemiology, family history, noninherited risk factors, and genetic mutations are important factors in the development of breast cancer. The pathologic characteristics of the primary breast carcinoma, however, are of paramount importance in determining the optimal treatment for breast cancer patients. For defining specific treatment options, breast cancer can be classified into the following clinically relevant categories: invasive/infiltrating carcinoma, ductal carcinoma *in situ,* microinvasive carcinoma, Paget's disease, inflammatory carcinoma, and lobular carcinoma *in situ.* These categories are based on the biologic behavior and prognosis of patients with these distinct types of breast cancer.

These clinically relevant categories provide a practical classification of breast cancer from which locoregional and systemic treatment decisions can be made. The histologic subtypes of invasive cancer play a relatively small role in affecting treatment decisions. For instance, histologic subtypes of invasive cancer associated with a slightly better prognosis than infiltrating ductal carcinoma include tubular, colloid or mucinous, papillary, and medullary carcinomas. Rarely does the presence of one of these more favorable histologic subtypes alter local treatment recommendations. However, other clinicopathologic factors such as multicentricity or unifocaly of disease, size of the primary tumor, presence or absence of regional lymph node involvement, and features of tumor aggressiveness (e.g., inflammatory carcinoma, histologic/nuclear grade, hormone receptor status, percent of S-phase cells, percent of aneuploid tumor cells, overexpression of her-2-*neu* oncogene, or *p53* mutations) are critical for making treatment decisions. For example, breast-conserving therapy is generally indicated for unifocal cancer with a primary tumor size of less than 5

From: *Current Clinical Oncology:*
Breast Cancer: A Guide to Detection and Multidisciplinary Therapy
Edited by: M. H. Torosian © Humana Press Inc., Totowa, NJ

cm. Clear surgical margins around the primary tumor site must be obtained prior to initiating radiation therapy; in addition, the tumor should be resected with an acceptable cosmetic result for the patient to be considered for breast-conserving therapy. Of course, mastectomy is always an option for treating patients with breast cancer and is generally indicated for patients with multifocal disease or a primary tumor larger than 5 cm in size or those who are not candidates or unwilling to receive radiation therapy. Because of the varied treatment options available, multidisciplinary treatment planning is encouraged, with input from surgical, medical, and radiation oncology to develop an optimal treatment plan for each breast cancer patient.

2. INVASIVE/INFILTRATING CARCINOMA

Approximately 75–80% of all cancers are invasive or infiltrating carcinomas. The invasive or infiltrating characteristic of cancer cells is biologically extremely important and gives these cells the ability to penetrate surrounding lymphatic and vascular channels. Penetration of lymphatic and vascular channels is clinically significant and can result in tumor metastasis to regional lymph nodes or distant organs. Microscopically, the invasive phenotype is characterized by penetration of breast cancer cells through the lining of their structure of origin (e.g., terminal duct for infiltrating ductal carcinoma, breast lobule for infiltrating lobular carcinoma). Preoperative metastatic evaluation of patients with invasive breast cancer typically consists of chest X-ray, bone scan, and blood tests including complete blood count and liver function tests. If liver function tests are elevated, abdominal computed tomography scan is performed to evaluate the liver for metastasis radiologically. Because bone scans are sensitive but not specific for detecting skeletal metastasis, in the absence of musculoskeletal symptoms, the necessity of routine of bone scans in patients with asymptomatic, early-stage (T1 and T2) breast cancer has been challenged. Nevertheless, bone scan is often obtained routinely in patients with breast cancer at initial diagnosis for use as a baseline study should skeletal symptoms develop in the future.

The general principle in treating patients with invasive breast cancer is to treat the breast and ipsilateral axillary lymph nodes. Two options exist for treating the primary tumor including breast-conserving therapy and modified radical mastectomy. Breast-conserving therapy consists of lumpectomy, axillary dissection, and radiation therapy. Ideal candidates for breast-conserving therapy include patients with a unifocal tumor that can be removed with clear resection margins. Our experience at Fox Chase Cancer Center indicates that optimal results are obtained if there is a margin of 2 mm or more from the tumor to the surgical margin of resection. If the margin of resection is less than 2 mm, the incidence of ipsilateral breast recurrence is increased, and reexcision is typically indicated prior to initiating radiation therapy. In general, primary tumor size should be less than 5 cm to obtain the best results with breast-conserving therapy. However, tumor size relative to breast size is relevant when considering breast-conserving therapy, as breast cosmesis and treatment success are both important goals. Depending on tumor location or relative tumor/breast size, patients with tumors less than 5 cm may not be ideal candidates for breast conservation. Other relative contraindications to breast-conserving therapy include diffuse calcifications or extreme density of breast tissue on mammography, rendering clinical and/or radiologic follow-up after breast conservation especially difficult.

Axillary lymph node surgery is indicated to determine whether or not metastasis has occurred to regional lymph nodes. The standard axillary lymph node dissection consists of removing level I and II lymph nodes. These lymph nodes are located lateral and posterior to the pectoralis minor muscle. Level III lymph nodes, which are located medial to the pectoralis minor muscle, are removed only if they are found to be grossly involved with tumor. The lymph node dissection should be performed inferior to the axillary vein and without cutting the pectoralis minor muscle, to minimize postoperative morbidity. The goal of standard axillary dissection is to remove at least 10 lymph nodes for accurate staging and prognosis. Sentinel lymph node mapping and biopsy has recently been introduced and, over the past few years, has been used with increasing frequency in patients with early breast cancer. The precise indications for this technique remain to be determined by clinical investigation. Nevertheless, the sentinel node mapping and biopsy procedure has great appeal to patients undergoing conservative surgery for its presumed decrease in postsurgical morbidity. However, long-term follow-up and incidence of complications (e.g., lymphedema, numbness of axilla and arm, arm pain) following sentinel lymph node mapping and biopsy in breast cancer patients remain to be determined.

The alternative to breast-conserving therapy is modified radical mastectomy. Modified radical mastectomy consists of removing the breast tissue, nipple/areola complex, and ipsilateral axillary lymph nodes. The extent of axillary dissection is the same whether breast-conserving therapy or modified radical mastectomy is used to treat the primary tumor. Skin-sparing incisions can be used for this procedure when mastectomy is performed with immediate breast reconstruction. Skin-sparing mastectomy allows more rapid expansion of the chest wall when the tissue expander/implant technique is used and requires less donor site skin when autologous tissue transfer is performed. The skin-sparing technique is typically not performed unless immediate reconstruction is done to avoid redundancy of skin and subcutaneous tissue at the surgical site.

Radiation therapy is typically initiated 2–4 weeks after breast-conserving surgery. Radiopaque clips can be placed at the lumpectomy site to assist with accurate delivery of the tumor boost to the primary tumor site. Radiation therapy may also be indicated after mastectomy for microscopically positive or close resection margins, for involvement of more than three axillary lymph nodes with the tumor, or for extracapsular extension of carcinoma in the axillary nodes.

3. DUCTAL CARCINOMA *IN SITU*

Ductal carcinoma *in situ* (DCIS) is a noninvasive carcinoma that remains confined to the ductal system of the breast without penetrating the basement membrane and extending into the surrounding stroma. The inability of these carcinoma *in situ* cells to penetrate the basement membrane renders them unable to penetrate lymphatic and vascular channels. Therefore, DCIS is a local disease of the breast and typically does not warrant regional lymph node dissection or metastatic evaluation.

Three treatment options exist for DCIS, including lumpectomy with radiation therapy, total (or simple) mastectomy, or lumpectomy without radiation therapy; however, lumpectomy without radiation therapy is not a standard treatment option and should be conducted on a study protocol except for very select patients. As indicated, treatment for DCIS is confined to the ipsilateral breast without the need for axillary lymph node dissection. Standard breast-conserving therapy consists of lumpectomy followed by radiation therapy to the entire breast. The subset of patients with microscopic DCIS for whom lumpectomy without radiation should be considered remains to be precisely defined. Adequate lumpectomy (i.e., removal of the entire area of DCIS with at least 2-mm margins on all aspects of the lumpectomy specimen) can be difficult. Although DCIS does not invade the basement membrane of the duct, it frequently presents as a diffuse biologic entity that extends for long distances along the ductal system. The extent of disease can sometimes be determined by the area of calcification seen on mammography. However, it is also possible for this disease to extend beyond the area of abnormality seen on mammography so that adequate lumpectomy cannot be accomplished. In instances of extensive DCIS, total (or simple) mastectomy is the treatment of choice. Although lymph node dissection is typically not indicated for patients with DCIS, removal of level I lymph nodes at the time of mastectomy is reasonable in patients with large areas of DCIS in case invasive cancer is identified in the mastectomy specimen. The role of sentinel lymph node mapping and biopsy in patients with DCIS is currently under investigation.

There are several proposed classifications for DCIS. The traditional classification utilized architectural growth pattern and cytologic characteristics but was limited in predicting clinical outcome. Three of the current, well-known systems for categorizing DCIS are the van Nuys, Nottingham, and European systems. Two-, three- and four-tiered classification systems have been proposed based on the presence or absence of necrosis, pattern of necrosis, nuclear grade, histologic grade, and other pathologic features. A simple and clinically relevant classification of DCIS separates comedo from all other subtypes (i.e., noncomedo) of DCIS. Comedo or high-grade DCIS typically exhibits central necrosis, aneuploidy, high proliferative rate, and increased microvessel density—features of increased tumor aggressiveness. Comedo tumors tend to be estrogen receptor-negative, overexpress her-2-neu protein, and exhibit *p53* gene mutations. In contrast, noncomedo DCIS is considered intermediate or low grade and exhibits less aggressive pathologic features and biologic behavior. The most critical difference is the finding of microinvasion, which is much more common in comedo versus noncomedo subtypes. The presence of microinvasion raises the possibility of regional or distant metastasis. Until a uniform classification for DCIS has been adopted, it is essential for clinicians to understand the histologic characteristics of DCIS and to be familiar with the classification system used by pathologists in their institution.

4. MICROINVASIVE CARCINOMA

Microinvasive carcinoma is a relatively recent description used for patients with breast cancer characterized by biologic and prognostic features midway between infiltrating carcinoma and DCIS. The term microinvasive carcinoma has been defined differently by different investigators. In various reports, microinvasion has been used to describe tumors with less than 1 mm, 5 mm or less, and even 10 mm or less of invasive carcinoma. It is the author's opinion that microinvasive carcinomas should be defined as lesions with no more than 5 mm and perhaps as little as 1–2 mm of invasive carcinoma. In addition to size of the invasive lesion, clinical investigation is needed to identify other biologic and prognostic characteristics that can define this patient population more accurately.

Primary tumor treatment in patients with microinvasive carcinoma is similar to that for patients with infiltrating carcinoma. Two treatment options exist including breast-conserving therapy (consisting of lumpectomy, axillary dissection, and radiation therapy) and modified radical mastectomy. The incidence of regional metastasis to axillary lymph nodes in patients with microinvasive carcinoma is 5% or less, depending on patient selection criteria. Although the incidence of axillary metastasis is low in this group of patients and the role of axillary lymph node dissection has been challenged, when the discovery of positive axillary lymph nodes will significantly alter systemic therapy, axillary dissection is indicated. For example, in most patients under 50 years of age or in patients with tumors exhibiting poor prognostic features, axillary dissection is generally indicated. As an alternative to the standard level I and II axillary dissection performed for more advanced carcinomas, a reasonable approach is to perform a level I lymph node dissection. Alternatively, studies are currently under way to define the role of sentinel lymph node mapping and biopsy. If the primary tumor site can be accurately localized, sentinel lymph node mapping and biopsy can be considered. If the sentinel lymph nodes are found on pathologic examination to contain metastatic carcinoma, a complete level I and II lymph node dissection is indicated. Although long-term outcome in breast cancer patients with breast cancer undergoing sentinel lymph node mapping and biopsy is not yet available, this technique appears to be a reliable method for detecting regional metastasis and the subsequent need for axillary dissection and systemic therapy.

5. PAGET'S DISEASE

Paget's disease represents approximately 1% of all breast carcinomas and typically presents with symptoms of the nipple/areolar complex. Persistent erythema, rash, ulceration, discharge, or retraction of the nipple/areolar complex are indications for biopsy and are typical symptoms of Paget's disease. On biopsy, the Paget's cell, which is a large, ovoid cell with abundant pale-staining cytoplasm and a large round or oval nucleus, is found within the epidermis of the nipple. Most patients with Paget's disease present with noninvasive carcinoma confined to the nipple. Two hypotheses have been proposed regarding the origin of the Paget's cell within the nipple epidermis. It has been proposed that Paget's cells originate from *in situ* malignancies within the nipple epidermis or, alternatively, that the cells migrate to the nipple from an underlying carcinoma. It is likely that Paget's disease can occur by either mechanism owing to the varied clinical and pathologic characteristics of patients with this disease.

Paget's disease has classically been treated with total (or simple) mastectomy. There has been little experience with breast-conserving therapy in patients with Paget's disease, although several case reports and small series have been reported in the literature. In patients with Paget's disease consisting exclusively of noninvasive carcinoma, axillary lymph node dissection is not indicated. However, a less common presentation of Paget's disease includes patients with Paget's cells seen on nipple/areolar biopsy but with an underlying invasive breast carcinoma. In such patients, the underlying mass may be detected on examination or seen as an area of increased density or microcalcifications on mammography. If invasive carcinoma is found to be associated with Paget's disease, modified radical mastectomy is indicated with standard level I and II lymph node dissection.

Thus, mastectomy is indicated for the treatment of patients with Paget's disease; *en bloc* level I and II lymph node dissection is performed if underlying invasive carcinoma is present. The extent of surgical treatment is based on the most aggressive component of the carcinoma. Patients with Paget's disease should be distinguished from patients with locally advanced, retroareolar tumors that involve the nipple/areolar complex by direct extension. These locally advanced breast carcinomas are centrally located infiltrating carcinomas and are not to be confused with Paget's disease.

6. INFLAMMATORY CARCINOMA

Inflammatory carcinoma is a fast growing aggressive carcinoma that presents with clinical signs and symptoms characteristic of inflammation or infection. This disease typically affects younger women and is characterized by diffuse erythema, breast enlargement, warmth and edema (peau d'orange) of the skin of the breast, and induration of the underlying breast tissue. There is usually no dominant mass detectable on physical examination. After the initial presentation of symptoms, rapid progression can occur over the course of several weeks. Typically these patients are initially treated with antibiotics for a clinical diagnosis of mastitis. If the symptoms persist despite antibiotic treatment, biopsy of the skin and underlying breast tissue is indicated. If a dominant mass is present, this mass should be biopsied with a portion of overlying skin and subcutaneous tissue. The skin biopsy should be performed in an area exhibiting peau d'orange to increase the accuracy of establishing a diagnosis of inflammatory breast cancer. Plugging of the dermal lymphatics with cancer causes skin and subcutaneous edema of the breast and is a classic finding in patients with inflammatory breast carcinoma. Mammography of the breast affected with inflammatory carcinoma can show increased density of the breast tissue and increased thickness of the skin and subcutaneous tissue from superficial edema and may reveal the presence of an irregular mass or malignant-appearing calcifications.

Because of the aggressive nature of inflammatory breast cancer and presumed distant spread of disease at the time of diagnosis, systemic chemotherapy is administered as the initial treatment. Both surgery and radiation therapy are typically indicated in patients with inflammatory carcinoma, with the timing of these therapies primarily dependent on the clinical response to chemotherapy. Resolution of the presenting symptoms of inflammatory carcinoma (including reduction of skin erythema, resolution of breast mass or induration, reduction in breast size, and disappearance of peau d'orange) are the best measures of tumor response to chemotherapy. Multidisciplinary treatment planning is recommended by the medical oncologist, radiation oncologist, and surgeon in order to design the optimal treatment regimen.

Surgery for patients with inflammatory carcinoma generally consists of total (or simple) mastectomy. Axillary dissection is typically not performed in patients with inflammatory carcinoma since treatment with systemic therapy is routinely administered in these patients. Axillary dissection is only performed if it will alter future treatment recommendations, is required for inclusion in a study protocol, or will remove gross axillary adenopathy. Routine axillary dissection is not indicated, as interruption of axillary lymphatics may initiate or exacerbate upper extremity lymphedema. Patients with inflammatory carcinoma are prone to develop lymphedema because significant plugging of dermal lymphatics has already occurred by the inherent nature of this disease. Pathologic evaluation of the mastectomy specimen is important to correlate with preoperative tumor response to chemotherapy and for determining whether or not additional chemotherapy should be administered after surgery.

7. LOBULAR CARCINOMA *IN SITU*

Lobular carcinoma *in situ* (LCIS) is a misnomer, as this entity is not a true breast carcinoma. Although technically classified as a Tis or *in situ* tumor, lobular carcinoma should be considered a tumor marker indicating an increased risk for future development of breast cancer. In women with LCIS, the lifetime risk of breast cancer is approximately 25–35%. An individual's specific lifetime risk of breast cancer may be significantly higher or lower than this average statistical incidence as modified by other familial and nonfamilial risk factors. Nevertheless, LCIS is an independent risk factor for future development of breast cancer in both the ipsilateral and contralateral breast to which LCIS was discovered.

Because of the bilateral risk of breast cancer conferred by the presence of LCIS, three treatment options exist for patients with this diagnosis. First, close observation and monitoring can be performed, which consists of self-breast examination monthly, breast examination by a physician every 4–6 months, and annual mammography. A low threshold for performing breast biopsies should exist for patients with LCIS, with surgical intervention indicated for significant changes noted on physical examination or mammography. A second option for treating patients with LCIS is bilateral prophylactic mastectomies. This surgical approach minimizes the risk of developing breast cancer by removing the end organ or target tissue. However, not every breast cell can be removed when performing total mastectomy and, although small, the risk of developing breast cancer after bilateral prophylactic mastectomies exists. To minimize this risk, subcutaneous mastectomies are not indicated in this situation as significant ductal tissue remains in the retroareolar and nipple regions. Unilateral mastectomy, quadrantectomy, and subtotal mastectomy with preservation of the nipple/areolar complex are contraindicated as prophylactic surgery in patients with LCIS.

A third treatment alternative is chemoprevention. The P1 chemoprevention trial conducted by the National Institutes of Health and the National Surgical Adjuvant Breast and Bowel Project clearly showed a role for tamoxifen in preventing breast cancer in women at high risk of developing this disease. In this prospective, randomized trial, women receiving tamoxifen exhibited a 50% reduction in subsequent development of invasive and *in situ* carcinomas. Specifically in women with LCIS, tamoxifen reduced the incidence of breast cancer by 56%. However, tamoxifen therapy is associated with significant side effects including an increased risk of endometrial cancer and deep venous thrombosis. A second chemoprevention trial (P2 trial) is currently underway in postmenopausal, high-risk women randomized to receive either tamoxifen or raloxifene. There is preliminary evidence indicating that raloxifene may inhibit breast cancer development without the risk of promoting endometrial cancer. Chemoprevention truly represents a compromise between the alternative options of close observation and bilateral prophylactic mastectomies.

The treatment options for women with LCIS span the entire spectrum from observation to bilateral total mastectomies. Obviously, this is a difficult decision to make, and such decisions should be made electively with physician and patient input. Individual risk determination of patients with LCIS should be performed so that additional familial and nonfamilial factors are taken into consideration. One clinically relevant model of individual risk assessment is the Gail Risk Assessment Model. This clinical risk assessment formula takes into account both familial and nonfamilial risk factors and determines an individual's 5-year and lifetime risk of developing breast cancer. Genetic testing for *BRCA-1* and *BRCA-2* genetic mutations can be performed in women with a strong family history of breast cancer. This additional information is frequently useful in helping both the physician and the patient with LCIS elect an appropriate treatment plan.

8. CONCLUSIONS

Breast cancer is a heterogeneous group of diseases capable of presenting with a wide range of clinical and pathologic features. It is important to understand the biologic behavior of different types of breast cancer in order to provide optimal oncologic management. As molecular and pathologic technology becomes more sophisticated, our diagnostic capability and treatment strategies will become ever more individualized. Multidisciplinary management with input from the surgeon, medical oncologist, radiation oncologist, and associated diagnostic and clinical physicians is necessary to provide optimal treatment for the patient with breast cancer.

BIBLIOGRAPHY

Bodian CA, Perzin KH, Lattes R (1996) Lobular neoplasia: long term risk of breast cancer and relation to other factors. *Cancer* **78,** 1024–1034.

Borger J, Kemperman H, Hart A, et al. (1994) Risk factors in breast-conserving therapy. *J. Clin. Oncol.* **12,** 653–660.

Cady B, Stone M, Wayne J (1993) New therapeutic possibilities in primary invasive breast cancer. *Ann. Surg.* **183,** 338.

Carlson GW, Bostwick J, Styblo TM, et al. (1997) Skin-sparing mastectomy. Oncologic and reconstructive considerations. *Ann. Surg.* May **225,** 570–575.

Fisher B, Anderson S, Redmond CK, Wolmark N, Wickerham DL, Cronin WM (1995) Reanalysis and results after 12 years of follow-up in a randomized clinical trial comparing total mastectomy with lumpectomy with or without irradiation in the treatment of breast cancer. *N. Engl. J. Med.* **333,** 1456–1461.

Fisher B, Costantino J, Redmond C, et al. (1993) Lumpectomy compared with lumpectomy and radiation therapy for the treatment of intraductal breast cancer. *N. Engl. J. Med.* **328,** 1581–1586.

Giuliano A, Kirgan D, Guenther J, et al. (1994) Lymphatic mapping and sentinel lymphadenectomy for breast cancer. *Ann. Surg.* **220,** 391.

Gump FE, Kinne DW, Schwartz GF (1998) Current treatment for lobular carcinoma in situ (LCIS). *Ann. Surg. Oncol.* **5,** 33–36.

Gwin JL, Eisenberg BL, Hoffman JP, Ottery FD, Boraas M, Solin LJ (1993) Incidence of gross and microscopic carcinoma in specimens from patients with breast cancer after re-excision lumpectomy. *Ann. Surg.* **218,** 729–734.

Holland R, Peterse JL, Millis RR, et al. (1994) Ductal carcinoma in situ: a proposal for a new classification. *Semin. Diagn. Pathol.* **11,** 167.

Hunter MA, McFall TA, Hehr KA (1996) Breast-conserving surgery for primary breast cancer: necessity for surgical clips to define the tumor bed for radiation planning. *Radiology* **200,** 281–282.

Jacobson JA, Danfort DN, Cowan KH, et al. (1995) Ten-year results of a comparison of conservation with mastectomy in the treatment of stage I and II breast cancer. *N. Engl. J. Med.* **332,** 907–911.

Lagios MD (1990) Duct carcinoma in situ: pathology and treatment. *Surg. Clin. North Am.* **70,** 853–871.

Lagios MD, Westdahl PR, Rose MR, et al. (1984) Paget's disease of the nipple: alternative management in cases without or with minimal extent of underlying breast carcinoma. *Cancer* **54,** 545.

Petrek JA, Blackwood MM (1995) Axillary dissection: current practice and technology. *Curr. Probl. Surg.* **32,** 256–323.

Schafter P, Alberto P, Formi M, et al. (1987) Surgery as a part of a combined modality approach for inflammatory breast carcinoma. *Cancer* **59,** 1063.

Schnitt SJ, Abner A, Gelman R, et al. (1994) The relationship between microscopic margins of resection and the risk of local recurrence in patients with breast cancer treated with breast-conserving surgery and radiation therapy. *Cancer* **74,** 1746–1751.

Silverstein MJ, Poller DN, Waisman JR, et al. (1995) Prognostic classification of breast ductal carcinoma in situ. *Lancet* **345,** 1154–1157.

Smitt MC, Nowels KW, Zdeblick MJ, et al. (1995) The importance of the lumpectomy surgical margin status in long term results of breast conservation. *Cancer* **76,** 259–267.

Solin LJ, Yeh IT, Kurt J, et al. (1993) Ductal carcinoma in situ (intraductal carcinoma) of the breast treated with breast-conserving surgery and definitive irradiation: correlation of pathologic parameters with outcome of treatment. *Cancer* **71,** 2532–2542.

Yeatman TJ, Cantor AB, Smith TJ, et al. (1995) Tumor biology of infiltrating lobular carcinoma. Implications for management. *Ann. Surg.* **222,** 549–561.

5

Breast-Conserving Surgery
Lumpectomy With or Without Axillary Dissection

Samuel W. Beenken, MD, and Kirby I. Bland, MD

CONTENTS

INTRODUCTION
HISTOPATHOLOGY OF EARLY BREAST CANCER
IMAGING AND DIAGNOSIS OF EARLY BREAST CANCER
INDICATIONS FOR BREAST-CONSERVING SURGERY
LUMPECTOMY AND AXILLARY DISSECTION
RADIATION THERAPY AFTER BREAST-CONSERVING SURGERY
BREAST-CONSERVING SURGERY AFTER NEOADJUVANT CHEMOTHERAPY
BREAST-CONSERVING SURGERY FOR OTHER BREAST TUMORS
BIBLIOGRAPHY

1. INTRODUCTION

There was an increase of more than 4% per year in breast cancer incidence between 1980 and 1987 in the United States. This increase was characterized by more frequent detection of early-stage cancers with small primary lesions. At the same time, incidence rates for regional metastatic disease dropped. Because of this, lumpectomy with or without axillary dissection is more frequently being utilized as definitive surgical therapy.

The clinical management of breast cancer depends on the stage of disease. Clinical stage is determined through 1) careful physical examination, including examination of skin, breast tissue, and lymph nodes (axillary, supraclavicular, and cervical); 2) mammography, chest X-ray, and other imaging studies; 3) pathologic examination of biopsy material; and 4) intraoperative findings (primary cancer size, chest wall invasion, etc.). Pathologic stage combines clinical stage data with findings from pathologic examination of the completely resected primary cancer and the resected axillary lymph nodes (at least level I).

2. HISTOPATHOLOGY OF EARLY BREAST CANCER

Decisions regarding the use of lumpectomy with or without axillary dissection as definitive surgical therapy for breast cancer depend on the specific histopathology of the cancer being treated. Malignant breast cells are described as *in situ* or invasive depending on whether or not there has been invasion of cells through the basement membrane. Ductal

From: *Current Clinical Oncology:*
Breast Cancer: A Guide to Detection and Multidisciplinary Therapy
Edited by: M. H. Torosian © Humana Press Inc., Totowa, NJ

Table 1
Classification of Breast Ductal Carcinoma *In Situ* (DCIS)

| Histology | Determining Characteristics | | DCIS grade |
	Nuclear grade	Necrosis	
Comedo	High	Extensive	High
Intermediate[a]	Intermediate	Focal or absent	Intermediate
Noncomedo[b]	Low	Absent	Low

[a] Often a mixture of noncomedo patterns.

[b] Solid, cribriform, papillary, or focal micropapillary.

carcinoma *in situ* (DCIS) arises predominantly in terminal duct lobular units (TDLUs) but also involves extralobular ducts. It carries a high risk for conversion to an invasive cancer. DCIS has traditionally been classified as comedo, cribriform, papillary, solid, and micropapillary on the basis of architectural features. DCIS is now frequently classified based on nuclear grade and the presence of necrosis (Table 1). The term lobular carcinoma *in situ* (LCIS) describes the distention, distortion, and filling of TDLUs by characteristic malignant cells. LCIS is a marker for increased risk of invasive cancer and that risk applies equally to both breasts.

Invasive breast cancers have also been described as lobular or ductal in origin. Early classifications used the term lobular to describe invasive cancers that were associated with LCIS. Other invasive cancers were referred to as ductal. In fact, most breast cancers originate in TDLUs. Because fewer than 10% of invasive cancers are of a pure lobular type, the term ductal has no specific meaning. Current histologic classifications recognize special types of breast cancers that are defined in terms of specific histologic criteria. To qualify as a special-type cancer, at least 90% of the cancer must contain the defining histologic features. Several of these special types are associated with a better prognosis than cancers that lack these specific histologic features. The special-type cancers (tubular, colloid, medullary, invasive lobular and invasive cribriform carcinoma) make up about 25% of all invasive cancers. The remaining cancers are described as invasive ductal or no special type (NST) cancers. Limited prognostic information is obtained from the histologic patterns of NST cancers. Instead, prognosis is determined primarily by cancer stage.

3. IMAGING AND DIAGNOSIS OF EARLY BREAST CANCER

Over the last 15 years, progressively more early-stage breast cancers with small primary lesions have been diagnosed (particularly in women older than 55 years), mostly because more older women have had breast imaging. Thus lumpectomy with or without axillary dissection is more frequently utilized as the definitive surgical therapy.

The most commonly used breast imaging procedure is mammography, and the two basic types are screening and diagnostic. Screening mammography is used to detect unexpected breast cancer in asymptomatic women. Diagnostic mammography is used to evaluate the breasts of patients with symptoms or with signs such as nipple discharge or nodule. Mammography is also used to guide interventional procedures involving the breast, including prebiopsy needle localization, needle aspiration, core needle biopsy, and ductography. Ultrasonography is the next most commonly used modality for diagnostic imaging of the breast. In the past, its use was primarily restricted to differentiating cystic from solid masses. However, ultrasonography is now also used to guide fine needle aspiration biopsy (FNAB), core needle biopsy, and prebiopsy needle localization of suspicious-appearing solid masses.

The increasing utilization of mammography has resulted in the need for image-guided biopsies to diagnose nonpalpable breast lesions. Ultrasound localization techniques are employed when a mass lesion is present. Stereotactic techniques are utilized when there is no mass lesion (e.g., microcalcifications only). The combination of diagnostic mammography, ultrasound or stereotactic localization, and FNAB for nonpalpable breast lesions produces an accurate diagnosis of malignancy in nearly 100% of cases. Whereas FNA biopsy permits cytologic evaluation, core needle biopsy also permits analysis of tissue architecture and allows the pathologist to determine whether or not invasive disease is present.

FNAB of a suspicious, palpable breast mass is performed in an outpatient setting. A $1^1/_2$-inch, 22-gage needle on a 20-mL syringe is used. The syringe is held within a syringe holder to enable the physician performing the FNAB to control the syringe and needle with one hand while positioning and holding the breast mass with the opposite hand. After the needle is placed in the mass, suction is applied while the needle is moved slowly back and forth within the mass. Once cellular material is seen at the hub of the needle, the suction is released and the needle is withdrawn. The cellular material is then expressed onto a microscope slide. Both air-dried and 95% ethanol-fixed slides are prepared for analysis. Core needle biopsy is performed using a 14-gage Trucut needle or the equivalent. Automated devices are available. Tissue specimens are placed into formalin and then processed to paraffin blocks.

Misdiagnosed breast cancer accounts for the greatest number of malpractice claims related to errors in diagnosis and also for the largest number of paid claims. Malpractice claims often involve younger women, in whom physical examination and mammography can be misleading. If a young patient (age less than 45 years) presents with a palpable breast mass and a negative mammogram, ultrasound examination and liberal use of biopsy techniques are indicated to avoid a delay in diagnosis.

4. INDICATIONS FOR BREAST-CONSERVING SURGERY

Breast-conserving surgery is indicated for stages 0, I, II, and IIIa breast cancer (Table 2).

4.1. In Situ Cancer of the Breast (Stage 0)

Both LCIS and DCIS may be difficult to distinguish from atypical hyperplasia or from cancers with early invasion. Expert pathologic review is required in all cases. Bilateral mammography is also performed to identify the presence of multiple primary tumors and to estimate the extent of the noninvasive lesion. LCIS does not require surgical therapy, only observation. Patients with DCIS and evidence of widespread disease (two or more quadrants) require total (simple) mastectomy. For patients with limited disease in whom negative margins are achieved by lumpectomy or by reexcision, ipsilateral breast radiotherapy completes therapy. Very small (<0.5 cm), low-grade DCIS of the solid, cribriform, or papillary subtypes can be managed by lumpectomy alone. For nonpalpable lesions, needle localization techniques are utilized to guide the surgical resection. Specimen mammography is performed to ensure that all visible evidence of disease has been excised.

Table 2
Extent of Surgery by Cancer Stage

Stage[a]	TNM[a]			Breast		Axilla	
				Lumpectomy	Mastectomy	Axillary dissection	Sentinel node biopsy
0	Tis	N0	M0	X	X		
I	T1[b]	N0	M0	X	X	X	X
IIa	T0	N1	M0		X[d]	X	
	T1	N1	M0	X	X	X	
	T2[b,c]	N0	M0	X	X	X	X
IIb	T2[c]	N1	M0	X	X	X	
	T3[c]	N0	M0	X	X	X	
IIIa	T0	N2	M0		X[d]	X	
	T1	N2	M0	X	X	X	
	T2[c]	N2	M0	X	X	X	
	T3[c]	N1	M0	X	X	X	
	T3[c]	N2	M0	X	X	X	

[a] The American Joint Committee on Cancer (AJCC) staging for breast cancer: T, primary cancer or tumor; N, regional lymph nodes; M, distant metastases.

[b] Some special-type cancers do not require axilary dissection or sentinel node biopsy.

[c] Consider lumpectomy after neoadjuvant chemotherapy for some cases.

[d] Consider mastectomy or breast radiotherapy.

4.2. Stage I, IIa, or IIb Invasive Breast Cancer

A number of randomized trials have documented that modified radical mastectomy or breast-conserving therapy (lumpectomy, axillary dissection, and breast radiotherapy for local control of disease) are equivalent treatments for stage I and II breast cancer. Relative contraindications to breast-conserving therapy include prior radiotherapy to the breast or chest wall, involved or unknown margin status following reexcision, multicentric disease, and scleroderma or other connective tissue disease.

Traditionally, elective axillary lymph node dissection (levels 1 and 2) has permitted pathologic assessment of axillary nodes when there was no palpable lymphadenopathy. Currently, sentinel lymph node biopsy can be performed in the elective situation to assess node status. Candidates for this procedure have clinically negative axillary lymph nodes and a T1 or T2 primary cancer and have not had neoadjuvant chemotherapy (Table 2). If the sentinel lymph node cannot be identified or is found to harbor metastatic disease, axillary dissection is performed. The performance of an elective axillary dissection or sentinel node biopsy is not warranted when the selection of adjuvant therapy will not be affected by the status of the axillary nodes, for some special-type cancers, in the elderly (more than 70 years of age), and in those with serious comorbid medical conditions.

4.3. Advanced Local and/or Regional Breast Cancer (Stage IIIa)

Patients with stage IIIa breast cancer have advanced local and/or regional disease but no clinically detected distant metastases. In an effort to provide optimal local and regional disease-free (as well as distant disease-free) survival for patients with advanced local and/or regional breast cancer, surgery is integrated with radiotherapy and chemotherapy.

Stage IIIa disease is divided into operable and inoperable categories. Surgical therapy for patients with operable stage IIIa disease is usually a modified radical mastectomy, followed by postoperative (adjuvant) chemotherapy, followed by adjuvant radiotherapy. Adjuvant chemotherapy is used to maximize distant disease-free survival, and radiotherapy is used to maximize local and regional disease-free survival. In selected stage IIIa patients, initial (neoadjuvant) chemotherapy is used to reduce the size of the primary cancer and permit breast-conserving surgery. Surgery is followed by adjuvant radiotherapy and additional chemotherapy.

5. LUMPECTOMY AND AXILLARY DISSECTION

Findings from the National Surgical Adjuvant Breast and Bowel Project B-06 indicated no significant difference in distant disease-free survival or overall survival among women treated by modified radical mastectomy or by lumpectomy and axillary dissection with or without breast radiotherapy. Patients receiving lumpectomy and axillary dissection with breast radiotherapy had significantly fewer "in-breast" recurrences than did patients receiving lumpectomy and axillary dissection without breast radiotherapy (35 versus 10%). Currently, lumpectomy and axillary dissection with adjuvant breast radiotherapy is standard treatment for the involved breast of patients with stage I and II invasive breast cancer. Women whose disease recurs locally following initial breast-conserving surgery undergo a total mastectomy.

A curvilinear incision, lying concentric to the areola, is made in the skin of the breast overlying the breast cancer. In the absence of a prior incisional biopsy, skin excision is not necessary, but skin encompassing any prior biopsy site is excised. The cancer is removed so that it is completely enveloped in normal fat or breast tissue. The aim is to remove an adequate amount of tissue to achieve specimen margins that are free of cancer. Once the specimen is removed from the wound, margins are identified (anterior, posterior, medial, lateral, superior, and inferior), and the specimen is sent directly to pathology for diagnostic studies, analysis of margins, and determination of hormone receptor status, S-phase fraction, Ki-67 expression and HER-2/neu expression. When closing the breast wound, it is not necessary to obliterate the dead space. Complete hemostasis is obtained, and no drains are placed. The subcutaneous fat of the breast is approximated with interrupted suture (absorbable), and the skin is approximated with a running subcuticular suture (absorbable) and Steri-strips.

For invasive disease, an axillary lymph node dissection is performed if a sentinel node biopsy has not been performed. Following lumpectomy, and after the surgeon's gloves are changed, the axillary dissection is performed through a curvilinear incision made just below the axillary hairline and separate from the incision used for removal of the breast cancer. The medial boundary of the dissection is the chest wall, and the superior boundary is the axillary vein; the lateral boundary is the latissimus dorsi muscle. Once the boundaries are defined, the loose areolar tissue of the lateral axillary space is elevated with identification of the lateral-most extent of the axillary vein. The vein is sharply exposed on its anterior and ventral surfaces in a lateral to medial direction. Caudal to the vein, the loose areolar tissue at the juncture of the axillary vein with the anterior margin of the latissimus dorsi is swept inferomedially to include the lateral and subscapular nodal groups (level 1) of the axilla. Care is taken to preserve the thoracodorsal neurovascular bundle, which is fully invested with the loose areolar tissue and nodes of the lateral group.

The dissection then continues medially with extirpation of the central nodal group (level 2). The long thoracic nerve (respiratory nerve of Bell) is identified and preserved as it travels in the deep investing (serratus) fascia of the axillary space along the lateral chest wall. If there is palpable lymphadenopathy in the apical (subclavicular) nodal group (level 3), the tendinous portion of the pectoralis minor muscle is divided near its insertion on the coracoid process (Patey procedure), allowing dissection of the axillary vein medially to the costoclavicular (Halsted's) ligament. Finally, the axillary contents are removed from the wound and sent to pathology.

5.1. Safe Margins for Lumpectomy

Local recurrence of breast cancer after lumpectomy is determined by the biology of the cancer and by the adequacy of surgical margins; cancer size and extent of skin excision are not significant factors in this regard. For T1NOMO cancers, a prospective study has shown that involvement of the surgical margins by microscopic disease and tumor grade are significant adverse prognostic features. For T1 and T2 breast cancer, tumor size does not influence the risk of local recurrence if the surgical margins are negative. For patients treated with skin-sparing mastectomy (excision of nipple-areola complex and 1 cm around prior biopsy sites), there is a recurrence rate of only 1–2% for T1–T3 cancers.

5.2. Sentinel Node Biopsy

Sentinel lymph node biopsy is now accepted as an appropriate diagnostic tool for determining whether breast cancer has spread to the regional lymph nodes. Its accuracy has been validated in large studies. The most commonly employed colloids for localizing the sentinel node are isosulfan blue (blue dye) and technetium-99m-labeled sulfur colloid. The risk of failing to identify a sentinel node is lowest when both a blue dye technique and a radioactive tracer technique are used. Peritumoral, subdermal, and/or subareolar injections of radioactive tracer and/or blue dye are appropriate. Radioactive tracer can be injected the day before or the day of surgery. In the operating room, a hand-held gamma counter is used to localize the sentinel node. Blue dye is injected after the patient is prepared for surgery and the surgical drapes have been placed. The breast is then massaged for 3–5 minutes, with the axillary incision being made immediately thereafter.

Successful sentinel node biopsy depends not only on an experienced surgeon, but also on an expert nuclear medicine physician and staff and an experienced pathologist. A sentinel lymph node biopsy team generally will have the necessary level of expertise to perform sentinel lymph node biopsy without axillary lymph node dissection after the team has performed 30 sentinel biopsies that were followed by an axillary dissection. Candidates for sentinel lymph node biopsy have clinically negative axillary lymph nodes and a T1 or T2 primary cancer and have not had neoadjuvant chemotherapy. If the sentinel lymph node cannot be identified or is found to harbor metastatic disease, formal axillary lymph node dissection is performed.

Many questions regarding sentinel lymph node biopsy remain to be answered. These include defining the optimal material and technique to identify the sentinel node, patient selection, the role of biopsy of nonaxillary sentinel nodes, the role of immunohistochemical and reverse transcriptase-polymerase chain reaction analysis of nodes to identify metastatic disease, and the situations under which complete axillary node dissection is indicated.

6. RADIATION THERAPY AFTER BREAST-CONSERVING SURGERY

6.1. In Situ Cancer of the Breast (Stage 0)

For patients with limited DCIS, in whom negative margins are achieved by lumpectomy or by reexcision, breast radiotherapy is given to reduce the risk of local recurrence. Very small (<0.5 cm), low-grade DCIS of the solid, cribriform, or papillary subtypes can be managed by excision alone.

6.2. Stage I, IIa, or IIb Invasive Breast Cancer

For patients in whom negative margins are achieved by lumpectomy or by reexcision, breast radiotherapy is given to reduce the risk of local recurrence. All women with four or more positive axillary lymph nodes and premenopausal women with one to three positive nodes are at increased risk for recurrence and are candidates for the use of chest wall and supraclavicular lymph node radiotherapy.

6.3. Advanced Local and/or Regional Breast Cancer (Stage IIIa or IIIb)

For patients in whom negative margins are achieved after neoadjuvant chemotherapy by lumpectomy or by reexcision, breast radiotherapy and supraclavicular radiotherapy are given to reduce the risk of local and regional recurrence.

7. BREAST-CONSERVING SURGERY
AFTER NEOADJUVANT CHEMOTHERAPY

The NSABP has evaluated the role of neoadjuvant chemotherapy in women with operable breast cancer (B-18). Patients entered into this study were randomized to surgery followed by chemotherapy or primary chemotherapy followed by surgery. There was no significant difference in estimated 5-year disease-free survival among patients in either group. Before randomization, lumpectomy was proposed for 3% of women with tumors larger than 5.0 cm. After neoadjuvant chemotherapy, there was a 175% increase in the number of lumpectomies performed in that group of women. It was suggested that neoadjuvant chemotherapy be considered for the initial management of breast cancers judged too large for lumpectomy.

Current recommendations for operable stage IIIa breast cancer are neoadjuvant chemotherapy with a doxorubicin (Adriamycin)-containing regimen, followed by lumpectomy and axillary dissection, if possible, followed by adjuvant radiotherapy, followed by additional chemotherapy.

8. BREAST-CONSERVING SURGERY FOR OTHER BREAST TUMORS

8.1. Cystosarcoma Phylloides

Cystosarcoma phylloides (CSP) of the breast is an uncommon fibroepithelial tumor that resembles benign fibroadenoma but has a definite potential to recur locally or to metastasize. The diagnosis of CSP is made by open biopsy. Lumpectomy with clear margins is curative in most cases, although mastectomy may be required. Elective axillary lymph node dissection is not warranted.

9.2. Paget's Disease

Paget's disease is a unique presentation of breast cancer characterized by an eczematous area on the nipple that may be subtle but can progress to an ulcerated, weeping lesion. Paget's disease is usually associated with extensive DCIS within the breast and can be associated with an invasive carcinoma. A palpable mass may or may not be present. Biopsy of the nipple will show a population of cells that are identical to the underlying DCIS; these are referred to as pagetoid features or pagetoid change. Surgical therapy can involve lumpectomy with or without axillary dissection, total (simple) mastectomy with or without axillary dissection, or modified radical mastectomy depending on the extent of involvement and the presence of invasive disease.

BIBLIOGRAPHY

American Joint Committee on Cancer (1997) *Manual for Staging of Cancer,* 5th ed. Lippincott-Raven, Philadelphia.

Bland KI, Chang HR, Copeland EM (1998) Modified radical mastectomy and total (simple) mastectomy. In: Bland KI, Copeland EM (eds.) *The Breast: Comprehensive Management of Benign and Malignant Diseases.* WB Saunders, Philadelphia, pp. 881–912.

Calle R, Pilleron JP, Schlienger P, Vilcoq JR (1978) Conservative management of operable breast cancer: ten years experience at the Foundation Curie. *Cancer* **42,** 2045–2053.

Cope O, Wang CA, Chu A, et al. (1976) Limited surgical excision as the basis of a comprehensive therapy for cancer of the breast. *Am. J. Surg.* **131,** 400–406.

Crile G Jr (1965) Treatment of breast cancer by local excision. *Am. J. Surg.* **109,** 400.

Fisher B (1995) Lumpectomy versus quadrantectomy for breast conservation: a critical appraisal. *Eur. J. Cancer* **31A, 10,** 1567–1569.

Fisher B, Anderson S, Redmond CK, Wolmark N, Wickerham DL, Cronin WM (1995) Reanalysis and results after 12 years of follow-up in a randomized clinical trial comparing total mastectomy with lumpectomy with or without irradiation in the treatment of breast cancer. *N. Engl. J. Med.* **333,** 1456–1461.

Fisher B, Bauer M, Margolese R, et al. (1985) Five-year results of a randomized clinical trial comparing total mastectomy and segmental mastectomy with or without radiation in the treatment of breast cancer. *N. Engl. J. Med.* **312,** 665–673.

Fisher B, Costantino J, Redmond C, et al. (1993) Lumpectomy compared with lumpectomy and radiation therapy for the treatment of intraductal breast cancer. *N. Engl. J. Med.* **328,** 1581–1586.

Fisher B, Ore L (1993) On the underutilization of breast-conserving surgery for the treatment of breast cancer. *Ann. Oncol.* **4,** 96–98.

Fisher B, Redmond C (1992) Lumpectomy for breast cancer: an update of the NSABP experience. *J. Natl. Cancer Inst. Monogr.* **11,** 7–13.

Fisher B, Redmond C, Fisher ER, et al. (1985) Ten year results of a randomized clinical trial comparing radical mastectomy and total mastectomy with or without radiation. *N. Engl. J. Med.* **312,** 674–681.

Fisher B, Wolmark N, Fisher ER, Deutsch M (1985) Lumpectomy and axillary dissection for breast cancer: surgical, pathological, and radiation considerations. *World J. Surg.* **9,** 692–698.

Kern KA (1998) The delayed diagnosis of symptomatic breast cancer. In: Bland KI, Copeland EM (eds.) *The Breast: Comprehensive Management of Benign and Malignant Diseases.* WB Saunders, Philadelphia, pp. 1588–1631.

Lazovich DA, White E, Thomas DB, Moe RE (1991) Underutilization of breast-conserving surgery and radiation therapy among women with stage I or II breast cancer. *JAMA* **266,** 3433–3438.

Margolese R, Poisson R, Shibata H, et al. (1987) The technique of segmental mastectomy (lumpectomy) and axillary dissection: a syllabus from the National Surgical Adjuvant Breast Project workshops. *Surgery* **102,** 828–834.

Montague ED, Gutierrez AE, Barker JL, Tapley N, Fletcher GH (1979) Conservative surgery and irradiation for the treatment of favorable breast cancer. *Cancer* **43,** 1058–1061.

National Comprehensive Cancer Network (1999) Oncology practice guidelines. *Oncology* **13,** 187–212.

Peters MV (1967) Wedge resection and irradiation, and effective treatment in early breast cancer. *JAMA* **200,** 134–135.

Veronesi U, Marubini E, Del Vecchio M, et al. (1995) Local recurrences and distant metastases after conservative breast cancer treatments: Partly independent events. *J. Natl. Cancer Inst.* **87,** 19–27.

Veronesi U, Saccozzi R, Del Vecchio M, et al. (1981) Comparing radical mastectomy with quadrantectomy, axillary dissection, and radiotherapy in patients with small cancers of the breast. *N. Engl. J. Med.* **305,** 6–11.

Veronesi U, Salvadori B, Luini A, et al. (1995) Breast conservation is a safe method in patients with small cancer of the breast. Long-term results of three randomised trials on 1,973 patients. *Eur. J. Cancer* **31A,** 1574–1579.

Vilcoq JR, Calle R, Stacey P, Ghossein NA et al. (1981) The outcome of treatment of tumorectomy and radiotherapy of patients with operable breast cancer. *Radiat. Oncol. Biol. Phys.* **7,** 1327.

6

Mastectomy

David R. Brenin, MD, and David W. Kinne, MD

CONTENTS

INTRODUCTION
HISTORY
INDICATIONS
TOTAL MASTECTOMY
MODIFIED RADICAL MASTECTOMY
RADICAL MASTECTOMY
SKIN-SPARING MASTECTOMY WITH IMMEDIATE BREAST
 RECONSTRUCTION
REFERENCES

1. INTRODUCTION

The appropriate local management of breast cancer has been a subject of controversy since the inception of breast surgery. The failure of radical surgery to cure many patients with breast cancer has resulted in a close examination of surgical procedures used to treat the disease as well as intense investigation of the disease itself. Over time, a new paradigm evolved for the treatment of breast cancer. This new thinking revolves around the systemic nature of breast cancer at the time of diagnosis. Appropriately, the procedures utilized by surgeons in the treatment of breast cancer have evolved in parallel with these changing concepts. From the mid-1990s onward, most patients with early invasive breast cancer or ductal carcinoma *in situ* have been treated with breast-conserving therapy (BCT) *(1,2)*. This change has come about slowly and was caused not only by the results of randomized trials but also by changes in our perception of the biology of breast cancer, the detection of smaller tumors, an increased understanding of radiotherapy, more use of systemic therapy, and the recognition of the importance of patient involvement in decision making. Mastectomy may no longer be considered the gold standard, but it still represents an important modality in the modern treatment of breast cancer patients.

This chapter addresses the appropriate role of mastectomy in the modern care of breast cancer patients. History, indications, technical aspects, postoperative management, and management of complications following mastectomy are presented.

2. HISTORY

The first mention of mastectomy for the treatment of breast cancer can be traced to Albucasis, a Spanish-Arabian surgeon who lived from 1013 to 1106. He wrote that if the tumor

From: *Current Clinical Oncology:*
Breast Cancer: A Guide to Detection and Multidisciplinary Therapy
Edited by: M. H. Torosian © Humana Press Inc., Totowa, NJ

was small and the entire organ could be removed, operation should be done. Albucasis, however, admitted that he had never, nor had he known of anyone who had, cured a patient of the disease *(3)*. Mastectomy appears to have been occasionally used in the treatment of breast cancer over the next 700 years. By the beginning of the 19th century, however, surgery was being taught in organized schools, and several experienced surgeons had accumulated large numbers of cases. On examination of their data, they found that survival rates for breast cancer patients who underwent mastectomy were as poor as those for untreated patients, ranging between 0 and 4%. Thus, mastectomy fell out of favor, and less radical treatments were advocated. The later half of the 19th century, however, saw the return of more radical procedures, with surgeons such as Joseph Pancoast, Charles Moore, Joseph Lister, and Volkmann becoming proponents of complete removal of the breast with or without some sort of axillary dissection.

In 1894, William Halsted *(4)* published data from 76 breast cancer patients in which he described the radical mastectomy. Utilizing this procedure, Halsted was able to achieve a local recurrence rate of 6%, a regional recurrence rate of 22%, and a 3-year cure rate of 45%. This represented a vast improvement over the results achieved by contemporary European surgeons, who typically reported local recurrence rates as high as 82% and 3-year cure rates of 4–20% *(5)*. By demonstrating these superior results, Halsted ushered in the "modern era" of breast cancer surgery. Mastectomy, radical or modified radical, remained the dominant surgical procedure used to treat breast cancer for approximately the next 100 years. Today, however, BCT is considered by most to be the standard of care for the treatment of breast cancer.

3. INDICATIONS

BCT is generally considered the procedure of choice for operable breast cancer. Therefore, the presence of contraindications to BCT are the indications for mastectomy. The absolute and relative indications for mastectomy are summarized in Table 1. The absolute indications have been minimally debated. Patients in the first or second trimester of pregnancy are not able to undergo radiation therapy in a timely fashion and are thus ineligible for BCT. In the presence of diffuse disease, characterized by the presence of more than one malignant tumor in separate quadrants of the breast or the detection of diffuse malignant-appearing mammographic findings, patients treated with BCT are at a higher than acceptable risk for local recurrence. Such patients should undergo mastectomy. Women who have had reasonable attempts at reexcision with continued positive margins should also be considered to have diffuse disease. Patients who have undergone prior radiotherapy to the region of the breast are usually not able to safely undergo the additional whole-breast radiation required for BCT, and therefore mastectomy is indicated. Mastectomy is also required for patients with no access to radiation therapy facilities.

The relative indications for mastectomy are somewhat controversial. Modern breast surgery has increased the treatment options available to patients with large tumor-to-breast size ratios and centrally located lesions. These patients were considered to be ineligible for BCT when it was first introduced. As experience with BCT has increased, large tumor-to-breast size ratios and centrally located tumors are no longer considered absolute contraindications to BCT. The wishes of the patient should always be considered when dealing with a large tumor-to-breast size ratio. A final cosmetic result unacceptable to the surgeon may not be unacceptable to the patient. Several studies have demonstrated that patients tend to score their cosmetic results more favorably than their treating physicians *(6,7)*. Preservation of a

Table 1
Indications for Mastectomy

Absolute indications
  First or second trimester of pregnancy
  Diffuse disease
  Prior radiotherapy to the region of the breast
  No access to radiation therapy facilities
  Patient preference for mastectomy over breast-conserving
      therapy
Relative indications
  Large tumor-to-breast size ratio
  Centrally located tumor
  History of collagen vascular disease
  Large breast size

sensate, but cosmetically imperfect breast may be preferable to some patients. The same is true for patients with centrally located tumors. Removal of the nipple-areola complex as part of a central lumpectomy leaves behind a sensate breast mound. If desired, a nipple may be reconstructed at a later date. The outcomes of patients with collagen vascular disease treated with BCT including whole breast radiotherapy are unclear. One study has demonstrated no significant increase in the incidence of complications following radiotherapy (8). Others have reported unacceptable postradiotherapy breast fibrosis in patients with lupus and scleroderma (9,10). Concerns regarding the inability to deliver radiotherapy effectively to the extremely large breast have been addressed by newer methods of breast immobilization, allowing for adequate dose homogeneity. If these techniques are available to the patient, mastectomy would not be required.

Finally, patient choice should play a significant role in treatment determination. A recent study conducted by physicians at a major tertiary care center found that up to 30% of patients who underwent mastectomy for the treatment of ductal carcinoma *in situ* (DCIS) did so by choice (11). These patients were felt to be good candidates for BCT by their treating physicians. A significant proportion of patients when apprised of the risks of local recurrence associated with BCT will simply opt for mastectomy.

4. TOTAL MASTECTOMY

Total mastectomy and simple mastectomy refer to the same procedure. A total mastectomy preserves both the pectoralis major and minor muscles and does not include a formal axillary dissection. This procedure is indicated for patients with operable disease who require the complete removal of the breast and no axillary dissection and who meet the criteria in Table 1. A simple mastectomy can also be utilized in conjunction with a sentinel lymph node biopsy in the treatment of patients with invasive breast cancer. Candidates for simple mastectomy include DCIS patients with minimal or no microinvasion who cannot be treated with BCT, patients undergoing prophylactic surgery, patients with invasive cancer who suffer local recurrence in the breast following BCT with prior axillary dissection, DCIS patients with local DCIS recurrence after BCT that had included radiotherapy, patients with metastatic disease undergoing toilet mastectomy, and patients with invasive breast cancer in whom pathologic axillary staging in not required.

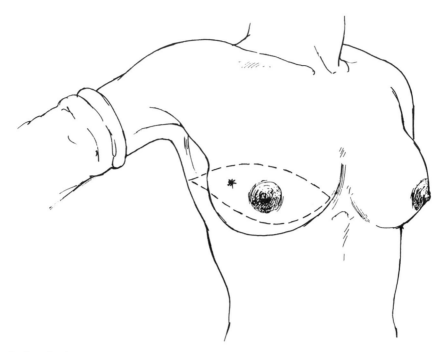

Fig. 1. Standard mastectomy incision, encompassing nipple-areola complex and prior biopsy site.

The use of total mastectomy in the treatment of patients with invasive breast cancer presupposes a minimal impact of regional lymphadenectomy on survival. In addition, the risk of axillary failure following total mastectomy for invasive breast cancer is much higher compared with the risk following modified radical mastectomy. The rate of axillary failure, however, can be significantly decreased by radiotherapy to the axillary nodal basin. The use of total mastectomy in the treatment of patients with invasive breast cancer should not be considered the standard of care. The elimination of axillary dissection in the treatment of invasive breast cancer patients is currently a hotly contested issue, beyond the scope of this chapter. This topic is well covered by Taneja and Gardner *(12)*.

Total mastectomy is typically performed under a general anesthetic. The choice of incision is based on the need for skin preservation and the location of the tumor and/or the previous biopsy site. The incision is typically elliptical in shape and must encompass both the nipple-areola complex and (if present) the previous biopsy site (Fig. 1). In some patients, the previous biopsy site may be well outside the usual mastectomy incision. In these patients, the skin from the prior biopsy site may be excised separately with a 1-cm margin, left attached the underlying breast parenchyma, and removed with the specimen. When this is attempted, care must be taken to preserve a well-vascularized intervening skin bridge. Another approach to the patient with a prior biopsy incision at the extreme periphery of the breast is the use of the inverted-T or T incision, (Fig. 2). The incision utilized for skin-sparing mastectomy is smaller in size but must still include the nipple-areola complex and prior biopsy site (Fig. 3). Skin-sparing mastectomy will be specifically dealt with later in this chapter.

Skin flaps are created in a plane between the subcutaneous fat and the underlying breast capsule. The thickness of the flaps is thus variable, depending on the amount of subcutaneous fat present. Flaps are dissected until the entire glandular breast is encompassed. Typi-

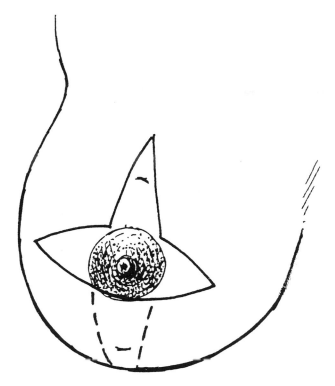

Fig. 2. Peripheral prior biopsy incisions in the upper inner or lower outer quadrants may be managed with inverted-T or T incisions (hatched line) respectively.

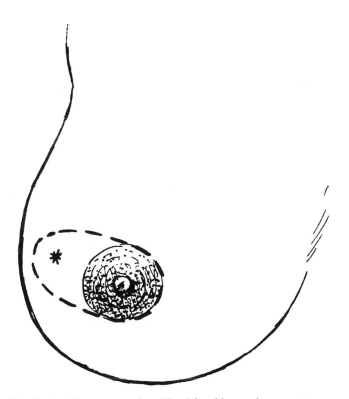

Fig. 3. Incision commonly utilized for skin-sparing mastectomy.

cally this requires dissection superiorly to the inferior boader of the clavicle, medially to the lateral border of the sternum, inferiorly to the superior portion of the rectus sheath, and laterally to the inferior part of the latissimus dorsi muscle. The lateral dissection is then carried superiorly along the latissimus dorsi until the first major intercostal brachial nerve is identified. This nerve is preserved. At this level, dissection of the lateral aspect of the superior flap is continued superiorly in a more superficial plane directly overlying the lateralmost extent of the latissimus dorsi muscle. In this way, the intercostal brachial nerves are spared, and the complete axillary tail of the breast (the tail of Spence) is included in the specimen.

The breast is then removed from the chest wall along with the underlying pectoralis major muscle fascia. The pectoralis fascia was thought to represent an anatomic barrier to the spread of cancer and thus its removal as the deep margin of resection was routinely advocated. This concept, however is invalid. Penetration of the pectoralis fascia by breast lymphatics has been well demonstrated, and this facia may be safely preserved when desired for immediate breast reconstruction *(13)*. Dissection of the plane superficial to the pectoralis fascia is, however, more difficult, and care must be taken to remove the overlying breast tissue in its entirety. The lateral margin of the specimen should be marked to assist the pathologist in identifying low axillary lymph nodes that may be present in the tail of the breast. The location, nature, and number of lesions suspected to be in the breast must be clearly conveyed to the pathologist.

After obtaining meticulous hemostasis, the incision is reapproximated over a single closed suction drain placed along the most dependent portion of the lower skin flap. Skin should be closed with a continuous subcuticular suture. Pressure dressings are not required.

Simple mastectomy may be performed as an outpatient procedure; however, most surgeons keep their patients in hospital until the first postoperative day. During the hospital stay, consultations with physical and occupational therapists are obtained, and the patient and family are instructed in drain care. Patients are discharged to home with the drain in place. The drain is removed when its output is less than 30mL over a 24-hour period. No attempt is made to limit use of the arm or shoulder. Postoperative complications are rare but include bleeding, hematoma, skin flap necrosis, seroma, and infection. Significant postoperative bleeding must be surgically controlled. Large hematomas, if noted early, should be evacuated. Skin flap necrosis is rare but is associated with denuding the subcutaneous fat from the flaps, closure under tension, infection, and use of pressure dressings. Skin necrosis occurring at the suture line can usually be managed conservatively, allowing the skin to demarcate, followed by debridement and closure by secondary intention. Seroma formation is common and is managed by repeated aspiration. Infections are managed with antibiotics and drainage where required. Functioning drains should be left in place in an infected mastectomy wound as they provide drainage of purulent material. Because no lymphadenectomy is preformed, the complications associated with axillary dissection, such as lymphedema, injury to the axillary vein, or injury of the long thoracic, thoracodorsal; or intercostal brachial nerves are avoided.

5. MODIFIED RADICAL MASTECTOMY

Modified radical mastectomy (MRM) refers to a collection of procedures all having in common the complete removal of the breast, the underlying fascia of the pectoralis major muscle, and the directed removal of axillary node-bearing tissue. The original technique is generally attributed to Patey *(14,15),* who modified Halsted's *(4)* operation by preserving the pectoralis major muscle. The Patey mastectomy included the removal of the pectoralis minor muscle to facilitate a complete level I, II, and III axillary lymphadenectomy. Based on his work in determining the incidence of skip metastasis, Auchincloss *(16,17)* modified Patey's operation so that both the pectoralis major and minor were preserved. A similar procedure was described by Madden *(18)*. The preservation of both pectoral muscles usually results in an incomplete level III axillary dissection. The clinical impact of limiting axillary dissection to levels I and II has been adequately evaluated. Limiting axillary dissection to levels I and II results in a decreased incidence of lymphadenectomy-related complications, including lymphedema *(19–21)*. As "skip metastases" to level III are rare, the negative impact of limiting dissection to levels I and II is minimal *(22–24)*. The operation, as described by Auchincloss and consisting of the complete removal of the breast along with a level I and II axillary dissection, with preservation of both the pectoralis major and minor muscles, is considered by most to be the standard form of MRM at this time.

MRM is indicated for patients with operable disease who require the complete removal of the breast and an axillary dissection and who meet the criteria in Table 1. Most patients with invasive breast cancer who are not eligible for BCT, or who opt not to have BCT, are good candidates for MRM. Patients who were treated for DCIS with BCT that included radiotherapy and no axillary dissection and then go on to suffer an invasive local recurrence must also undergo MRM. DCIS patients with large palpable tumors (>4 cm) and those with multiple areas of microinvasion (>2 mm) should also be considered for MRM. All other women with DCIS who are not eligible for BCT should be treated with a simple mastectomy, not MRM.

Likewise, patients with invasive breast cancer in whom pathologic axillary staging is not required, and in whom the issue of local control of axillary disease is to be addressed otherwise, should also undergo simple mastectomy and not MRM. Such patients might include those with metastatic disease at the time of diagnosis, the elderly in whom adjuvant chemotherapy will not be considered regardless of pathologic axillary status, and those with short life expectancies. As mentioned previously, the elimination of axillary dissection in the treatment of invasive breast cancer patients is currently a hotly contested topic involving issues of local control and the possible therapeutic nature of axillary lymphadenectomy. The use of total mastectomy in the treatment of patients with invasive breast cancer should not be considered the standard of care. This topic is well covered by Taneja and Gardner *(12)*.

MRM is typically performed under a general anesthetic. The patient is positioned supine, at the edge of the operating table. A folded towel is placed under the ipsilateral hemithorax and shoulder in order to lift the axillary contents further into the operative field and to allow for greater arm mobility during the procedure. The ipsilateral arm should be "free-prepped" to allow for its manipulation during the procedure. The choice of incision is based on the need for skin preservation and the location of the tumor and/or the previous biopsy site. The incision is typically elliptical in shape and must encompass the nipple-areola complex and, if present, the previous biopsy site (Fig. 1). In some patients, the previous biopsy site may be well outside the usual mastectomy incision. Planning of skin incisions for these patients is similar to that discussed previously for simple mastectomy.

Skin flaps are created in a plane between the subcutaneous fat and the underlying breast capsule. The thickness of the flaps is thus variable, depending on the amount of subcutaneous fat present. Flaps are dissected until the entire glandular breast is encompassed. Typically this requires dissection superiorly to the inferior border of the clavicle, medially to the lateral border of the sternum, inferiorly to the superior portion of the rectus sheath, and laterally to the inferior part of the latissimus dorsi muscle. The lateral dissection is then carried superiorly along the latissimus dorsi muscle belly to its white tendon; superior to this, the axillary vein is identified. During the dissection along the latissimus, several major intercostal brachial nerves should be identified and preserved.

The breast is then removed from the chest wall along with the underlying pectoralis major muscle fascia in a superior-to-inferior fashion. As mentioned in the section on simple mastectomy, removal of the breast just deep to the pectoralis fascia merely represents a convenient plane for the deep margin of resection. If preferred, as may be the case in patients undergoing immediate breast reconstruction, the pectoralis fascia may be left in place. Dissection of the plane superficial to the pectoralis fascia is, however, more difficult, and care must be taken to remove all the overlying breast tissue.

Axillary dissection is begun with the breast still attached inferiorly and laterally. Dissection is continued along the lateral aspect of the pectoralis major muscle to the level of the pectoralis minor where the medial pectoral nerve is identified and preserved. The lateral aspect of the pectoralis minor muscle is dissected down to the chest wall so that the muscle may be retracted, allowing easy access to level II of the axilla. At this point the axillary vein is identified at either the medial or lateral limits of the dissection. Medially, the axillary vein may be found just posterior to the neurovascular bundle containing the medial pectoral nerve. Laterally, the vein will be found crossing the latissimus dorsi muscle belly just superior to its white tendon. Dissection then continues along the inferior border of the axillary vein, where multiple venous tributaries entering the specimen may be encountered and divided. The largest such vessel to be divided is the thoracoepigastric vein, serving as a landmark to the thoracodorsal neurovascular bundle, which is to be identified deep and inferior to it. Attention is then returned to the lateral chest wall. With the pectoralis minor retracted medially, the tissue underlying it is removed and several major intercostal brachial nerves are identified. The most superior two or three intercostal brachial nerves are traced along their medial to lateral course and freed from the axillary specimen when possible. This is accomplished by splitting the axillary specimen and retracting the freed nerves upward, out of the operative field. The long thoracic nerve is then identified along the chest wall, approximately 2.5 cm deep to where intercostal brachial nerves emerge from the chest wall. The lateral aspect of the long thoracic nerve is then freed from the specimen along its entire course and returned to the chest wall. With the thoracodorsal neurovascular bundle and the long thoracic nerve under direct vision, the areolor connective tissue between them is clamped at the inferior aspect of the axillary vein and divided. This tissue is freed from the underlying subscapularis muscle with downwardly directed blunt dissection. The entire specimen is then reflected laterally, the thoracodorsal neurovascular bundle is dissected along its course, and several small venous tributaries entering the specimen from the thoracodorsal vein are ligated and divided at their origins.

At this point all major axillary structures that are to be preserved have been identified and protected. The specimen can now be amputated from the lateral border of the latissimus dorsi muscle. The removed breast and axillary contents are then clearly labeled and laterality indicated. The location, nature, and number of lesions thought to be in the breast are clearly conveyed to the pathologist.

At the conclusion of the procedure, closed suction drains are placed in the apex of the axilla and in the most dependent portion of the lower skin flap. Skin should be closed in two layers with interrupted inverted deep dermal sutures followed by a continuous subcuticular suture. Pressure dressings are not required.

MRM may be performed as an outpatient procedure; however, most surgeons keep their patients in hospital until the first postoperative day. During the hospital stay, consultations with physical and occupational therapists are obtained, and the patient and family are instructed in drain care. Patients are discharged to home with the drains in place. The drains are removed serially when their output is less than 30 mL over a 24-hour period. We make no attempt to limit use of the arm or shoulder on the operated side.

Postoperative complications are rare but include bleeding, hematoma, skin flap necrosis, seroma, and infection. The management of these early postoperative complications is similar to that discussed previously for simple mastectomy. The long-term complications of MRM are related to axillary dissection and include loss of sensation in the upper inner aspect of the arm, shoulder dysfunction, chronic upper extremity pain, and lymphedema of the arm. Factors contributing to the incidence of these long-term and sometimes devastating complications are widely debated. However, most investigators agree that the extent of axillary dissection does impact on their incidence. For a more complete discussion of the complications of axillary dissection, the reader is referred to Brenin and Morrow *(25)*.

6. RADICAL MASTECTOMY

Although rarely performed today, the radical mastectomy was a major step forward in its time. Popularized by Halsted, the radical mastectomy was the first therapy to be offered that made breast cancer a potentially survivable disease. In 1894 and 1907 Halsted *(4,26)* reported on two series of breast cancer patients treated with radical mastectomy. These patients were reported to have a 6% local recurrence rate and a 45% 3-year survival. Three-year survivals reported by other surgeons of that era ranged from 4.7 to 28.5%. Local recurrence rates were in the 50–80% range. Prior to the radical mastectomy, patients and physicians alike perceived breast cancer to be an incurable and routinely fatal disease.

The end of the 19th century witnessed a new understanding of cancer biology as well as significant advances in anesthesia. These changes, along with an understanding of statistics, allowed Halsted to incorporate the techniques described by surgeons before him and to clearly demonstrate and explain the improved results he achieved. The technique of radical mastectomy advocated by Halsted included:

1. Wide skin excision
2. Removal of both the pectoralis major and minor muscles
3. Complete level I, II, and III axillary dissection
4. Removal of the entire breast *en bloc* with the pectoral muscles and axillary tissue
5. Skin graft to cover the remaining defect.

The operation outlined above is significantly deforming. Modified radical mastectomy and BCT have both been clearly demonstrated to have survival equal to radical mastectomy. Therefore, radical mastectomy is to be avoided.

Radical mastectomy has few, if any, indications in the treatment of breast cancer. Patients with tumors invading the pectoral fascia or involving a small portion of the pectoral muscle are best treated by resecting a small portion of the muscle directly beneath the tumor in order to obtain a negative margin. Large tumors fixed to the pectoral muscles are best treated with neoadjuvant chemotherapy or radiation therapy. Most of these patients will have an adequate response so that they may safely undergo MRM, with negative margins and primary skin closure.

7. SKIN-SPARING MASTECTOMY
WITH IMMEDIATE BREAST RECONSTRUCTION

Skin-sparing mastectomy with immediate reconstruction is feasible for most patients undergoing mastectomy. The technical aspects of reconstruction are presented in a subsequent chapter. Issues related to the oncologic impact of immediate reconstruction are as follows: 1) increased risk of local recurrence; 2) delay of adjuvant therapy; and 3) hindrance of detection of chest wall recurrence. These issues have been addressed in several recent publications *(27–29)*.

Most studies evaluating skin-sparing mastectomy followed by immediate breast reconstruction indicate no increase in either local recurrence or delay in its detection. In the hands of an experienced plastic surgeon, the risk of complications associated with immediate reconstruction is small. Thus, the delay of adjuvant therapy resulting from an uncomplicated immediate reconstruction is minimal. The potential need for postoperative radiotherapy, however, should be considered in selecting the type of breast reconstruction offered. Patients who are expected to require postoperative chest wall irradiation should not undergo implant reconstruction. Postoperative radiation results in a significantly increased incidence of implant capsular contracture and loss. The use of postmastectomy radiotherapy is also associated with an increased risk of fat necrosis in patients who have undergone myocutaneous flap reconstruction *(30)*. However, the degree of necrosis is usually minimal, with only a small effect on the final cosmetic result.

In summary, it is reasonable to offer immediate reconstruction to most patients undergoing mastectomy. Implant reconstruction should be avoided in patients who are expected to require postoperative chest wall irradiation. However, such patients are good candidates for myocutaneous flap reconstruction.

REFERENCES

1. Bland KI, Menck HR, Scott-Conner CE, Morrow M, Winchester DJ, Winchester DP (1998) The National Cancer Data Base 10-year survey of breast carcinoma treatment at hospitals in the United States. *Cancer* **83,** 1262–1273.
2. Winchester DJ, Menck HR, Winchester DP (1997) National treatment trends for ductal carcinoma in situ of the breast. *Arch. Surg.* **132,** 660–665.
3. Degenshein GA, Ceccarelli F (1977) The history of breast cancer surgery. Part 1. Early beginning to Halsted. *Breast* **3,** 28–35.
4. Halsted WS (1894) The results of operations for the cure of cancer of the breast performed at the Johns Hopkins Hospital from June, 1889, to January, 1894. *Ann. Surg.* **20,** 497–555.
5. Bland K, Copeland III, E (1998) Halsted radical mastectomy. In Bland K, Copeland E III (eds.) *The Breast.* WB Saunders, Philadelphia, pp. 856.
6. Clarke D, Martinez A, Cox RS (1983) Analysis of cosmetic results and complications in patients with stage I and II breast cancer treated by biopsy and irradiation. *Int. J. Radiat. Oncol. Biol. Phys.* **9,** 1807–1813.
7. Harris JR, Levene MB, Svensson G, Hellman S (1979) Analysis of cosmetic results following primary radiation therapy for stages I and II carcinoma of the breast. *Int. J. Radiat. Oncol. Biol. Phys.* **5,** 257–261.
8. Ross JG, Hussey DH, Mayr NA, Davis CS (1993) Acute and late reactions to radiation therapy in patients with collagen vascular diseases. *Cancer* **71,** 3744–3752.
9. Robertson JM, Clarke DH, Pevzner MM, Matter RC (1991) Breast conservation therapy. Severe breast fibrosis after radiation therapy in patients with collagen vascular disease. *Cancer* **68,** 502–508.
10. Fleck R, McNeese MD, Ellerbroek NA, Hunter TA, Holmes FA (1989) Consequences of breast irradiation in patients with pre-existing collagen vascular diseases. *Int. J. Radiat. Oncol. Biol. Phys.* **17,** 829–833.
11. Brenin, DR, Morrow, M (1998) Is mastectomy over-treatment for ductal carcinoma in situ? *Breast Cancer Res. Treat.* **50,** 250.
12. Taneja C, Gardner B (1998) Therapeutic value of axillary lymph node dissection for breast cancer. In Bland K, Copeland E III (eds.), *The Breast.* WB Saunders, Philadelphia, pp. 943–961.
13. Turner-Warwick R (1958) The lymphatics of the breast. *Br. J. Surg.* **46,** 574–582.
14. Patey DH, Dyson WH (1948) The prognosis of carcinoma of the breast in relation to the type of operation performed. *Br. J. Cancer* **2,** 7–13.
15. Patey DH (1967) A review of 146 cases of carcinoma of the breast operated on between 1930 and 1943. *Br. J. Cancer* **21,** 260–269.
16. Auchincloss H (1963) Significance of location and number of axillary metastases in carcinoma of the breast. *Ann. Surg.* **158,** 37–46.
17. Auchincloss H (1970) Modified radical mastectomy: why not? *Am. J. Surg.* **119,** 506–509.
18. Madden JL (1965) Modified radical mastectomy. *Surg. Gynecol. Obstet.* **121,** 1221–1230.

19. Ivens D, Hoe AL, Podd TJ, et al. (1992) Assessment of morbidity from complete axillary dissection. *Br. J. Cancer* **66,** 136–138.

20. Kiel KD, Rademacker AW (1996) Early-stage breast cancer: arm edema after wide excision and breast irradiation. *Radiology* **198,** 279–283.

21. Liljegren G, Holmberg L (1997) Arm morbidity after sector resection and axillary dissection with or without postoperative radiotherapy in breast cancer stage I. Results from a randomized trial. *Eur. J. Cancer* **33,** 193–199.

22. Rosen PP, Lesser ML, Kinne DW, et al. (1983) Discontinuous or "skip" metastases in breast carcinoma. Analysis of 1228 axillary dissections. *Ann. Surg.* **197,** 276–283.

23. Boova RS, Bonanni R, Rosato FE (1982) Patterns of axillary nodal involvement in breast cancer, predictability of level one dissection. *Ann. Surg.* **196,** 642–644.

24. Veronesi U, Rilke F, Luini A, et al. (1987) Distribution of axillary node metastases by level of invasion. *Cancer* **59,** 682–687.

25. Brenin, DR, Morrow, M (1998) Conventional axillary dissection: extent, local control, and morbidity. *Semin. Breast Dis.* **1,** 118–124.

26. Halsted WS (1907) The results of radical operations for the cure of cancer of the breast. *Trans. Am. Surg. Assoc.* **25,** 61–79.

27. Carlson GW, Bostwick J 3rd, Styblo TM, et al. (1997) Skin-sparing mastectomy. Oncologic and reconstructive considerations. *Ann. Surg.* **225,** 570–578.

28. Kroll SS, Schusterman MA, Tadjalli HE, Singletary SE, Ames FC (1997) Risk of recurrence after treatment of early breast cancer with skin-sparing mastectomy. *Ann. Surg. Oncol.* **4,** 193–197.

29. Newman LA, Kuerer HM, Hunt KK (1998) Presentation, treatment, and outcome of local recurrence after skin-sparing mastectomy and immediate breast reconstruction. *Ann. Surg. Oncol.* **5,** 620–626.

30. Harris JR, Morrow M (1996) Treatment of early-stage breast cancer. In Harris JR, Lippman ME, Morrow M, Hellman S (eds.), *Diseases of the Breast.* Lippincott-Raven, Philadelphia, pp. 529.

7 Breast Reconstruction

Louis P. Bucky, MD, and Gary A. Tuma, MD

CONTENTS

INTRODUCTION
THE INITIAL CONSULTATION
GENERAL CONSIDERATIONS FOR RECONSTRUCTIVE SURGERY
RECONSTRUCTIVE OPTIONS
ALTERNATIVE CHOICES TO RECONSTRUCTION
CONTROVERSIES IN BREAST RECONSTRUCTION
BIBLIOGRAPHY

1. INTRODUCTION

The evolution of breast cancer treatment has led to the development of numerous breast reconstructive options for women. In years past, breast reconstruction was an afterthought following definitive oncologic treatment. Currently, surgical trends favor immediate breast reconstruction. Today, patients are presented with many different options at the initial consultation. The critical components of the consultation include the timing of reconstruction, the type of mastectomy (partial, unilateral, bilateral, skin-sparing), adjuvant therapy, patient anatomy, patient motivation, and family support. This chapter focuses on many of these issues and their impact on the options for breast reconstruction.

2. THE INITIAL CONSULTATION

The several options for breast reconstruction are reviewed and discussed during the initial consultation. In most cases, the patient has been recently diagnosed. This creates a challenge for the plastic surgeon to be clear, comprehensive, and concise, in order to help the patient make the appropriate decision. The critical component of the initial consultation is to describe the goals of breast reconstruction accurately. The goal is to allow patients to look good in clothes. Postoperatively, the patient should be able to wear a bra, a bathing suit, and eveningwear comfortably and thus avoid the difficulties associated with an external prosthesis (Fig. 1). It is important that, following reconstructive surgery, patients be able to participate in the normal activities of daily life just as they did prior to receiving treatment for breast cancer. This allows patients to avoid the persistent and often daily reminder that they have had breast cancer. It is critical, however, that the most satisfactory outcomes for breast reconstruction do not compromise oncologic safety.

From: *Current Clinical Oncology:*
Breast Cancer: A Guide to Detection and Multidisciplinary Therapy
Edited by: M. H. Torosian © Humana Press Inc., Totowa, NJ

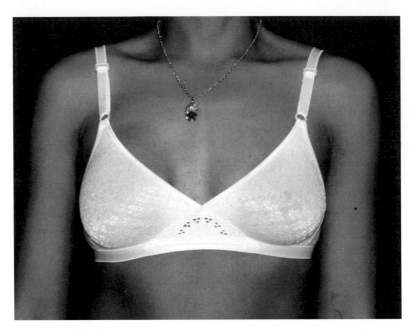

Fig. 1. A 40-year-old woman 1 year after expander placement followed by implant reconstruction with good symmetry in a brassiere.

The first issue, beyond the goals of treatment, is the timing of reconstruction. The advantages of immediate reconstruction far outweigh the disadvantages. Beyond the obvious savings of an additional operation, immediate reconstruction allows the patient to avoid a mourning period over the absent breast. In addition, the avoidance of scarring and distortion of tissue allows the surgeon to achieve an improved cosmetic result more easily (Fig. 2). Lastly, the development of the skin-sparing mastectomy technique enables the surgeon to preserve the entire skin envelope, which greatly enhances the cosmetic result of immediate breast reconstruction (Figs. 3 and 4). Other advantages of immediate reconstruction include reduced morbidity owing to a reduction in the number of operations, fewer secondary operations owing to superior cosmetic results, and an overall cost savings. In years past, concerns regarding immediate reconstruction included the delay of adjuvant therapy secondary to wound healing considerations. However, owing to the improvements in technique, any significant delay for postoperative chemotherapy or radiation therapy is indeed unusual.

The indications for delayed breast reconstruction are either psychological or oncologic. Examples include the patient who is unable to make a clear decision owing to the emotional stress of the initial diagnosis or is not comfortable with her plastic surgeon. In addition, some patients' need for adjuvant therapy is unclear and therefore delayed reconstruction is warranted. This subject is controversial and will be discussed in detail later in the text.

Once a patient chooses to undergo immediate reconstruction, several options need to be presented and discussed regarding the type of reconstruction. Immediate breast reconstruction can be divided into three types: 1) tissue expansion followed by breast implant placement; 2) a combination of tissue flaps with the use of an immediate breast implant; and 3) the use of autogenous tissue only. The use of tissue expansion followed by a breast implant has the advantage of utilizing no other patient donor site. It is also the simplest option with the shortest recovery. At the other end of the spectrum, the use of a patient's autogenous

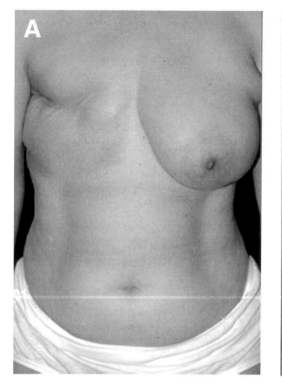
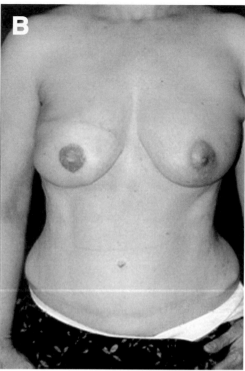

Fig. 2. (A) A 54-year-old woman 1 year after right modified radical mastectomy. Note the asymmetry and distortion of the right chest wall. (B) Same patient 4 months after right transverse rectus abdominis myocutaneous (TRAM) flap and nipple areola reconstruction.

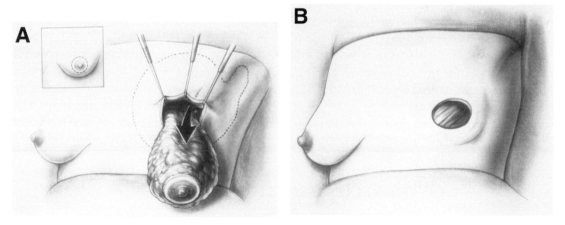

Fig. 3. Schematic of skin-sparing mastectomy

tissue for reconstruction requires the greatest surgical commitment and concomitant recovery for the patient. However, the use of autogenous tissue eliminates implant issues and/or maintenance considerations. The combination of autogenous tissue and implant reconstruction has some of the advantages and disadvantages of the other two options combined. At the time of initial consultation, the three types of reconstruction are presented.

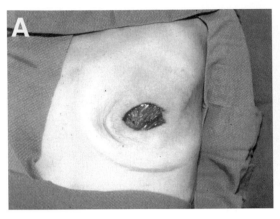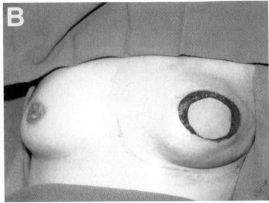

Fig. 4. Intraoperative view of reconstruction after skin-sparing mastectomy. Note the absent breast tissue with skin envelope on the right and the replacement with autogenous transverse rectus abdominis myocutaneous (TRAM) tissue and a skin paddle on the left.

3. GENERAL CONSIDERATIONS FOR RECONSTRUCTIVE SURGERY

The important anatomic features include the size of the surgically treated breast, the abundance of donor tissue for autogenous reconstruction, and the shape of the opposite breast. These features will help determine the appropriate reconstruction for each individual patient. The potential oncologic program, especially with regard to postoperative irradiation, is also an important consideration. In addition, unilateral versus bilateral mastectomies may influence the type of reconstruction with regard to symmetry and donor site morbidity. Finally, many patients have young children at home who require additional support during a lengthy convalescence. The patient's motivation and family support are critical in the determination of the reconstructive program, as more lengthy surgery and a concomitant longer recovery may be required.

The length of surgery ranges from 1 hour for a tissue expander placement to approximately 5 hours for transverse rectus abdominis myocutaneous (TRAM) flap reconstruction. Although length of surgery is a consideration, candidates for any type of reconstruction are typically healthy and are able to undergo additional surgery at the time of mastectomy. Historically, reconstruction was reserved for patients with T1 or T2 tumors. However, reconstruction is now being offered to select patients with larger tumors owing to improvements in quality of life and the absence of oncologic compromise.

4. RECONSTRUCTIVE OPTIONS

4.1. Tissue Expander and Implant Reconstruction

The sequence of events for tissue expansion reconstruction includes immediate placement of a tissue expander followed by a secondary operation and placement of a permanent breast implant. The technique involves the creation of a subpectoral/subserratus pocket followed by the placement of an empty tissue expander securely into the pocket. Certain surgeons perform a variation of the technique by allowing subcutaneous placement of the expander at the inframammary crease. Once the expander is in place and the overlying tissue is approximated, the tissue expander is filled with a variable amount of saline, and the wound is immediately closed. This procedure takes approximately 1 hour

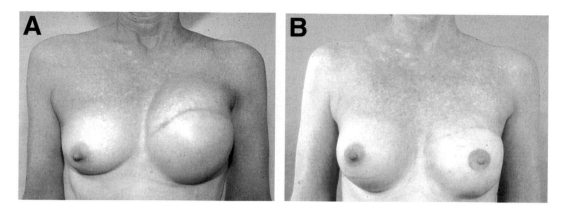

Fig. 5. (A) A 50-year-old woman after left modified radical mastectomy with tissue expander reconstruction. Note the overexpansion to allow for a soft result. **(B)** Same patient 6 months after implant exchange and nipple areola reconstruction.

after the completion of the mastectomy. A drain is placed, and the patient spends 24–48 hours in the hospital. Typically, 2 weeks after the procedure the patient begins a series of tissue expansions in the office. The technique involves serial expansion utilizing percutaneous injection of a designated amount of saline, until the tissue is taught but not ischemic. The injections are placed into a built-in port within the implant. Currently, tissue expanders come in a variety of shapes and sizes to enable the surgeon to best match the shape of the opposite breast. The expansion process typically takes 6–8 weeks. The patient is overexpanded by approximately 50% of the opposite breast and allowed to accommodate for an additional month, allowing for a softer result (Fig. 5).

The technique of overexpansion as well as the duration of expansion is variable, since there is some rebound contraction over a prolonged period. At the completion of the expansion process, roughly 3 months after the initial surgery, a second procedure is performed. This involves removal of the tissue expander and replacing it with a permanent breast implant. There are long-term maintenance issues with permanent implants. Implants need to be replaced roughly every 10–12 years to prevent implant rupture. Over time, implants have an increasing potential for leakage and capsular contracture, thus compromising the cosmetic result. Replacement of an intact implant can be performed on an outpatient basis with limited morbidity and minimal recovery. The early complications associated with implant reconstruction are a higher incidence of infection and a varying degree of rippling or wrinkling around the prosthesis. Rippling may be palpated or visualized in certain patients and results in a compromised cosmetic result.

The ideal patient for expander/implant reconstruction is the patient with a modest sized breast whose opposite breast is not ptotic or droopy. The patient often desires the "simplest" reconstruction without the use of any donor site tissue, thus making the recovery process shorter. Although this process requires weekly or biweekly visits to the physician's office for expansion, it is not associated with significant discomfort or morbidity. The most significant contraindication to tissue expander and implant reconstruction is the preoperative/postoperative use of radiation treatment. In general, radiation is severely limiting to both expansion and ultimately the result of a soft implant reconstruction. It is the author's experience that 8 of 10 patients do not expand to completion after receiving radiation to the chest wall. In the

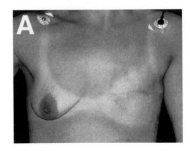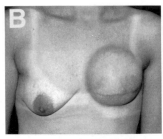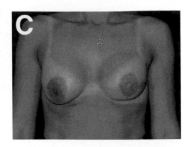

Fig. 6. (A) A 38-year-old woman after left modified radical mastectomy. Staged reconstruction with expander and implant. Note that her right breast is small and she will require augmentation to achieve symmetry. **(B)** After expander placement and overexpansion of left tissues. **(C)** Four months postoperatively. Expander and implant exchange on left and saline implant on right for augmentation with nipple areola reconstruction.

other two patients, in whom expansion is completed, the result is a rather firm and unsatisfactory breast replacement.

The selection of an implant is very important, and there are many options from which to choose for varying cosmetic results. These include different surface textures, different anatomic shapes and sizes, and different filler materials ranging from saline to silicone gel or a combination of both. In general, the saline-filled implants feel firmer; their silicone-filled counterparts are softer and more viscous, closely mimicking autogenous tissue. There are horizontal shaped implants with lower pole fullness as well as a gradual slope to the implant to help give a tapered appearance to the breast. The expander/implant sequence is less frequently used today than in years past owing to the advent of the very reliable autogenous tissue reconstruction techniques.

The older patient with a slightly ptotic opposite breast who desires a tissue expander sequence has the option either to accept the asymmetry or to have a mild reduction or mastopexy of the opposite breast. Lastly, the patient with a very small opposite breast may often choose to have a small implant placed in the opposite breast to achieve symmetry (Fig. 6).

Expander/implants are more favorable in bilateral mastectomy; because bilateral reconstruction is utilized, the difference in symmetry and maturation is minimized. In addition, other flap techniques required for bilateral reconstruction require additional donor sites, which may increase the donor morbidity and therefore become less advantageous. Bilateral expander/implant reconstruction allows the patient the choice of size and shape while maintaining a more youthful appearing breast throughout the years (Fig. 7).

Lastly, the advantages of skin-sparing mastectomy do not apply to expander/implant reconstruction. The redundancy of skin is not advantageous since the expander is placed beneath muscle. There is a redundancy of skin relative to the underlying muscle in the early postoperative period. The incision, therefore, can be modified to limit its length.

4.2. Latissimus Dorsi Flap Reconstruction with Breast Implant

The development of the skin-sparing mastectomy technique has reintroduced the use of immediate latissimus reconstruction with an implant as a popular option for immediate breast reconstruction (Fig. 8).

The latissimus myocutaneous flap is a standard workhorse flap in reconstructive surgery and was utilized many years ago for breast reconstruction. Owing to the early requirements

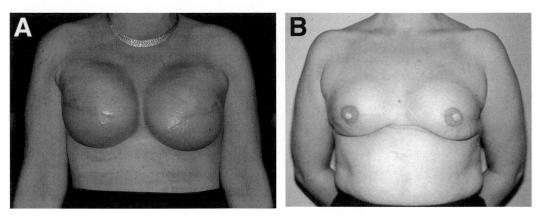

Fig. 7. (**A**) A 53-year-old woman with bilateral expanders after bilateral mastectomies. Note the overexpansion for a soft result. (**B**) Same patient with bilateral expanders followed by implant placement and nipple areola reconstruction.

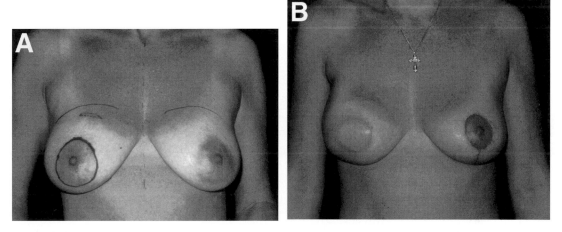

Fig. 8. (**A**) A 50-year-old woman before right skin-sparing mastectomy and latissimus flap with an implant for reconstruction. Note the large left breast that will require mastopexy for symmetry. (**B**) Three months after right skin-sparing mastectomy and immediate latissimus flap with an implant and left mastopexy for symmetry.

of significant skin and soft tissue after standard mastectomy, the donor site morbidity was considered too significant. The TRAM flap had replaced the latissimus flap as the most popular technique for partial or complete autogenous reconstruction. However, because skin-sparing mastectomy preserves most of the breast skin envelope, the skin requirement from the myocutaneous flap is minimized. Therefore, this technique has become more popular as an immediate reconstructive option. A disc of skin can be carried with the muscle flap, allowing the incision to be placed along the bra line. This technique is most often utilized with an implant for volume augmentation.

It has an advantage over tissue expander reconstruction in that it can be performed as a single-stage immediate reconstruction. In addition, latissimus reconstruction can create a more ptotic breast than the expander/implant sequence. The latissimus muscle itself is an accessory muscle of the back and is a favorable donor site (Fig. 9). Recovery from a latis-

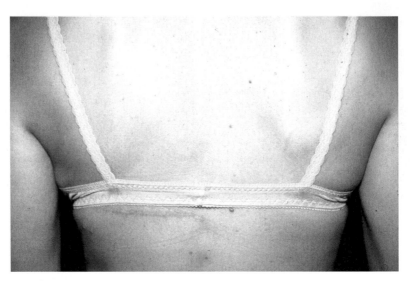

Fig. 9. Six months after right latissimus flap reconstruction. Note how well the incision is hidden by the bra strap for an aesthetic result.

simus flap with implant reconstruction is shorter than that from a TRAM flap reconstruction. The broad nature of the latissimus muscle requires the use of drains to the back and chest. Seroma formation is probably the most significant complication. The operation typically takes 4 hours to complete, and one must reposition the patient many times. The patient starts in the supine position for the mastectomy, is placed in the lateral decubitus position during the muscle harvest, and is finally placed back in the supine position for the flap and implant placement.

The vascular supply to this flap is the thoracodorsal artery and vein, which may be injured with an axillary lymph node dissection. If a complete lymph node dissection needs to be performed, it is important to decide whether this is a good option for reconstruction. This may increase the risk of injury to the blood supply of the latissimus flap. One way to avoid this is to perform the sentinel lymph node biopsy 2 weeks prior to mastectomy to determine whether a full lymph node dissection is necessary.

The latissimus muscle is a well-vascularized muscle, and the use of this flap avoids the incidence of fat necrosis occasionally found in TRAM flap reconstruction. In addition, by providing well-vascularized tissue into the field, the incidence of skin flap loss is also diminished. The latissimus muscle flap is also commonly utilized as a "bail-out" procedure for failed tissue expander reconstruction, usually because of compromise of the skin flaps owing to either ischemia or infection. It can also be used for treatment of complications from postoperative irradiation. By providing healthy vascularized muscle with additional skin, one is typically able to place a tissue expander underneath the latissimus and proceed with the expansion process. Latissimus reconstruction with an implant is not the first choice reconstruction for a patient who is going to need postoperative irradiation. There is a higher incidence of capsule formation around the implant, and firmness is associated with this reconstruction after irradiation. However, acceptable results have been achieved with this technique, and it certainly is an option in those patients who are not candidates for total autogenous reconstruction like the TRAM flap. The complications associated with this operation are seroma or hematoma formation owing to the large surface area of the latissimus donor

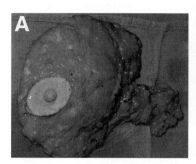
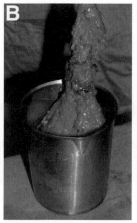
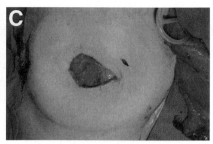

Fig. 10. (A) Breast specimen after a skin-sparing mastectomy. **(B)** Volume displacement using a sterile bucket and saline to measure the volume of the specimen. **(C)** After skin-sparing mastectomy with latissimus muscle prior to placement in the defect. The appropriate volume implant will be used to replace the volume lost by the mastectomy.

site, hypertrophic or widened scarring on the back, and obvious asymmetry or malposition of the implant at the time of reconstruction.

Estimating the appropriate size of implant for volume can be difficult, and a suggested technique that has been helpful is to utilize volume displacement. This technique involves placing the mastectomy specimen in saline and measuring the volume displaced. This can give an estimate of the volume of implant to use for reconstruction (Fig. 10).

The cosmetic result using this flap with a skin-sparing mastectomy is superb. It is the author's choice of immediate unilateral breast reconstruction with skin-sparing mastectomy if the patient is not a TRAM flap candidate. It is also an excellent choice for the older patient who may not tolerate the abdominal morbidity and recovery associated with the TRAM flap or other reconstructive choices (Fig. 11).

4.2. TRAM Flap Reconstruction

The most popular choice of total autogenous breast reconstruction is the TRAM flap breast reconstruction, which has gained significant popularity over the last 20 years. Technical advances and modifications have also made it more reliable, with diminished patient morbidity. It has the advantage of replacing breast tissue with abdominal tissue, which is similar in feel, weight, and contour to a natural breast (Fig. 13).

There are many technical variations in terms of the tissue transfer based on the rectus muscle, ranging from the bipedicle TRAM flap (the use of both rectus muscles) to a unipedicle (a single rectus muscle) and finally to the free TRAM or microvascular transplanted rectus muscle. The blood supply to the rectus muscle is bipedicle: inferiorly based on the inferior epigastric vessels and superiorly on the superior epigastric vessels. The standard unilateral pedicle TRAM flap divides the inferior epigastric vessels and bases the flap entirely on the superior pedicle system. The superior pedicle system is a secondary blood supply, and therefore its ability to provide an adequate blood supply to the rectus muscles and surrounding tissues needs to be assessed. Specifically, old scars in the abdomen that interrupt this blood supply or radiation to the internal mammary vessels are compromising

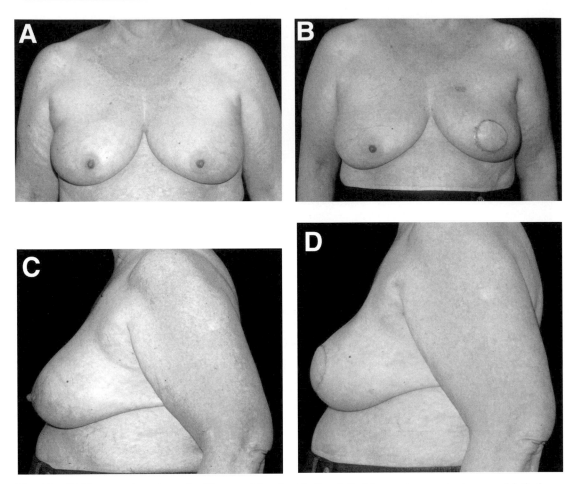

Fig. 11. **(A)** Preoperative view of a 68-year-old patient before left skin-sparing mastectomy and latissimus flap reconstruction. **(B)** Postoperative view. Note the skin paddle. **(C)** Lateral preoperative and **(D)** postoperative views. Note the similar position of the inframammary fold and position of the reconstructed breast on the lateral views.

factors that limit the use of this muscle in a pedicle fashion. A surgeon typically has the choice of a contralateral or ipsilateral rectus muscle.

Surgeons have various preferences regarding use of the free TRAM flap. The advantages are based on utilization of the inferior epigastric system, for microvascular anastomosis to the thoracodorsal system or the internal mammary vessels. By utilizing the dominant vascular supply, in theory one can provide for a greater amount of tissue with less incidence of fat necrosis. Fat necrosis results from ischemia caused by either arterial or venous insufficiency, ultimately leading to firmness of the flap and a poor aesthetic result. The incidence of fat necrosis in the pedicle flaps ranges from 5 to 30%. The microvascular TRAM flap reconstruction has a lower fat necrosis rate. In addition, the microvascular TRAM flap surgery has less abdominal morbidity. However, once any significant amount of muscle is utilized, this muscle is denervated and thus loses its continuity. The greatest disadvantage of the microvascular TRAM flap surgery lies in the fact that if there is a complication or thrombosis to the vessels, 100% flap loss can occur. This devastation after a failed reconstruction is significant to the patient, and therefore the author does not utilize free TRAM reconstruction

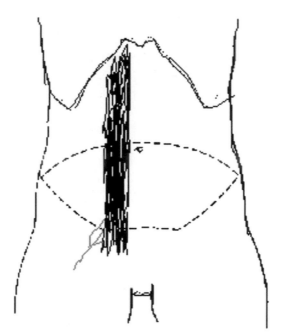

Fig. 12. Diagram of unipedicle transverse rectus abdominis myocutaneous (TRAM). The rectus muscle receives its blood supply from the inferior epigastric vessels. These are the vessels that are ligated when the tissue is harvested. The rectus has a dual blood supply and survives from the superior epigastric artery.

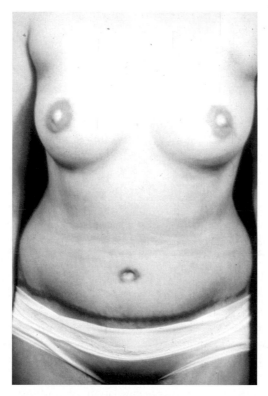

Fig. 13. A 43-year-old patient 6 months after bilateral skin-sparing mastectomies and immediate transverse rectus abdominis myocutaneous (TRAM) reconstruction. The patient has also undergone nipple areola reconstruction.

121

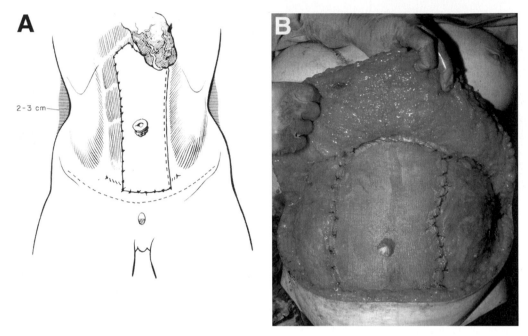

Fig. 14. (A) Diagram illustrating the use of mesh after the rectus has been harvested for a unipedicle transverse rectus abdominis myocutaneous (TRAM) flap. This is to add strength to the abdominal wall and decrease the risk of hernia postoperatively. **(B)** Intraoperative photo of Marlex mesh after the rectus has been harvested and the TRAM flap is in place.

as a routine procedure but uses it instead in anatomically select patients. The reported incidence of TRAM flap failure is roughly 2–5%. However, the monitoring and number of "take-backs" during this time is significantly higher.

Recent studies have shown some benefit to dividing or ligating the inferior epigastric vessels 2 weeks before ultimate transfer, to provide for a more robust superior epigastric system. This is known as the "delay" phenomenon. This technique has become more popular, in attempts to provide for a more robust blood supply. With the advent of sentinel lymph node biopsy, one can coordinate the delay technique with the sentinel lymph node biopsy to limit the number of trips to the operating room. This has decreased the cost as well as the logistical problems for the patient. Specifically, if a patient has sentinel lymph node biopsy prior to her ultimate mastectomy, then the plastic surgeon can simultaneously divide the inferior epigastric vessels at this time 2 weeks before surgery. A delay procedure can be done under local anesthesia with sedation, and 3-cm incisions are utilized to divide the unilateral inferior epigastric vessel and the superfical inferior epigastric systems bilaterally.

The pedicle TRAM flap procedure typically takes 4–5 hours and can be performed simultaneously with mastectomy. Hospital stay is typically 4 days, with a 4–5-week recovery period before the patient can be fully upright, standing straight, walking comfortably, and performing many of her routine activities.

Abdominal donor site morbidity is associated with the TRAM operation. Studies show that bilateral TRAM has the highest associated abdominal wall weakness. Patient dissatisfaction with unilateral TRAM is unusual. It is associated with a long lower abdominal incision. We utilize Marlex mesh reconstruction to provide for balance and support to the abdomen (Fig. 14).

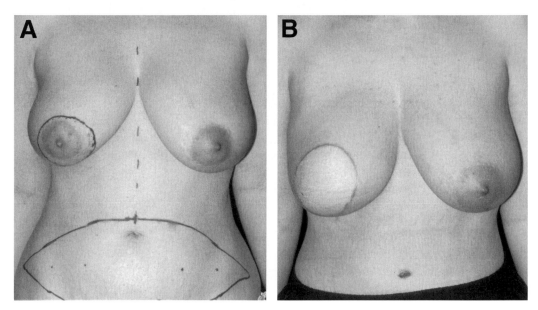

Fig. 15. (A) A 42-year-old patient before right skin-sparing mastectomy and transverse rectus abdominis myocutaneous (TRAM) reconstruction. (B) Postoperative view.

Fewer complaints about back pain or abdominal laxity are heard when abdominal balance for the missing rectus muscle and fascia is maintained. Bipedicled and bilateral TRAM flap reconstruction seems to increase abdominal weakness significantly. Therefore, the author reserves bilateral TRAM reconstruction for bilateral mastectomy patients. We do not use the bipedicle TRAM for unilateral breast reconstruction because of this factor. A significant advantage of the TRAM flap lies not only in the fact that unilateral cosmetic match is achievable but that there is a greater flexibility in shape contouring. Moreover, there is no future implant maintenance. A combination of skin-sparing mastectomy and TRAM flap reconstruction has allowed for significantly better cosmetic results with less surgical time (Fig. 15). Preoperative planning can be made with the patient in a standing position, and the small disc of abdominal skin can essentially replace the missing nipple/areola tissue. Therefore, total autogenous tissue replacement can be made effectively. The skin envelope with maintenance of the inframammary crease allows one to maintain the general anatomy of the breast, and therefore one can consider simply stuffing the breast with volumetric accuracy. The patient who has a mildly protuberant abdomen benefits from the use of this tissue by improving the contour of the abdomen (Fig. 16).

Some risk factors are associated with TRAM flap reconstruction, all of them involving the viability of the transferred tissue. Therefore, factors that compromise wound healing and blood supply such as cigarette smoking, previous radiation therapy, and prior abdominal surgery must be considered. Obesity, diabetes, and collagen vascular diseases are significant compromising factors as well. In current practice, the TRAM flap is the procedure of choice for unilateral breast reconstruction in the patient with the appropriate recovery ability. This flap allows for the best immediate contour and developmental changes, as well as better tissue for nipple reconstruction (Fig. 17).

Secondary contour can be performed simply by outpatient liposuction at the time of nipple reconstruction. The main complications of TRAM flap reconstruction are fat necrosis

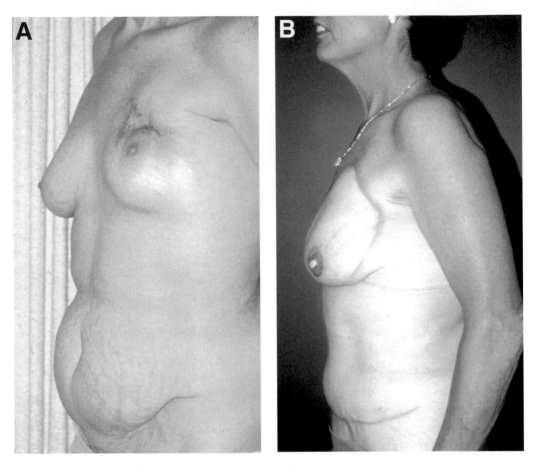

Fig. 16. (A) A 68-year-old woman after left lumpectomy and radiation with recurrence of her breast cancer. Note the excess abdominal tissue. **(B)** One year after TRAM and nipple areola reconstruction. The lower abdomen is flatter and asethetically pleasing.

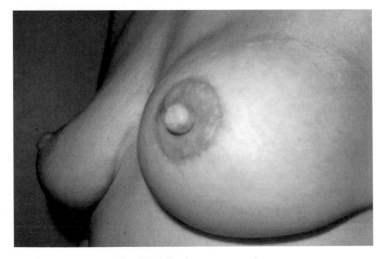

Fig. 17. Nipple reconstruction.

and infection of the breast. Hernia rates range from 1.5 to 6% but have diminished over the years. Abdominal skin necrosis is a rare problem. The need to remove Marlex mesh is extremely rare; however, other prosthetic materials are less forgiving. The authors use the entire muscle for transfer, but many authors only use partial muscle and fascia, to avoid the use of prosthetic material for abdominal repair.

Future attempts to improve reliability and diminish donor site morbidity should focus on understanding and refining the delay phenomenon. In addition, careful dissection of the vascular supply of the inferior epigastric vessel without utilizing any muscle is currently being performed. These flaps are called perforator flaps and have the advantage of avoiding the need to harvest the rectus muscle at all. They are microvascularly transferred and thus have some of the potential risks associated with microvascular breast reconstruction; however, they have the advantage of improved donor site morbidity.

5. ALTERNATIVE CHOICES TO RECONSTRUCTION

There are other anatomic donor sites that can be considered for breast reconstruction, the next most common being the gluteal-based flap. Both the superior artery and the inferior gluteal artery flaps are used for breast reconstruction. They are the appropriate flaps for a patient who has inadequate abdominal tissue and does not want to utilize any prosthetic material. They are performed via microvascular repair. The gluteal vessels are shorter and therefore do not have much flexibility in terms of pedicle length and ease of microvascular repair.

Lastly, the so-called Ruben's flap is a third choice flap for a patient who does not desire the abdominal or gluteal donor site deformity. It is based on the iliac vessels, and the donor site can be acceptable in a patient with appropriate lateral hip tissue. However, this dissection is more tedious and should be reserved for surgeons who perform many of these flaps routinely.

6. CONTROVERSIES IN BREAST RECONSTRUCTION

Immediate breast reconstruction with the use of skin-sparing mastectomy and autogenous tissue reconstruction has taken the aesthetic results of breast reconstruction to the next level. The physical and psychological benefits for patients are improved and have led to the increased use of these techniques. Although the increase in satisfaction for women after immediate reconstruction has improved, there are questions regarding the oncologic safety. Specifically, does immediate reconstruction with skin-sparing mastectomy lead to a delay in adjuvant treatments? Does immediate reconstruction with skin-sparing mastectomy diminish the efficacy of adjuvant chemotherapy or radiation therapy? Can immediate reconstruction be limited to only patients with T1 or T2 tumors? Does immediate reconstruction delay the detection of recurrences?

Previous studies have clearly shown that administration of adjuvant therapy is not delayed with immediate breast reconstruction compared with mastectomy alone. Typically, the initiation of treatment is around 3–4 weeks, and most patients after mastectomy and reconstruction are able to tolerate the initiation of chemotherapy. The most significant treatment delay occurs in patients who have mastectomy skin slough or perioperative infection and a prosthetic reconstruction. This can potentially require the removal of the prosthesis. However, the placement of a tissue expander in a complete submuscular pocket helps diminish any problems associated with skin breakdown in the mastectomy skin flaps. In addition, an appropriately performed skin-sparing mastectomy does not appear to cause any higher incidence of skin flap necrosis than mastectomy and no reconstruction. There is no question that patients who have had previous radiation therapy to the chest wall may require a modification of the skin-sparing technique owing to the viability of their skin flaps. Additionally, patients who have had previous radiation do not tolerate tissue expansion or implant placement as readily. These patients most commonly receive autogenous tissue reconstruction, and the vascular supply from these flaps tends to help the healing process.

Two significant studies from Emory University and the M.D. Anderson Cancer Center comparing the recurrence rate of skin-sparing mastectomy and reconstruction with mastectomy alone show no increased incidence of tumor recurrence or delay in the diagnosis of recurrence. The local recurrence that occurs from breast cancer tends to reside in the dermal lymphatics or skin, and therefore these potential lesions are readily palpable in the skin-sparing technique. In addition, lymph node recurrences are also easily palpable. Patients with advanced disease or indications that there may be a high incidence of chest wall recurrence are not good candidates for immediate reconstruction. These are typically patients with fixed masses to the chest wall or lesions involving the pectoralis major. Lastly, the use of immediate reconstruction in patients with larger lesions seems to be most acceptable on an individual basis. Several studies now show that patients with T3 lesions have had a satisfactory outcome after skin-sparing mastectomy and immediate reconstruction. Patients who are at high risk of systemic disease do not appear to have any complications associated with immediate reconstruction, and certainly these patients have an improved quality of life during their disease-free period. The chance of a systemic recurrence is much higher than a local recurrence, and therefore, when clearly informed, many patients and physicians will choose to perform immediate reconstruction.

The effectiveness of postoperative irradiation does not appear to be reduced in patients who have had immediate reconstruction. It seems that TRAM flaps tolerate radiation quite well and undergo changes similar to those of native breast tissue. There appears to be some temporary discoloration, firmness, and shrinkage of the TRAM flap. We tend to leave the TRAM flap slightly fuller in patients who are going to need postoperative irradiation, to account for the postoperative shrinkage. Latissimus flap and implant reconstructions also appear to tolerate irradiation well, although the incidence of capsular contracture is indeed higher.

In summary, immediate breast reconstruction utilizing skin-sparing techniques has afforded women with the diagnosis of breast cancer the opportunity to have breast reconstruction that most closely mimics their natural breast. In addition, it allows patients to have their surgery at one time and not undergo the traumatic, emotionally difficult period with significant breast deformity and body image changes. The concept of tissue maintenance with skin-sparing mastectomy and similar tissue replacement that is afforded by the use of autogenous tissues can almost be thought of as autogenous tissue treatment for patients with breast cancer and mastectomy. We believe that the avoidance of irradiation and the diminution of recurrence with a superior cosmetic result may swing the pendulum back toward mastectomy and immediate reconstruction for many patients versus lumpectomy and radiation treatment (Fig. 18).

It is our experience that these recent developments have expanded the indications for immediate reconstruction and have left patients with a higher degree of postoperative satisfaction.

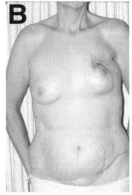
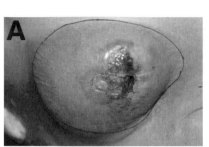
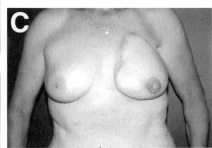

Fig. 18. (A) Radiation-induced changes after lumpectomy and radiation with recurrent cancer. **(B)** Status post lumpectomy and radiation. **(C)** One-year follow-up after TRAM and nipple areola reconstruction. Note the more extensive reconstruction.

BIBLIOGRAPHY

Albo RJ, Gruber R, Kahn R (1980) Immediate breast reconstruction after modified mastectomy for carcinoma of the breast. *Am. J. Surg.* **140,** 131–136.

Artz JS, Dinner MI, Foglietti MA, et al. (1991) Breast reconstruction utilizing subcutaneous tissue expansion followed by polyurethane-covered silicone implants: a 6-year experience. *Plast. Reconstr. Surg.* **88,** 635–639.

Baldwin BJ, Schusterman MA, Miller MJ, et al. (1994) Bilateral breast reconstruction: conventional vs free TRAM. *Plast. Reconstr. Surg.* **93,** 1410.

Banic A, Boeckx W, Gruelich M, et al. (1995) Late results of breast reconstruction with free TRAM flaps: a prospective multicentric study. *Plast. Reconstr. Surg.* **95,** 1195–1204; discussion 1205–1206.

Carlson GW, Bostwick J, Styblo TM, et al. (1997) Skin-sparing mastectomy: oncologic and reconstructive considerations. *Ann. Surg.* **225,** 570–575.

Dean C, Chetty U, Forrest AP (1983) Effects of immediate breast reconstruction on psychosocial morbidity after mastectomy. *Lancet* **1,** 459–462.

Dowden RV (1991) Selection criteria for successful immediate breast reconstruction. *Plast. Reconstr. Surg.* **88,** 628–634.

Elberlein TJ, Crespo LD, Smith BL, et al. (1993) Prospective evaluation of immediate reconstruction after mastectomy. *Ann. Surg.* **218,** 29–36.

Evans GRD, Schusterman MA, Kroll SS, et al. (1995) Reconstruction and the radiated breast: is there a role for implants? Discussion: Spear SL, Maxwell GP. *Plast. Reconstr. Surg.* **96,** 1111–1118.

Furey PC, Macgillivray DC, Castiglione CL, et al. (1994) Wound complications in patients receiving adjuvant chemotherapy after mastectomy and immediate breast reconstruction for breast cancer. *J. Surg. Oncol.* **55,** 194–197.

Grotting JC, Urist MM, Maddox WA, Vasconez LO (1989) Conventional TRAM flap versus free microsurgical TRAM flap for immediate breast reconstruction. *Plast. Reconstr. Surg.* **83,** 828–841.

Handel N, Jenson JA, Black Q, et al. (1995) The fate of breast implants: a critical analysis of complications and outcomes. *Plast. Reconstr. Surg.* **96,** 1521.

Hartrampf CR Jr, Bennet GK (1987) Autogenous tissue reconstruction in the mastectomy patient: a critical review of 300 patients. *Ann. Surg.* **205,** 508.

Khoo A, Kroll SS, Reece GP, et al. (1998) A comparison of resource costs of immediate and delayed breast reconstruction. *Plast. Reconstr. Surg.* **101,** 964–968.

Kroll SS, Evans GRD, Reece GP, et al. (1996) Comparison of resource costs between implant-based and TRAM flap breast reconstruction. *Plast. Reconstr. Surg.* **97,** 364.

McGraw JB, Papp C, Edwards A, et al. (1994) The autogenous latissimus breast reconstruction. *Clin. Plast. Surg.* **21,** 279.

Miller MJ, Rock CS, Robb GL (1996) Aesthetic breast reconstruction using a combination of free transverse rectus abdominus musculocutaneous flaps and breast implants. *Ann. Plast. Surg.* **37,** 258–264.

Noguchi M, Kitagawa H, Kinoshita K, et al. (1993) Psychologic and cosmetic self-assessments of breast conserving therapy compared with mastectomy and immediate breast reconstruction. *J. Surg. Oncol.* **54,** 260–266.

O'Brien W, Hasselgren PO, Hummel RP, et al. (1993) Comparison of postoperative wound complications and early cancer recurrence between patients undergoing mastectomy with or without immediate breast reconstruction. *Am. J. Surg.* **166,** 1–5.

8   Radiation Therapy

Barbara Fowble, MD, and Gary Freedman, MD

CONTENTS

INTRODUCTION
DUCTAL CARCINOMA *IN SITU*
BREAST CONSERVATION THERAPY FOR STAGE I AND II INVASIVE
    BREAST CANCER
THE ROLE OF RADIATION FOLLOWING CONSERVATIVE SURGERY
    IN WOMEN WITH EARLY-STAGE INVASIVE BREAST CANCER
RADIATION FOLLOWING MASTECTOMY FOR STAGE I–II
    BREAST CANCER
INTEGRATION OF ADJUVANT SYSTEMIC THERAPY WITH CONSERVATIVE
    SURGERY AND RADIATION OR POSTMASTECTOMY RADIATION
LOCALLY ADVANCED BREAST CANCER
COMPLICATIONS OF RADIATION THERAPY
LOCAL REGIONAL RECURRENCE FOLLOWING MASTECTOMY
RADIATION FOR THE PALLIATION OF METASTATIC BREAST CANCER
CONCLUSIONS
BIBLIOGRAPHY

1. INTRODUCTION

Radiotherapy has played an important role in the treatment of breast cancer. It is frequently given following conservative surgery for ductal carcinoma *in situ* (DCIS) or stage I and II invasive breast cancer. Its role as adjuvant therapy following mastectomy in selected patients with stage I and II disease is currently being defined, and it is an essential component of the combined modality approach for stage III disease. Radiation represents an important therapeutic option for the palliation of metastases to sites such as bone and brain and may be used alone or in combination with surgery to control recurrent disease in the chest wall or regional nodes following mastectomy. This chapter discusses the role of radiation in the treatment of DCIS, stage I and II breast cancer, locally advanced breast cancer, local-regional recurrence, and metastatic disease (Table 1).

2. DUCTAL CARCINOMA *IN SITU*

The success of conservative surgery and radiation for stage I and II invasive breast cancer prompted its evaluation in the treatment of DCIS. The rationale for treatment directed to the

From: *Current Clinical Oncology:*
Breast Cancer: A Guide to Detection and Multidisciplinary Therapy
Edited by: M. H. Torosian © Humana Press Inc., Totowa, NJ

Table 1
Indications for Radiation in the Treatment of Breast Cancer

Breast conservation therapy
  Ductal carcinoma *in situ*
    1. Excision with negative margins
    2. Radiation to the intact breast
  Stage I–II Invasive Cancer
    1. Excision with negative margins
    2. Axillary dissection or sentinel node biopsy
    3. Radiation to the intact breast ± regional nodes
    4. Systemic therapy as indicated
Postmastectomy
  Stage I–II
    1. Mastectomy and axillary dissection
    2. Adjuvant systemic therapy
    3. Radiation to the chest wall and regional nodes if:
       Primary tumor >5 cm
       ≥4 positive nodes
       Close or positive mastectomy margin
       1–3 positive nodes with extracapsular extension
  Stage III
    1. Neoadjuvant chemotherapy
    2. Mastectomy and axillary dissection
    3. Further systemic therapy if indicated by response
    4. Radiation to the chest wall and regional nodes
Recurrent disease
    1. Local-regional recurrence following mastectomy
    2. Surgical resection where possible
    3. Radiation to involved sites ± uninvolved sites
Metastases
  Palliation for bone or brain metastases including spinal cord compresion

entire breast with radiation is related to the potential for multifocal DCIS or the presence of an occult invasive cancer. Multifocality, i.e., two or more foci of DCIS in the same quadrant, or multicentricity, i.e., two or more foci of DCIS in separate quadrants, has been correlated with low nuclear grade, micropapillary architectural pattern, DCIS greater than 2.5 cm, and the clinical presentation of a palpable or mammographically detected mass. The presence of an occult invasive cancer with DCIS has been correlated with presentation as a palpable mass, the comedo architectural pattern, and more than 5 cm of DCIS.

Ten to 20% of DCIS patients treated with conservative surgery and radiation will subsequently develop another cancer in the treated breast. Approximately 50% of these recurrences are invasive cancer, and 50% are DCIS. Factors that minimize the risk of an ipsilateral breast tumor recurrence (IBTR) include wide surgical excision with negative margins generally defined as greater than 2 mm and a postbiopsy mammogram with magnification views in patients presenting with mammographic calcifications demonstrating no residual calcifications. The nuclear grade and architectural pattern of DCIS do not appear to influence ipsilateral breast tumor recurrence rates in patients treated with conservative surgery and radiation. Patient age may impact on outcome since several series have reported higher breast recurrence rates in younger (i.e., ≤40 years of age) compared with older women. Ten-year survival rates following conservative surgery and radiation for DCIS range from 98 to 100%.

DCIS may have various clinical presentations including the presence of a palpable mass, bloody nipple discharge, mammographic finding of calcifications, or a mass with or without calcifications. Most of the series reporting results of conservative surgery and radiation for DCIS included patients with all clinical presentations. There is more limited information regarding the long-term results of conservative surgery and radiation for DCIS detected solely as a mammographic finding. For these patients, the 5-year rate of ipsilateral breast tumor recurrence has ranged from 5 to 10%, with 10-year rates of 10 to 20%. Negative margins of resection diminish the risk of an ipsilateral breast tumor recurrence; in a collaborative study from multiple institutions in the United States and Europe, patients with mammographically detected DCIS and negative resection margins (>2 mm), had a 7% ipsilateral breast tumor recurrence rate with a median follow-up of 9.3 years. The risk of a contralateral breast cancer at 15 years in patients treated with conservative surgery and radiation for DCIS has been reported to be 9%.

The prognosis for patients who develop an ipsilateral breast tumor recurrence following conservative surgery and radiation for DCIS has been favorable. Virtually all of such patients have been salvaged with mastectomy, and approximately 75% of invasive occurrences are salvaged with additional therapy, usually mastectomy, with or without adjuvant systemic therapy depending on the extent of the disease.

The role of radiation following conservative surgery for DCIS has been evaluated by two prospective randomized trials. The National Surgical Adjuvant Breast Project (NSABP) B17 trial randomized 818 women with ductal carcinomas (80% of which were mammographically detected) to conservative surgery or conservative surgery and radiation. The addition of radiation decreased the 8-year cumulative incidence of an ipsilateral breast tumor recurrence from 26.8 to 12.1%. The cumulative incidence of an invasive recurrence was reduced from 13.4 to 3.9% with radiation and that of a noninvasive recurrence from 13.4 to 8%. There were no differences in survival between these two groups. In this randomized trial, young age did not predict for an increased risk of an ipsilateral breast tumor recurrence in either group of patients. The results of this trial support the addition of radiation in all patients with DCIS. However, patients who had scattered mammographic calcifications experienced a significant breast tumor recurrence rate when they were treated with either conservative surgery or conservative surgery and radiation. These patients, therefore, should not be considered candidates for breast conservation therapy. (The European Organization for Research and Treatment of Cancer (EORTC) randomized 1010 women with DCIS less than 4–5 cm to wide excision with or without radiation. With a median follow-up of 4.2 years, the addition of radiation decreased the ipsilateral breast tumor recurrence rate from 16 to 10%, invasive recurrences from 8 to 5%, and noninvasive recurrences from 8 to 5%. Overall survival was 99% in both groups.)

An analysis of pathologic features correlating with ipsilateral breast tumor recurrence in the NSABP B17 trial found that significant factors included margin status and the presence of moderate to marked comedo necrosis. For patients with negative resection margins and absent to slight necrosis, radiation decreased ipsilateral breast tumor recurrence rates from 7 to 4% compared with 16 to 4% for those with moderate to marked necrosis. These results would suggest that patients who may benefit least from radiation are those with negative margins and none or slight necrosis. The pathologic analysis of the EORTC trial confirmed growth pattern (solid and cribriform) and margin status as factors predicting recurrence, in addition to young age and detection as a physical finding.

The Van Nuys prognostic classification was based on a retrospective review of patients with DCIS treated by either mastectomy, conservative surgery and radiation, or conservative surgery alone. The formulation of this index represented an attempt to establish guidelines for clinical decision making in patients with DCIS. The classification includes tumor size, margin status, and nuclear grade. There are three categories for each of the factors, with a score ranging from 1 to 3. The size categories are: 1.5 cm or less, 1.6–4 cm, and 4.1 cm or more. The margin categories include ≥1 cm, 1–9 mm, and less than 1 mm. The pathologic categories are divided into low grade without necrosis, low grade with necrosis, and high grade with or without necrosis. A total score is achieved by summing each of the individual scores. The clinical application of this scoring system is often limited by the inability to determine the extent of DCIS accurately. Size is frequently determined by the area on a given slide; however, this assessment does not evaluate the three-dimensional extent. The most accurate way of assessing the extent of the DCIS is by serially and sequentially sectioning the entire biopsy specimen and determining the number of blocks in which DCIS is present out of the total number and their location. This detailed pathologic correlation is not commonly performed. In series in which excellent clinical and pathologic correlation of the size of DCIS has been found, patients with scores of 3–4 in the Van Nuys Prognostic Index appear to have little benefit from radiation in terms of an ipsilateral breast tumor recurrence, whereas those with scores of 5–7 have a definite benefit. Scores of 8–9 are associated with high ipsilateral breast tumor recurrence rates with or without radiation, and these patients are advised to undergo mastectomy.

The role of tamoxifen following radiation in the treatment of DCIS has been evaluated by a single prospective randomized trial. The NSABP B24 trial randomized 1804 patients with DCIS to radiation with or without 5 years of tamoxifen. With a mean follow-up of 5.1 years, the addition of tamoxifen to radiation decreased the ipsilateral breast tumor recurrence rate from 8.6 to 6.4%, invasive ipsilateral breast tumor recurrences from 3.4 to 2.1%, and noninvasive ipsilateral breast tumor recurrences from 5.2 to 4.3%. Tamoxifen also decreased the cumulative incidence of a contralateral breast cancer. Although the results of this trial favor the use of tamoxifen in patients with DCIS, it should be noted that patients in this trial were not required to have negative margins of resection or the removal of all malignant calcifications prior to treatment. The absolute benefit from tamoxifen was relatively small. At the present time, there is no general consensus regarding which patients with DCIS should be treated with tamoxifen.

Radiation for ductal DCIS includes treatment initially directed to the entire breast for a total dose of 4600–5000 cGy over a period of $4^1/_2$–5 weeks with treatment given 5 days a week. A supplemental boost of radiation may be directed to the initial tumor site. Treatment is not directed to the regional nodes since the risk of positive axillary nodes is less than 5%. The expected side effects of treatment include erythema to the skin of the breast and possible fatigue; these changes resolve upon completion of treatment. A postbiopsy mammogram with magnification views of the excision site is essential prior to the initiation of radiation in patients presenting with mammographic calcifications. This mammogram should demonstrate no residual malignant-appearing calcifications.

The American College of Radiology, the American College of Surgeons, the Society of Surgical Oncology, and the College of American Pathologists recently reported standards for the evaluation and treatment of patients with DCIS. Patients who are candidates for conservative surgery and radiation include those with DCIS whose extent is 4 cm or less determined pathologically, those for whom there is no clinical evidence of gross multifocal or multicentric disease, and those for whom negative margins of excision can be obtained following a reasonable surgical excision. Mastectomy is the recommended treatment for patients with extensive DCIS, i.e., tumor larger than 4 cm, those in whom negative margins cannot be achieved after a reasonable attempt at surgical excision, and those with clinical evidence of gross multifocal or multicentric disease.

The Eastern Cooperative Oncology Group has initiated a prospective single-arm study of wide excision alone for selected patients with DCIS. Patients who have mammographically detected DCIS of low to intermediate nuclear grade (2.5 cm or less) or high DCIS grade (1 cm or less; both measured pathologically) and margins of 3 mm or more are eligible for the study. It is anticipated that this study will provide further information regarding which patients with DCIS may be treated with wide excision alone.

3. BREAST CONSERVATION THERAPY FOR STAGE I AND II INVASIVE BREAST CANCER

Six prospective randomized trials have compared conservative surgery, axillary dissection, and radiation with radical mastectomy or modified radical mastectomy in selected patients with stage I–II breast cancer. The eligibility for these trials included patients with primary tumors less than 4–5 cm and clinically negative or positive (nonfixed) axillary nodes. Despite variations in the degree of surgical resection, the technical aspects of radiation, and the use of adjuvant systemic therapy, the trials have consistently demonstrated no significant difference in terms of local-regional recurrence, distant metastasis, or long-term survival for the two treatments. Patients with positive axillary nodes had a similar outcome whether treated by breast conservation therapy or mastectomy. The trials also demonstrated no increased risk of contralateral breast cancer or second nonbreast cancer malignancy in patients who received radiation.

Although most patients with stage I–II breast cancer are candidates for breast conservation therapy, a number of clinical and pathologic factors should be considered before advising a patient of this treatment option. These factors include past medical history, patient age, family history, clinical presentation, tumor size and location, breast size, the presence or absence of DCIS and its extent, histology, the presence or absence of lymphatic invasion, the axillary nodal status, and the resection margin status. A recommendation for mastectomy may be prompted by the potential risk for a unacceptable cosmetic result, significant complications, or a substantial risk of ipsilateral breast tumor recurrence. Contraindications to breast conservation therapy with radiation include prior history of collagen vascular disease, i.e., lupus, scleroderma, or mixed connective tissue disease, a history of prior chest or mantle radiation, or pregnancy. A prior history of collagen vascular disease has been associated with an increased incidence of severe fibrosis or soft tissue or bone necrosis in patients treated with conventional radiation. Reirradiation of the soft tissues and ribs in patients who have previously received mantle or chest irradiation may increase the risk of severe complications but, more importantly, may also increase the risk of a radiation-induced sarcoma. Radiation should be avoided in pregnant women because of the potential for scatter radiation to the fetus.

Certain factors have been associated with an increased risk of ipsilateral breast tumor recurrence. However, this risk may not be of sufficient magnitude to recommend mastectomy or may be similar to the risk of local-regional recurrence with mastectomy. Young women, i.e., younger than 35–40 years, have been reported to have a 10–25% 5-year risk of ipsilateral breast tumor recurrence when they are treated with conservative surgery and radiation. Some of this increased risk has been attributed to a greater prevalence of invasive cancers with an extensive intraductal component or certain adverse histologic features including high nuclear and histologic grade or the presence of necrosis. The risk of an ipsilateral breast tumor recurrence in young women can be decreased by the addition of adjuvant systemic chemotherapy and also by ensuring that resection of the primary tumor achieves pathologically negative margins. Young women have also been reported to have an increased risk of local-regional recurrence when treated with mastectomy. A positive family history of breast cancer has not been associated with an increased risk of ipsilateral breast tumor recurrence in patients treated with breast conservation therapy and radiation. There are few data regarding outcome in women with hereditary breast cancer. However, several recent series suggest that these women do not have a significantly increased risk of ipsilateral breast tumor recurrence within 5 years when they are treated with conservative surgery and radiation. There is an increased incidence of contralateral breast cancer, which has also been observed in women with hereditary breast cancer treated with mastectomy.

The clinical presentation of more than one area of malignancy in a single breast is considered a contraindication to breast conservation therapy. These women have been reported to have ipsilateral breast tumor recurrence rates in the range of 35–40% despite radiation, and this increased risk has been related to a significant residual tumor burden as demonstrated by pathologic studies of mastectomy specimens. The increased risk of recurrence has been observed for two or more lesions in the same quadrant as well as two or more lesions in separate quadrants.

Tumor size and location may also impact on treatment recommendations. In general, breast conservation therapy has been limited to patients whose primary tumor size is less than 5 cm. Patients with invasive cancers of more than 5 cm have been found to have a significant risk of multicentric disease. The role of breast conservation therapy in patients with T3 primary tumors following neoadjuvant chemotherapy is currently being evaluated. Patients with tumors located in the subareolar region (i.e., within 1–2 cm of the nipple-areolar complex) may require resection of the nipple-areolar complex to achieve negative margins. The subsequent cosmetic appearance may be unacceptable to the patient. Breast size is another important consideration in selecting patients for breast conservation therapy. Patients with very small breasts who require a significant resection of breast tissue may prefer mastectomy with reconstruction. Obese women or those with large pendulous breasts require special modifications in radiation technique to achieve a good cosmetic result.

The following pathologic factors have been associated with an increased risk of ipsilateral breast tumor recurrence in patients undergoing conservative surgery and radiation: the presence of an extensive intraductal component, defined as DCIS comprising 25% or more of the primary tumor and present in the normal surrounding breast tissue, the presence of lymphatic/vascular invasion, and positive or close resection margins. Patients with an extensive intraductal component have been reported to have an increased risk of ipsilateral breast tumor recurrence, primarily when attention has not been paid to the microscopic status of the resection margin. These patients have not been noted to have an increased risk of ipsilateral breast tumor recurrence if resection margins are negative. The presence of lobular carcinoma *in situ* has not been associated with an increased risk of ipsilateral breast tumor recurrence. The presence of lymphatic or vascular invasion has been associated with an increased risk of both ipsilateral breast tumor recurrence and distant metastasis. Patients with positive margins, i.e., tumor cells at the resection margin who are young (40 years of age or less) or who have an extensive intraductal component or an invasive lobular cancer have been reported to have ipsilateral breast tumor recurrence rates in the range of 25–40% despite radiation. It is important to achieve negative margins in these patients, to minimize the risk of a breast recurrence. The extent of the margin positivity has also been correlated with ipsilateral breast tumor recurrences. Diffuse margin involvement, i.e., more than 3 low power fields, or involvement of more than one margin have resulted in ipsilateral breast tumor recurrence rates in the range of 30–35%. Ideally, negative margins of resection should be achieved in all patients undergoing breast conservation therapy with radiation to minimize the risk of an ipsilateral breast tumor recurrence. However, the significance of a focally positive margin in elderly women with estrogen receptor-positive tumors in the absence of lymphatic or vascular invasion or an extensive intraductal component remains unknown.

Radiation is generally initiated within 4–6 weeks after surgical resection of the primary tumor and an axillary node dissection or sentinel node biopsy. Treatment is initially directed to the entire breast for a total dose of 4500–5000 cGy over a period of $4^1/_2$–$5^1/_2$ weeks. A supplemental dose of radiation termed *the boost* may be given to the excisional biopsy site with either a radioactive implant, electrons, or photons. The role of the boost in patients with negative margins of resection has been questioned. Two prospective randomized trials have evaluated the role of the boost in these patients; both confirmed a decreased ipsilateral breast tumor recurrence rate at 8 years with the addition of the boost. Irradiation of the regional nodes in patients with early-stage invasive breast cancer remains controversial in patients with histologically positive axillary nodes. There is general agreement that regional node radiation is not indicated in women with negative axillary nodes. For patients with one to three positive axillary nodes who have undergone an adequate axillary dissection, regional node failures are uncommon. There is an increasing trend to avoid radiation to the supraclavicular, apical axillary, and internal mammary nodes in these women. For patients with four or more positive nodes, radiation is recommended to the supraclavicular region in addition to the breast. The role of internal mammary node irradiation again remains controversial.

4. THE ROLE OF RADIATION FOLLOWING CONSERVATIVE SURGERY IN WOMEN WITH EARLY-STAGE INVASIVE BREAST CANCER

Six prospective randomized trials have evaluated the role of radiation following wide excision or quadrantectomy and axillary dissection for stage I–II breast cancer. All of the trials have demonstrated a significant reduction in the incidence of ipsilateral breast tumor recurrence with the addition of radiation. For axillary node-negative patients who did not receive radiation, ipsilateral breast tumor recurrence rates ranged from 12 to 40%, compared with 2 to 12% with radiation, and for axillary node-positive patients, ipsilateral breast tumor recurrence rates ranged from 27 to 41% without radiation to 4 to 20% with radiation. These trials have demonstrated that patients with invasive cancers who should not be considered candidates for conservative surgery alone because of a significant risk of ipsilateral breast tumor recurrence include those with primary tumors greater than 2 cm, young age, and the presence of an extensive intraductal component, lymphatic invasion, or positive axillary nodes. Even in the most favorable subgroup of patients (i.e., those with primary tumors 2 cm or less in diameter, negative margins, pathologically negative nodes, older age, and the absence of an extensive intraductal component or lymphatic or vascular invasion and who are estrogen receptor-positive), the addition of radiation appears to decrease the risk of an ipsilateral breast tumor recurrence; however, the absolute benefit may be relatively small. The Cancer and Leukemia Group B recently completed a randomized trial of women older than 70 years with T1 tumors, negative resection margins, and a clinically negative axilla comparing breast irradiation and tamoxifen or tamoxifen alone. Axillary dissection was optional. The early results of this trial have demonstrated no signigicant differences in local-regional control or deaths from breast cancer with addition of radiation in this select group of women.

Although radiation has diminished the risk of an ipsilateral breast tumor recurrence in women with stage I–II breast cancer, it has resulted in a survival benefit of only 1–4% in axillary node-negative patients and 8% in axillary node-positive patients. None of these differences was statistically significant; however, none of the trials had enough patients to demonstrate that this modest benefit would be statistically significant. At the present time, patients who may be considered candidates for wide excision alone without radiation, with or without tamoxifen, include elderly women those who are pathologically node negative without an extensive intraductal component or lymphatic invasion, those with primary tumor size 1 cm or less and negative margins, and those who are estrogen receptor-positive.

5. RADIATION FOLLOWING MASTECTOMY FOR STAGE I–II BREAST CANCER

Thirty-three prospective randomized trials involving 15,000 women have evaluated the role of radiation following mastectomy. The earliest of these trials did not include adjuvant systemic therapy and although radiation decreased the risk of a local-regional recurrence (chest wall, axilla, supraclavicular, or internal mammary nodes), a benefit in survival was uncommon. Subsequent analyses demonstrated that the decrease in breast cancer mortality associated with radiation was offset by an increase in cardiac mortality, especially for women older than 60 years of age and for those with left-sided primary tumors. The increased risk of cardiac mortality was associated with radiation technique. With the development of effective adjuvant systemic therapy regimens, interest in and the use of postmastectomy radiation declined. It was anticipated that adjuvant chemotherapy or hormonal therapy would decrease both local and regional as well as distant recurrences and obviate the need for postmastectomy irradiation.

Recent studies have suggested that adjuvant systemic therapy does not significantly impact on the overall incidence or pattern of local regional recurrence following mastectomy. Patients who have been reported to have a significant risk of local-regional recurrence, i.e., 25–35%, despite adjuvant systemic therapy include those with primary tumor size over 5 cm, four or more positive nodes, and positive or close mastectomy margin, as well as those who have had an inadequate axillary dissection. The incidence of local regional recurrence following mastectomy in axillary node-positive patients does not appear to be influenced by the use of multiagent chemotherapy compared with single-agent, longer versus shorter duration of therapy, the use of doxorubicin-based regimens, sequential versus alternating regimens, or dose-intensive regimens with autologous bone marrow transplant or peripheral stem cell reinfusion. Two prospective randomized trials have demonstrated that postmastectomy radiation is more effective than chemotherapy or tamoxifen alone in the prevention of local-regional recurrence.

Ten prospective randomized trials have evaluated the role of postmastectomy radiation and adjuvant chemotherapy in axillary node-positive patients. Nine of these 10 trials have demonstrated a decrease in the incidence of local-regional recurrence from approximately 15–30% without radiation to approximately 10% with radiation. Two recent trials have demonstrated that this improvement in local-regional recurrence has also translated into a statistically significant survival benefit in premenopausal women receiving cyclophosphamide, methotrexate, and 5-fluorouracil chemotherapy. At the present time, indications for postmastectomy radiation include primary tumor size larger than 5 cm, the presence of four or more positive axillary nodes, a close or positive mastectomy margin, i.e., 5 mm or less, and an inadequate axillary dissection in patients with one to three positive nodes. In these patients, the survival benefit with the addition of radiation to chemotherapy is 6–12%. Postmastectomy radiation is considered an essential component of the treatment in women with 10 or more positive nodes receiving dose-intensive chemotherapy with autologous bone marrow transplant or peripheral stem cell rescue. The role of postmastectomy radiation in patients with one to three positive nodes who have had an adequate axillary dissection is controversial; some investigators recommend treatment based on the results of the Danish and British Columbia prospective randomized trials, and others do not, based on the observation that inadequate axillary surgery contributed to the local-regional recurrence rates in patients who did not receive radiation. A recent update of the British Columbia trial has demonstrated a benefit for postmastectomy radiation in patients with one to three positive nodes only in those with extracapsular extension.

Postmastectomy radiation includes the chest wall and supraclavicular region for a total dose of 4600–5000 cGy over a period of $4^{1}/_{2}$–$5^{1}/_{2}$ weeks. Bolus material is used over the chest wall every other day to treat the skin and subcutaneous tissues adequately. Daily bolus or a boost to the mastectomy scar is not routinely needed. A posterior axillary field may be used to supplement the dose to the axilla; however, it is generally not necessary if an adequate dissection has been performed. The role of internal mammary node radiation in early-stage invasive breast cancer remains controversial. The potential for late cardiac mortality related to treatment of the internal mammary nodes may offset any benefit, especially in patients receiving chemotherapy. Clinical internal mammary node recurrences are infrequent and occur in less than 5% of patients undergoing mastectomy for stage I–II breast cancer.

6. INTEGRATION OF ADJUVANT SYSTEMIC THERAPY WITH CONSERVATIVE SURGERY AND RADIATION OR POSTMASTECTOMY RADIATION

In clinical practice, radiation either as part of conservative surgery or as an adjuvant postmastectomy has been delayed until the completion of all adjuvant systemic chemotherapy. This delay has raised the theoretical concern of the potential for an increased risk of local regional recurrence. However, delays in the initiation of systemic therapy may result in an increased risk of distant disease. A single prospective randomized trial in patients undergoing conservative surgery and radiation has demonstrated that delays of up to 4 months do not result in an increased risk of ipsilateral breast tumor recurrence provided that margins of resection are negative. The concurrent use of chemotherapy and radiation in patients undergoing conservative surgery and radiation has been evaluated by several institutions. However, depending on the chemotherapy agents used, there may be an increased risk of symptomatic pneumonitis, moist desquamation, skin erythema, and diminished cosmesis. Therefore, the sequential use of radiation or chemotherapy is favored rather than concurrent regimens.

For patients undergoing mastectomy, radiation is generally delayed until the completion of chemotherapy, and a recent study has demonstrated that delays of 6 months or longer may not compromise local-regional recurrence rates.

7. LOCALLY ADVANCED BREAST CANCER

Locally advanced breast cancer can be subdivided into three separate clinical entities: operable, inoperable, and inflammatory disease. Operable locally advanced breast cancer includes tumors that are resectable at presentation but are greater than 5 cm (T3) in size and/or have positive axillary lymph nodes fixed to each other (N2). The standard initial management of these tumors is modified radical mastectomy, postoperative adjuvant systemic therapy, and radiation. Local-regional control rates range from 85 to 95% with 10-year survival of 40–45% for operable stage III breast cancer treated in this manner. In prospective randomized trials, patients with operable IIIA disease randomized to receive postmastectomy radiation had a local-regional recurrence rate of less than 15%, compared with 25–60% after mastectomy and adjuvant systemic chemotherapy alone. Absolute improvements in survival of 7–25% after radiation have been reported. The technical aspects of radiation are similar to those previously described for postmastectomy radiation for stage I and II disease.

Neoadjuvant chemotherapy has been used for operable T3 tumors to permit breast conservation. The recurrence rates in the preserved breast with initial T3 disease generally have exceeded those observed in early-stage breast cancer or those observed on the chest wall after mastectomy. Despite a high rate of clinical response to induction therapy, few patients overall will have a pathologic complete response. Even in a favorable subgroup (the fewer than 20–25% with a clinical complete response to induction chemotherapy), the 5-year recurrence rate in the breast after radiation alone can be 20% or higher. A low risk of breast recurrence has been observed in small numbers of patients with a clinical complete response and a negative repeat breast biopsy after neoadjuvant chemotherapy. The recurrence rate after breast-conserving surgery and radiation for T3 tumors after a partial response to induction has been reported to be 4–20%. The ultimate rates of breast recurrence at 10 years or more after radiation for breast conservation in this setting are unknown. The optimal patient selection and surgical and radiation techniques are also uncertain. At the present time, breast conservation in operable locally advanced disease remains investigational.

Inoperable locally advanced breast cancer includes tumors that present with ulceration of the skin, edema, satellite skin nodules, or chest wall fixation (T4) and/or unresectable positive axillary nodes (N2). Internal mammary node disease (N3) is also considered in this category although it is rarely diagnosed at presentation. Induction chemotherapy is the standard management for inoperable patients and will be successful in rendering most tumors resectable. The response of inoperable tumors to induction chemotherapy is prognostic for subsequent disease-free and overall survival. Second-line chemotherapy or preoperative radiation therapy may be used to increase the response rates and resectability after a less than complete response to induction chemotherapy.

After induction systemic therapy, patients with initially inoperable disease are treated with modified radical mastectomy and postmastectomy radiation. In patients with a complete clinical response to chemotherapy who are to receive chest wall irradiation, a more radical resection of the prechemotherapy volume of involved skin and chest wall may not be necessary. Adjuvant systemic therapy may be considered before radiation if less than a pathologic complete response was achieved with the neoadjuvant regimen. This combined modality approach is associated with local-regional control rates of 80–95%. Breast conservation should not be considered in patients with inoperable locally advanced disease. Radiation alone after induction chemotherapy is associated with local-regional recurrence rates of 30–40%. Even after a rare complete clinical and pathologic response to induction chemotherapy, breast irradiation is associated with failure rates of 20–30% or more with initially inoperable disease. Although mastectomy in these patients may not significantly improve survival, it will enhance local-regional control as opposed to radiation alone.

Inflammatory carcinomas (T4d) present with clinical findings of erythema greater than one-third of the breast, increased warmth, skin edema, and induration. Dermal lymphatic invasion is a pathologic hallmark of inflammatory disease but is not required for the diagnosis in the presence of clinical findings. The diagnosis should not be based on secondary inflammatory changes immediately associated with neglected locally advanced tumors or dermal lymphatic invasion alone. Regardless of their apparent resectability, inflammatory breast cancers should be considered inoperable at time of presentation. These patients will have a high incidence of local-regional recurrence and rapid interval to failure after initial attempts at surgery alone.

Neoadjuvant systemic therapy (chemotherapy with or without tamoxifen), modified radical mastectomy, and radiation are all important elements of the treatment of inflammatory breast cancer treatment. The response rates to induction doxorubicin-based chemotherapy range from 50 to 90%, with complete clinical responses in as many as 50% or more. Most patients with a complete clinical response to induction chemotherapy will have microscopic residual disease at subsequent surgery. Sequential administration of second-line chemotherapy or local-regional radiation should be employed prior to surgery for those not initially achieving a complete clinical response. The degree of response to neoadjuvant chemotherapy, particularly the subsequent finding of a pathologic complete response, is prognostic for locoregional control and survival for inflammatory breast cancers. The 5-year survival after combined modality therapy is generally 40–50% for inflammatory tumors. For those obtaining a complete response to induction chemotherapy, 5-year disease-free survivals of over 60% have been reported. The local-regional control rates for inflammatory breast cancers treated by mastectomy in addition to radiation and chemotherapy are 85% or more. Breast conservation should not be considered in patients with inflammatory breast cancer. The rate of locoregional failure after induction chemotherapy and radiation without mastectomy is over 30–40%. Even in the setting of a complete clinical response and negative repeat biopsy after neoadjuvant chemotherapy, the breast recurrence rates are over 20–40% for inflammatory disease.

Postmastectomy radiation is indicated in all patients with nonmetastatic inoperable locally advanced or inflammatory breast cancer to the chest wall and supraclavicular regions. The sequential delivery of radiation after chemotherapy and mastectomy is preferable. This is due to concerns of significant toxicity with concurrent radiation and chemotherapy, the need for dose reductions or avoidance of doxorubicin with previous or concurrent radiation, and the increase in perioperative morbidity after chemoradiation. Axillary irradiation may be considered in the preoperative setting to improve resectability of nodes that remain fixed after chemotherapy. Otherwise, axillary irradiation is not necessary after an adequate axillary lymph node dissection. Internal mammary irradiation is indicated only for patients with biopsy-proven internal mammary metastases to improve their local-regional control.

8. COMPLICATIONS OF RADIATION THERAPY

The potential complications following radiation either as part of breast-conserving surgery or mastectomy include arm edema, symptomatic pneumonitis, rib fracture, radiation-related heart disease, brachial plexopathy, soft tissue or bone necrosis, and second malignancy.

The incidence of lymphedema ranges from 2 to 37% and is related to the extent of the axillary surgery and the regions treated with radiation. In patients undergoing an axillary dissection who did not receive radiation to the axilla, the incidence of arm edema is approximately 10%. The addition of radiation to the axilla and supraclavicular regions increases this incidence to 15–30%. Radiation to the axilla in the absence of an axillary dissection is associated with a less than 5% incidence of lymphedema.

Symptomatic pneumonitis is characterized by a clinical syndrome of dry cough, dyspnea, and low-grade fever developing within 6–12 weeks after radiation. The overall incidence is 5% or less. The incidence of symptomatic pneumonitis is increased by the use of regional node irradiation as well as concurrent chemotherapy and in these patients may be as high as 9%.

Cardiac morbidity related to radiation includes the development of coronary artery disease and ischemic heart disease. The initial trials of postmastectomy radiation demonstrated an increased cardiac mortality in patients with left-sided tumors who received orthovoltage or cobalt 60 radiation to the regional nodes and were older than 50–60 years. Improvements in radiation technique have decreased the long-term cardiac morbidity. The combination of radiation to the left breast or chest wall as well as doxorubicin-based regimens may also result in increased cardiac morbidity.

Brachial plexopathy is an uncommon event and is characterized by pain in the ipsilateral shoulder and arm, paresthesias, and subsequent weakness. The incidence of brachial plexopathy is less than 1%. It is increased by the use of regional node radiation with doses of more than 5000 cGy and the use of adjuvant chemotherapy.

Rib fractures occur in less than 5% of patients receiving radiation, and the incidence is related to total radiation dose, the use of adjuvant chemotherapy, and the type of radiation.

Second malignancies following radiation for breast cancer include contralateral breast cancer, second nonbreast cancer malignancies, and bone or soft tissue sarcomas. Four of the prospective randomized trials comparing conservative surgery and radiation with mastectomy and two prospective randomized trials evaluating postmastectomy radiation have demonstrated no increased incidence of contralateral breast cancer or second nonbreast cancer malignancy in patients who received radiation. Several case-control studies, however, have reported an elevated risk of contralateral breast cancer in patients receiving radiation. This risk has been primarily seen in women younger than 45 years. The cumulative incidence of a radiation-induced sarcoma, in either the breast or soft tissues, has been estimated to be 0.2% at 10 years, i.e., an extremely small risk. The median interval to a radiation-induced sarcoma is approximately 10 years, with the most frequent site being in the treated breast or chest wall and the most common histology being angiosarcoma, fibrosarcoma, or malignant fibrous histiocytoma. Several recent studies have reported an increased risk of lung cancer in smokers who received radiation as part of their breast cancer treatment. Therefore, these patients should be advised to cease smoking.

9. LOCAL REGIONAL RECURRENCE FOLLOWING MASTECTOMY

Approximately 10–15% of patients who undergo a modified radical mastectomy for stage I–II breast cancer will experience a local-regional recurrence defined as recurrent disease in either the chest wall, axilla, supraclavicular nodes, or internal mammary nodes. The most frequent site of failure is the chest wall, followed by the supraclavicular region. As previously stated, clinical internal mammary node recurrences are uncommon. The term "isolated local-regional recurrence" implies recurrent disease in the absence of distant metastasis. Treatment of an isolated local-regional recurrence following mastectomy involves surgical excision when possible with the goal of achieving complete gross and microscopic excision of the recurrent disease. The use of an excisional biopsy prior to radiation results in improved local control rates and also diminishes the dose of radiation required. Despite surgical resection and radiation, approximately 50% of these patients will subsequently experience further disease in the chest wall or regional nodes. The long-term control rates are higher, i.e., in the range of 70% for patients who present with an isolated chest wall recurrence that is completely excised, is estrogen receptor-positive, and has been associated with a long disease-free interval from initial treatment, i.e., more than 2 years. Radiation has been employed for patients who present with unresectable isolated local-regional recurrences, and long-term control is in the range of 30–50%.

For patients experiencing an isolated chest wall recurrence, radiation is directed to the chest wall and supraclavicular region. For those experiencing a recurrence in the supraclavicular region, radiation is directed to this area as well as the chest wall. For patients experiencing either an isolated axillary or internal mammary node recurrence, radiation may be restricted to this regional site and may also include the chest wall and supraclavicular region. The dose to the area of recurrent disease is generally in the range of 6000–6600 cGy and that to prophylactic regions is 4600–5000 cGy delivered over a period of $4^1/_2$–7 weeks.

10. RADIATION FOR THE PALLIATION OF METASTATIC BREAST CANCER

Radiotherapy has an important role in the palliation of distant metastases from breast cancer. Brain and bone metastases are clinically the most commonly involved sites that require radiation. Spinal cord compression is a special consequence of bony metastases to the spine and is an indication for immediate radiotherapy. Radiation may also be used in the palliation of metastases to the lung, lymph nodes, choroid of the eye, or skin.

Indications for palliative radiotherapy for bony metastases are pain, decreased function, risk of pathologic fracture, consolidation after surgical stabilization, or soft tissue extension causing nerve compression. Over 80–90% of patients treated with 30 Gy in 10 fractions or 20 Gy in 5 fractions will have a response to radiotherapy. For the debilitated patient with a peripheral bony lesion, 8 Gy in a single fraction may be adequate for short-term palliation. Most patients will require analgesic or steroid medication for immediate palliation, but this can often be reduced as tolerated after radiation. Patients with metastases of weight-bearing bones, particularly the proximal femur, may benefit from surgical stabilization prior to radiotherapy. Significant pain or degree of cortical erosion are common but not reliable signs predicting the risk of fracture. Radiation alone may improve pain, but not decrease the risk of fracture, in these patients.

Presenting symptoms of spinal cord compression from bony metastases include back pain, leg weakness, sensory loss or paresthesias, and loss of bladder and bowel function. Radiation, high-dose steroids, and bed rest with spinal precautions should begin emergently once the diagnosis is made, to stabilize the patient and prevent further neurologic compromise. The duration of neurologic deficits at presentation and their response to steroids are prognositc for the response to radiation. Neurosurgical intervention may be indicated in selected patients with compression owing to retropulsed bone fragments, history of prior irradiation, spinal instability, or tumors not responding to radiation.

Radiotherapy is indicated for palliation of brain metastases from breast cancer. The primary goal of treatment is reduction in size of the metastases, resulting in stabilization or reversal of the patient's neurologic symptoms. Secondary goals include prevention of seizures or steroid dependency and reduction in risk of immediate death from the brain metastases. Approximately 80% of patients treated with 30 Gy in 10 fractions or 20 Gy in 5 fractions will have a response to whole brain radiation. The median survival following treatment is 6 months. The prognostic factors include the extent of extracranial disease, age, performance status, and number of brain metastases. Selected patients with solitary brain metastases may benefit from an aggressive approach with surgical resection followed by whole brain radiation. Stereotactic radiosurgery is presently under investigation for the treatment of brain metastases and may prove to be an alternative to surgery for selected patients.

11. CONCLUSIONS

The indications for radiation in the treatment of breast cancer are outlined in Table 1. Current areas of research include the identification of patients with DCIS or early-stage invasive breast cancer for whom radiation may not be a necessary component of breast conservation therapy. In addition, postmastectomy radiation in patients with stage I–II disease receiving contemporary chemotherapy regimens requires further investigation. Radiation will continue to be an important component of the treatment of stage III disease. The increasing use of biphosphonates in the treatment of bone metastases may diminish the need for palliative radiation.

BIBLIOGRAPHY

Arriagada R, Le MG, Rochard F, Contesso G, for the Institut Gustave-Roussy Breast Cancer Group (1996) Conservative treatment versus mastectomy in early breast cancer: patterns of failure with 15 years of follow-up data. *J. Clin. Oncol.* **14,** 1558–1564.

Blichert-Toft M, Rose C, Andersen JA, et al. (1992) Danish randomized trial comparing breast conservation therapy with mastectomy: six years of life-table analysis, Danish Breast Cancer Cooperative Group. *Monogr. Natl. Cancer Inst.* **11,** 19–25.

Bartelink H, Horiot JC, Poortmans P, et al. (2001) Recurrence rates after treatment of breast cancer with standard radiotherapy with or without additional radiation. *N. Engl. J. Med.* **345,** 1378–1387.

Bijker N, Peterse JL, Duchateau L, et al. (2001) Risk factors for recurrence and metastasis after breast-conserving therapy for ductal carcinoma-in-situ: Analysis of European Organization for Research and Treatment of Cancer Trial 10853. *J. Clin. Oncol.* **19,** 2263–2271.

Bonadonna G, Valagussa P, Brambilla C, et al. (1998) Primary chemotherapy in operable breast cancer: eight-year experience at the Milan Cancer Institute. *J. Clin. Oncol.* **16,** 93–100.

Clark RM, Whelan T, Levine M, et al. (1996) Randomized clinical trial of breast irradiation following lumpectomy and axillary dissection for node-negative breast cancer: an update. *J. Natl. Cancer Inst.* **88,** 1659–1664.

Coia LR, Aaronson N, Linggood R, et al. (1996) A report of the consensus workshop panel on the treatment of brain metastases. *Int. J. Radiat. Oncol. Biol. Phys.* **23,** 223–227.

Danforth Jr DN, Zujewski J, O'Shaughnessy J, et al. (1998) Selection of local therapy after neoadjuvant chemotherapy in patients with stage IIIA,B breast cancer. *Ann. Surg. Oncol.* **5,** 150–158.

Early Breast Cancer Trialists' Collaborative Group (2000) Favorable and unfavorable effects on long-term survival of radiotherapy of early breast cancer: an overview of the randomised trials. *Lancet* **335,** 1757–1770.

Fisher B, Dignam J, Wolmark N, et al. (1999) Tamoxifen in treatment of intraductal breast cancer: National Surgical Adjuvant Breast and Bowel Project B-24 randomised controlled trial. *Lancet* **353,** 1993–2000.

Fisher B, Anderson S, Redmond CK, Wolmark N, Wickerham DL, Cronin WM (1995a) Reanalysis and results after 12 years of follow-up in a randomized clinical trial comparing total mastectomy with lumpectomy with or without irradiation in the treatment of breast cancer. *N. Engl. J. Med.* **333,** 1456–1461.

Fisher B, Dignam J, Wolmark N, et al. (1998) Lumpectomy and radiation therapy for the treatment of intraductal breast cancer: Findings from the National Surgical Adjuvant Breast and Bowel Project B-17. *J. Clin. Oncol.* **16,** 441–452.

Fisher ER, Costantino J, Fisher B, Palekar AS, Redmond C, Mamounas E (1995b) Pathologic findings from the National Surgical Adjuvant Breast Project (NSABP) protocol B-17. Intraductal carcinoma (ductal carcinoma in situ). *Cancer* **75,** 1310–1319.

Fleming RYD, Asmar L, Buzdar AU, et al. (1997) Effectiveness of mastectomy by response to induction chemotherapy for control in inflammatory breast carcinoma. *Ann. Surg. Oncol.* **4,** 452–461.

Forrest AP, Stewart HJ, Everington D, on behalf of Scottish Cancer Trials Breast Group (1996) Randomized controlled trial of conservation therapy for breast cancer: 6 year analysis of the Scottish trial. *Lancet* **348,** 708–713.

Fowble B (1997) Postmastectomy radiation: then and now. *Oncology* **11,** 213–239.

Fowble B, Glover D (1991) Locally advanced breast cancer. In: Fowble B, Goodman RL, Glick JH, Rosato EF (eds.) *Breast Cancer Treatment. A Comprehensive Guide to Management.* Mosby-Year Book, St. Louis, MO, pp. 345–372.

Fowble B, Gray R, Gilchrist K, et al. (1988) Identification of a subgroup of patients with breast cancer and histo-logically positive axillary nodes receiving adjuvant chemotherapy who may benefit from postoperative radio-therapy. *J. Clin. Oncol.* **6,** 1107–1117.

Fowble B, Hanlon AL, Fein DA, et al. (1997) Results of conservative surgery and radiation for mammographi-cally detected ductal carcinoma in situ (DCIS). *Int. J. Radiat. Oncol. Biol. Phys.* **38,** 949–957.

Freedman GM, Fowble BL, Hanlon AL, et al. (1997) Postmastectomy radiation and adjuvant systemic therapy: outcomes in high-risk women with stage II–III breast cancer and assessment of clinical, pathologic, and treat-ment-related factors influencing local-regional control. *Breast J.* **3,** 337–344.

Gaspar L, Scott C, Rotman M, et al. (1997) Recursive partitioning analysis (RPA) of prognostic factors in three Radiation Therapy Oncology Group (RTOG) brain metastases trials. *Int. J. Radiat. Oncol. Biol. Phys.* **37,** 745–751.

Hughes KS, Schnaper L, Berry D, et al. (2001) Comparison of lumpectomy plus tamoxifen with or without radio-therapy in women 70 years of age or older who have clinical stage I, estrogen receptor positive breast carci-noma. *Proc. Am. Soc. Clin. Oncol.* **20,** 24a (abst.).

Jacobson JA, Danforth DN, Cowan KH, et al. (1995) Ten year results of a comparison of conservation with mas-tectomy in the treatment of stage I and II breast cancer. *N. Engl. J. Med.* **332,** 907–911.

Liljegren G, Holmberg L, Bergh J, et al. (1999) 10-Year results after sector resection with or without postopera-tive radiotherapy for stage I breast cancer: A randomized trial. *J. Clin. Oncol.* **17,** 2326–2333.

Loblaw DA, and Laperriere NJ (1998) Emergency treatment of malignant extradural spinal cord compression: an evidence-based guideline. *J. Clin. Oncol.* **16,** 1613–1624.

National Comprehensive Cancer Network (1999) Practice guidelines for the treatment of breast cancer. *Oncology* **13,** 41–66.

Overgaard M, Hansen PS, Overgaard J, et al. (1997) Postoperative radiotherapy in high-risk premenopausal women with breast cancer who receive adjuvant chemotherapy. *N. Engl. J. Med.* **337,** 949–955.

Perez CA, Fields JN, Fracasso PM, et al. (1994) Management of locally advanced carcinoma of the breast. II. Inflammatory carcinoma. *Cancer* **74,** 466–476.

Ragaz J, Jackson S, Le M, et al. (1999) Postmastectomy radiation outcome in node positive breast cancer patients among N1–3 versus N4 and subset: impact of extracapsular spread. Update of the British Columbia random-ized trial. *Proc. Am. Soc. Clin. Oncol.* **18,** 73a.

Ragaz J, Jackson SM, Nhu L, et al. (1997) Adjuvant radiotherapy and chemotherapy in node-positive pre-menopausal women with breast cancer. *N. Engl. J. Med.* **337,** 956–962.

Recht A, Bartelink H, Fourquet A, et al. (1998) Postmastectomy radiotherapy: questions for the twenty-first cen-tury. *J. Clin. Oncol.* **16,** 2886–2889.

Recht A, Come SE, Henderson IC, et al. (1996) The sequencing of chemotherapy and radiation therapy after con-servative surgery for early-stage breast cancer. *N. Engl. J. Med.* **334,** 1356–1361.

Renton SC, Gazet J-C, Ford HT, Corbishley C, Sutcliffe R (1996) The importance of the resection margin in con-servative surgery for breast cancer. *Eur. J. Surg. Oncol.* **22,** 17–22.

Romestaing P, Lehingue Y, Carrie C, et al. (1997) Role of a 10-Gy boost in the conservative treatment of early breast cancer: Results of a randomized clinical trial in Lyon, France. *J. Clin. Oncol.* **15,** 963–968.

Rutqvist LE, Cedermark B, Glas U, et al. (1990) Randomized trial of adjuvant tamoxifen combined with post-operative radiotherapy or adjuvant chemotherapy in postmenopausal breast cancer. *Cancer* **66,** 89–96.

Silverstein MJ (1997) *Ductal Carcinoma In Situ of the Breast.* Williams & Wilkins, Baltimore.

Solin LJ, Kurtz J, Fourquet A, et al. (1996a) Fifteen year results of breast conserving surgery and definitive breast irradiation for the treatment of ductal carcinoma in situ (intraductal carcinoma of the breast). *J. Clin. Oncol.* **14,** 754–763.

Solin LJ, Fourquet A, Vicini FA, et al. (2001) Mammographically detected ductal carcinoma in situ of the breast treated with breast-conserving surgery and definitive breast irradiation: long-term outcome and prognostic sig-nificance of patient age and margin status. *Int. J. Radia. Oncol. Biol. Phys.* **50,** 991–2001.

Tennrall-Nittby L, Tengrup J, Landberg T (1993) The total incidence of loco-regional recurrence in a randomized trial of breast cancer TNM stage II. The South Sweden Breast Cancer Trial. *Acta Oncol.* **32,** 641–646.

Tong D, Gillick L, Hendrickson FR (1982) The palliation of symptomatic osseous metastases. Final results of the study by the Radiation Therapy Oncology Group. *Cancer* **50,** 893–899.

Valagussa P, Zambetti M, Bonadonna G, et al. (1990) Prognostic factors in locally advanced noninflammatory breast cancer. Long term results following primary chemotherapy. *Breast Cancer Res. Treat.* **15,** 137–147.

van Dongen JA, Voogd AD, Fentiman IS, et al. (2000) Long-term results of a randomized trial comparing breast-conserving therapy with mastectomy: European Organization for Research and Treatment of Cancer 10801 trial. *J. Natl. Cancer Inst.* **92,** 1143–1150.

Veronesi U, Marubini E, Mariani L, et al. (2001) Radiotherapy after breast-conserving surgery in small breast car-cinoma: Long-term results of a randomized trial. *Ann Oncol.* **12,** 997–1003.

Veronesi U, Salvadori B, Luini A, et al. (1995) Breast conservation is a safe method in patients with small cancer of the breast. Long-term results of three randomized trials on 1973 patients. *Eur. J. Cancer* **31A,** 1574–1579.

Winchester DP, JD C (1998) Standards for diagnosis and management of invasive breast carcinoma. *CA Cancer J. Clin.* **48,** 83–107.

Winchester DP, Strom EA (1998) Standards for diagnosis and management of ductal carcinoma in situ (DCIS) of the breast. *CA Cancer J. Clin.* **48,** 108–128.

Wolmark N, Dignam J, Fisher B (1998) The addition of tamoxifen to lumpectomy and radiotherapy in the treatment of ductal carcinoma in situ (DCIS): preliminary results of NSABP Protocol B-24. *Breast Cancer Res. Treat.* **50,** 227.

9   Chemotherapy in Breast Cancer

Michael P. Russin, MD, and Lori J. Goldstein, MD

CONTENTS

INTRODUCTION
ADJUVANT CHEMOTHERAPY
TREATMENT OF METASTATIC DISEASE
TOXICITY OF CHEMOTHERAPY
CONCLUSIONS
REFERENCES

1. INTRODUCTION

At the time of diagnosis, breast cancer is generally thought of as a systemic disease. For many years, chemotherapy has been considered one of the cornerstones of treatment and has evolved over the past 20 years. Chemotherapy has shown benefit in both early and advanced disease. The decision of when to administer cytotoxic therapy and which agents to utilize is often a complex and challenging dilemma for clinicians and their patients.

2. ADJUVANT CHEMOTHERAPY

Adjuvant systemic therapy for breast cancer is defined as the administration of chemotherapy or other potentially cytotoxic agents after primary surgery has been performed. In this situation, all clinically evident cancer has been removed. The goal of systemic therapy in this setting is to eliminate any potential microscopic foci of disease that may remain. The clinician must determine, therefore, which patients are at significant risk for occult disease and weigh this against the risks of chemotherapy. In general, adjuvant therapy is recommended for any woman with a greater than 10% chance of relapse at 10 years.

2.1. Node-Positive Disease

The single most important factor predicting risk of future relapse is the presence of axillary nodal metastases and the number of involved axillary nodes. The greater the number of involved nodes, the greater the risk of recurrence. In addition to axillary nodal disease, tumors that do not express hormonal receptors have a worse prognosis. The use of adjuvant chemotherapy has been standard in this group for almost 20 years. In general, agents that have shown a high degree of activity in advanced disease are then evaluated in randomized clinical trials and incorporated into the standard of care in the adjuvant setting.

From: *Current Clinical Oncology:*
Breast Cancer: A Guide to Detection and Multidisciplinary Therapy
Edited by: M. H. Torosian © Humana Press Inc., Totowa, NJ

Several large randomized trials utilizing both single- and multiagent regimens have been performed in patients with axillary nodal disease and hormone receptor-negative tumors. At the time of original publication, these trials demonstrated improvement in disease-free survival only *(1)*. The largest benefit was seen in women with four or more positive lymph nodes *(2)*. Every 5 years, the Early Breast Cancer Trialists' Collaborative Group (EBCTCG) publishes a comprehensive metaanalysis of all trials involving chemotherapy in early breast cancer. Subsequent analysis by the EBCTCG of these trials and many like them has substantiated the notion that adjuvant chemotherapy improves disease-free survival and reduces mortality *(3)*.

Further trials were carried out in women previously thought not to benefit from cytotoxic therapy, specifically postmenopausal women with estrogen receptor (ER)-positive tumors. These women were considered at high risk for relapse but were previously offered only adjuvant hormonal manipulation. In a large randomized clinical trial, patients older than 50 years with node-positive, ER-positive breast cancer were randomized to receive either adjuvant tamoxifen or adjuvant polychemotherapy plus tamoxifen *(4)*. This study showed a benefit in disease-free survival, but overall survival did not reach statistical significance in favor of chemotherapy at 3 years of follow-up. Longer follow-up has shown an improvement in overall survival for the chemotherapy plus tamoxifen group when compared with the tamoxifen alone group *(3)*.

In general, polychemotherapy in women with node-positive disease results in an absolute improvement in survival at 10-year follow-up of approximately 11% for women younger than 50 years and 3.3% for women aged 50–69 years. These results are slightly smaller for patients with ER-positive tumors. Considering the large number of women diagnosed with breast cancer each year, small improvements in overall survival translate into a significant number of lives saved. Most studies have few patients over the age of 70 years and, therefore, the exact benefit of chemotherapy in this group is difficult to assess *(3)*. Regardless of age, state of the art treatment recommendations should be given. The current recommendations for adjuvant treatment of node-positive patients are shown in Table 1.

2.2. Node-Negative Disease

Although most women with node-negative breast cancer are cured by local therapy alone, a significant number of patients have recurrence, and some ultimately succumb to disease. As with node-positive disease, women with ER-negative tumors were chosen for the early trials. These women were considered to be at the greatest risk of recurrence. Three large randomized trials of adjuvant polychemotherapy versus observation for women with ER-negative, node-negative breast cancer were simultaneously published and dramatically changed clinical practice. Each of these trials demonstrated improvement in disease-free survival for this subgroup of patients and led the way to further trials involving node-negative patients *(5–7)*. As with node-positive disease, longer follow-up showed a survival advantage with the administration of adjuvant chemotherapy in these patients *(3)*.

Patients with node-negative, ER-positive early breast cancer were also studied. The National Surgical Adjuvant Breast and Bowel Project (NSABP) B-14 demonstrated the benefit of tamoxifen alone over placebo in ER-positive, node-negative patients *(8)*. In a large subsequent trial, patients similar to those in the NSABP B-14 were randomized to adjuvant tamoxifen versus adjuvant polychemotherapy and tamoxifen. This study demonstrated a benefit in both disease-free and overall survival in favor of the combined chemotherapy and tamoxifen group over tamoxifen alone for both pre- and postmenopausal women *(9)*.

Table 1
Guidelines for Adjuvant Treatment
of Node-Positive Breast Cancer

Patient group	Treatment
Premenopausal	
ER or PR positive	Chemotherapy + tamoxifen
ER and PR negative	Chemotherapy
Postmenopausal	
ER or PR positive	Tamoxifen + chemotherapy
ER and PR negative	Chemotherapy
Elderly	
ER or PR positive	Tamoxifen ± chemotherapy
ER and PR negative	Consider chemotherapy

ER, estrogen receptor; PR, progesterone receptor.

Adapted from ref. *40.*

When considering all patients with early-stage breast cancer, polychemotherapy results in an absolute improvement in survival at 10-year follow-up of approximately 7% for women younger than 50 years and 2% for women aged 50–69 years. Patients with ER-positive tumors gain a slightly smaller benefit than those with ER-negative tumors, but the improvement is still significant. Most studies have few patients over the age of 70 years and, again, the exact benefit of chemotherapy in this group in difficult to assess *(3).*

Although chemotherapy has shown benefit to all subgroups under the age of 70 years, a significant number of women (particularly node-negative patients) are cured by local therapy alone. If adjuvant chemotherapy was arbitrarily given to all patients, a large number of women would be exposed unnecessarily to the potential toxicities of chemotherapy. In women with a lower risk of relapse, prognostic factors related to the patient or tumor often help the physician and patient determine the risk/benefit ratio of adjuvant chemotherapy for that individual. These prognostic factors include size of the primary tumor, hormonal receptor status, nuclear grade, histologic grade, presence of angiolymphatic invasion, percent cells in S-phase, ploidy status, and Her-2/neu overexpression. Trials continue to investigate which factors are clinically relevant and which women may not require adjuvant treatment *(10).* In 1998, the International Consensus Panel on the Treatment of Primary Breast Cancer devised a risk stratification system for node-negative patients based on age, hormonal receptor status, tumor size, and histologic and/or nuclear grade (Table 2). This stratification has led to the recommendations for adjuvant therapy shown in Table 3.

2.3. Standard Adjuvant Regimens

Once the decision to administer adjuvant chemotherapy has been made, the regimen and duration of treatment must be determined. A multitude of regimens and treatment durations have been studied. Bonadonna and colleagues *(2,11)* originally showed the benefit of 12 months of cyclophosphamide, methotrexate, and 5-fluorouracil (CMF), but a subsequent trial demonstrated that 6 months of therapy was equally effective. More recently, four cycles of doxorubicin/cyclophosphamide (AC) was found to be at least as effective as six cycles of CMF and resulted in a shorter total treatment time *(12).*

Table 2
Risk Stratification for Node-Negative Breast Cancer

Factor	Minimal/low risk (has all listed factors)	Intermediate risk (risk classified between the other two categories)	High risk (has at least one listed factor)
Tumor size	≤1 cm	>1–2 cm	>2 cm
ER and/or PR status	Positive	Positive	Negative
Grade	Grade 1	Grade 1–2	Grade 2–3
Age (yr)	≥35		<35

ER, estrogen receptor; PR, progesterone receptor.

Adapted from ref 40.

Table 3
Guidelines for Adjuvant Treatment of Node-Negative Breast Cancer

Patient group	Minimal/low risk	Intermediate risk	High risk
Premenopausal			
ER or PR positive	None or tamoxifen	Tamoxifen ± chemotherapy	Chemotherapy + tamoxifen
ER and PR negative	Not applicable	Not applicable	Chemotherapy
Postmenopausal			
ER or PR positive	None or tamoxifen	Tamoxifen ± chemotherapy	Tamoxifen + chemotherapy
ER and PR negative	Not applicable	Not applicable	Chemotherapy
Elderly			
ER or PR positive	None or tamoxifen	Tamoxifen	Tamoxifen
ER and PR negative	Not applicable	Not applicable	Consider chemotherapy

ER, estrogen receptor; PR, progesterone receptor.

Adapted from ref. 40.

In general, four to six cycles of chemotherapy is considered the standard duration for adjuvant therapy. However, since taxanes have shown significant activity in the metastatic setting, interest has grown for their use in the adjuvant setting. Preliminary data suggest that the addition of paclitaxel alone for four cycles after standard AC provides benefit to high-risk, node-positive patients (13). Ongoing clinical trials are attempting to define the role of taxanes in the treatment of early-stage breast cancer.

Several recent trials have suggested that anthracycline-based regimens may offer improved outcomes compared with CMF, although they are associated with slightly more toxicity (14,15). Although these results favor increased administration of anthracyclines in the adjuvant setting, many patients are medically unable to receive these drugs or do not find their toxicity profile acceptable. In these cases, CMF is still a reasonably effective regimen. Women should also be encouraged to enroll in clinical trials investigating new therapeutic approaches or optimizing current regimens. The most common clinically relevant adjuvant regimens are shown in Table 4.

Table 4

Adjuvant Chemotherapy Regimens for Early-Stage Breast Cancer

Drugs	Regimen
CMF	
Cyclophosphamide	100 mg/m^2 po on days 1–14
Methotrexate	40 mg/m^2 iv on days 1 and 8
5-Fluorouracil	600 mg/m^2 iv on days 1 and 8
Repeat every 28 days, for 6 cycles	
AC	
Doxorubicin	60 mg/m^2 iv on day 1
Cyclophosphamide	600 mg/m^2 iv on day 1
Repeat every 21 days, for 4 cycles	
CAF	
Cyclophosphamide	100 mg/m^2 po on days 1–14
Doxorubicin	30 mg/m^2 iv on days 1 and 8
5-FU	500 mg/m^2 iv on days 1 and 8
Repeat every 28 days, for 6 cycles	
AC + paclitaxel	
Doxorubicin	60 mg/m^2 iv on day 1
Cyclophosphamide	600 mg/m^2 iv on day 1
Repeat every 21 days, for 4 cycles, followed by:	
Paclitaxel	175 mg/m^2 iv over 3 hr on day 1
Repeat every 21 days, for 4 cycles	
CEF	
Cyclophosphamide	75 mg/m^2 po on days 1–14
Epirubicin	60 mg/m^2 iv on days 1 and 8
5-Fluorouracil	500 mg/m^2 iv on days 1 and 8
Repeat every 28 days, for 6 cycles	

2.4. Dose Intensity

Despite improvements in survival through the use of adjuvant chemotherapy, a significant number of women relapse after primary therapy. Evidence exists that adjuvant chemotherapy, given at doses less than standard, results in suboptimal outcomes (16). These data suggest a dose-response relationship in the treatment of early breast cancer. Studies testing the intensification of current standard cytotoxics (cyclophosphamide and doxorubicin) utilizing doses that are non-myeloablative have not proved that such doses increase disease-free or overall survival and have shown greater treatment-related toxicity (13,17).

Recently, results from several randomized trials evaluating the role of adjuvant high-dose chemotherapy with peripheral blood stem cell support/autologous bone marrow transplant in patients with 10 or more positive lymph nodes have been reported. Although these results are still quite preliminary, they suggest that myeloablative doses of chemotherapy should not be utilized outside the setting of a clinical trial for the treatment of high-risk early-stage breast cancer (18–20). Current adjuvant trials are exploring dose density, chemotherapy scheduling, and the role of novel new agents. All eligible patients should be offered participation in clinical trials in order to improve survival for patients with early-stage breast cancer.

2.5. Clinical Monitoring

Once a woman has completed adjuvant therapy, close follow-up is necessary. The exact schedule of evaluation has evolved over many years. Posttreatment intensive monitoring of

Table 5
Most Active Cytotoxic Agents for Metastatic
Breast Cancer (>50% response rate)

| Taxanes |
| Anthracyclines |

blood work and radiographic studies in asymptomatic patients have not impacted on overall survival. The National Comprehensive Cancer Network (NCCN) recommends the following schedule for physical examinations: monthly patient self-examinations and physician examinations every 4 months for 2 years and then every 6 months for the next 3 years, followed by yearly exams thereafter. In terms of studies, mammograms are recommended yearly. Otherwise, further evaluation and testing should be symptom-directed *(21)*.

3. TREATMENT OF METASTATIC DISEASE

Once clinically evident systemic disease develops, breast cancer, unfortunately, is no longer curable. The median survival for advanced disease is approximately 3 years. In this setting, the goals of therapy become quite different from those of adjuvant treatment. Chemotherapy is used to alleviate symptoms, improve quality of life, and (hopefully) prolong survival. In general, chemotherapy is recommended as initial therapy for patients with ER/PR-negative tumors or symptomatic visceral disease. Patients with ER/PR-positive tumors who have failed hormonal therapy or who have extremely symptomatic visceral disease should also be considered for cytotoxic therapy.

The 1990s have witnessed the introduction of several new agents with activity in advanced breast cancer. In the past, the most active drugs in this disease were the anthracyclines. Taxanes have now demonstrated activity comparable to that of the anthracyclines. The current agents with greater than 50% activity are shown in Table 5. In addition, many drugs have shown 20–50% response rates as single agents (Table 6). The combination regimens used in adjuvant therapy are also very effective in metastatic disease (Table 1).

The clinician must address several issues in determining the proper treatment for each patient: 1) combination versus single-agent therapy; 2) dose intensity; 3) schedule of drug administration; 4) agents to be used as first-line versus second-line therapy; and 5) duration of treatment.

3.1. Combination versus Single-Agent Therapy

Polychemotherapy is effective in the treatment of metastatic breast cancer. The regimens used in the adjuvant setting were originally evaluated in advanced disease. The issues of toxicity and impact on quality of life from these regimens are very important considerations in a situation in which palliation of symptoms is the primary aim. Combination chemotherapy does result in improved response rates and time to progression. These advantages, however, do not translate to improved overall survival when compared with sequential single-agent therapy *(22)*. Multidrug regimens also tend to have more treatment-related toxicity. Combination chemotherapy is best utilized when a rapid disease response is required, i.e., for patients with symptomatic visceral metastases. In most situations, however, sequential single-agent therapy is very effective and is associated with less toxicity.

Table 6
Moderately Active Agents for Metastatic
Breast Cancer (20–50% response rate)

Capecitabine
Cisplatin
Cyclophosphamide
5-Fluorouracil
Methotrexate
Mitomycin-C
Mitoxantrone
Thiotepa
Vinblastine
Vincristine
Vinorelbine

3.2. Dose Intensity

As in adjuvant therapy, the issues of dose response and dose intensity of chemotherapy are areas of great interest. Increasing the dose of paclitaxel as a single agent has failed to demonstrate an improvement in response rates or overall survival. The higher doses of paclitaxel may increase time to disease progression. This benefit is, however, at the cost of increased treatment-related toxicity (23). The use of myeloablative levels of chemotherapy with peripheral blood stem cell support/autologous bone marrow transplant has also been studied in metastatic breast cancer. The results from several trials have recently been reported and are controversial. A large randomized trial was unable to demonstrate a difference in time to progression or overall survival between standard doses of chemotherapy and high-dose chemotherapy (24). Although these data are still preliminary, they suggest that consolidative high-dose chemotherapy after induction therapy will not be considered the standard of care for advanced breast cancer.

3.3. Schedule of Drug Administration

Recent data have indicated that varying the administration schedule of certain agents can alter their pharmacokinetics, tumor-killing activity, and toxicity profile. This is most notable of the taxanes. The optimal dosing schedule has yet to be determined. Paclitaxel was originally delivered on a 21-day cycle utilizing infusion durations of 3, 24, and 96 hours. Although 96-hour infusions of paclitaxel are more effective in metastatic breast cancer, the need for either inpatient administration or adequate home care services to administer the drug as an outpatient makes this schedule inconvenient and costly. Direct comparison of fixed doses of pacitaxel given every 21 days as either a 3-hour or 24-hour infusion has been carried out. These data suggest that the 24-hour infusion regimen produces higher response rates with no difference in event-free or overall survival. The 24-hour infusion was associated with increased toxicity and, as with the 96-hour infusion, the inconvenience of prolonged infusion (25). The shorter 3-hour infusions, therefore, have been adopted by most clinicians.

More recently, the concept of dose density has become popular. Under this paradigm, lower doses of chemotherapy are given more frequently to reach a higher total dose of drug per cycle. Weekly 1-hour infusions increase the exposure of the cell to drug and recapitulate a continuous infusion. Both paclitaxel and docetaxel have been given on a weekly schedule. These regimens have produced response rates that are at least comparable to those seen with every 3-week dosing and result in lower incidences of hematologic and neurologic toxicity *(26,27)*. The improved toxicity profile and apparent high level of activity make these regimens attractive alternatives to the standard every 3-week dosing schedule. Formal direct comparison between the two dosing schedules is currently being evaluated in a CALC+B study.

3.4. First-versus Second-Line Therapy

Anthracyclines, taxanes, and vinorelbine have all shown significant response rates as single agents in metastatic breast cancer. The choice of the initial therapeutic agent is often a difficult decision. Anthracyclines have been used most frequently in the past. Now that more women are receiving adjuvant therapy, an increasing number of patients will have received prior anthracycline treatment when they develop metastatic disease. The taxanes, as well as vinorelbine, have been quite effective in women who have previously received anthracyclines *(28–30)*.

Debate has occurred over initial use of an anthracycline versus a taxane in previously untreated women. Both drug classes have been found effective as first-line therapy *(31)*. The choice of the initial and subsequent treatment regimens should be based on the individuals' comorbid conditions and the toxicity profile of the chemotherapeutic agent. All patients with metastatic breast cancer should also be considered for enrollment in clinical trials exploring new therapeutic approaches or optimizing current therapies.

3.5. Duration of Treatment

The final decision in the treatment strategy of metastatic breast cancer is the length of therapy. Since advanced breast cancer is not currently curable, the goal of therapy is palliation of symptoms. Cytotoxic chemotherapy has the potential for significant toxicity; therefore, issues of quality of life must be balanced against response rates and potential survival benefit.

Intermittent versus continuous therapy has been studied in metastatic breast cancer. Under the intermittent treatment paradigm, a set course of induction chemotherapy is given. Once the predetermined number of treatments has been reached, therapy is stopped until disease progression is evident. At that time, a set number of cycles of chemotherapy is given again. The regimen chosen may be different from the original, or the same drug or drugs may be utilized if a marked response and a prolonged progression-free interval were obtained. Continuous therapy entails the administration of a chemotherapy regimen until disease progression is evident. A new regimen is then instituted without a significant break in therapy, except for reasons of toxicity. Continuous treatment with chemotherapy has been associated with significant prolongation of the time to progression compared with intermittent therapy. No difference in overall survival has been noted between the two strategies *(32)*. Continuous treatment has also been associated with improved quality of life compared with intermittent therapy *(33)*.

3.6. New Agents

The next step forward in the treatment of advanced breast cancer will probably be the use of biologically targeted therapy in conjunction with chemotherapy. The first major breakthrough in this area has been trastuzumab (Herceptin®), a humanized anti-Her-2 antibody. Trials have shown that trastuzumab, when given as a single agent, has significant activity against breast tumors that overexpress Her-2/neu *(34)*. When combined with chemotherapy, synergistic activity has been noted, confirming preclinical data. Trastuzumab has been evaluated in combination with doxorubicin/cyclophosphamide and also paclitaxel. When it was used with a doxorubicin-containing regimen, an unacceptable incidence of cardiac toxicity was noted, and this combination is not recommended for routine usage *(35)*. Trastuzumab is used routinely as a single agent or in combination with paclitaxel. It is currently being studied in combination with other therapies. Further investigation utilizing molecular and immunotherapeutic approaches may continue to improve outcomes in this difficult disease.

3.7. Supportive Therapy

In addition to chemotherapy, noncytotoxic palliative agents have shown improvements in quality of life for patients with metastatic breast cancer. Bisphosphonates have been used widely for the treatment of malignant hypercalcemia. More recently, these agents have been used to decrease morbidity from skeletal metastases. In patients with bony metastases, monthly pamidronate has been shown to delay the occurrence of first skeletal complications, decrease bone pain, and decrease deterioration of performance status compared with placebo *(36)*. Pamidronate offers a simple adjunctive therapy to chemotherapy for palliation of symptoms in skeletal disease without significant negative side effects. Bisphosphonates are now being investigated in the adjuvant setting.

4. TOXICITY OF CHEMOTHERAPY

Although chemotherapy has proved beneficial to a large number of patients with breast cancer, it does carry the risk of serious toxicity. Some of these toxicities are typical of all chemotherapeutic agents, whereas others are specific to a particular drug or drug class. The intensity of a particular toxicity may also vary greatly within a drug class. Toxicities are usually categorized as acute or long term and can involve a multitude of organ systems, including hematologic, gastrointestinal, neurologic, pulmonary, renal, and dermatologic systems.

4.1. Acute Toxicity

Acute toxicities are those that occur in the period immediately surrounding or within a short time after the administration of chemotherapy. Table 7 shows the most common acute toxicities of the chemotherapeutic agents used in the treatment of breast cancer and their severity compared with one another. These toxicities may be additive if chemotherapeutic agents are used in combination.

4.1.1. ACUTE HEMATOLOGIC TOXICITY

The most common and potentially most serious acute toxicity is myelosuppression. Leukopenia generally occurs by days 7–14 after chemotherapy is given and usually reverts by days 21–28. Patients are considered neutropenic when the absolute neutrophil count falls below 500. During this period, patients are at greatly increased risk for infection, and fever is considered a medical emergency. Thrombocytopenia can also occur within 1–2 weeks after chemotherapy. Patients should be monitored very closely for any signs of bleeding. Anemia may also result as a cumulative effect of repeated cycles of chemotherapy. The hemoglobin level may gradually decrease, causing significant fatigue and other associated symptoms. Management of these problems has been improved with new extended spectrum antibiotics and the development of recombinant hematopoietic growth factors. Patients should, however, have frequent monitoring of blood counts. The physician may need to delay or dose

Table 7

Relative Frequency/Intensity of Acute Toxicities for Agents Commonly Used in Treatment of Breast Cancer [a]

Drug	Hematologic	Nausea/vomiting	Stomatitis	Diarrhea	Alopecia	Neurologic	Genitourinary
Doxorubicin	+++	++	++	+	+++	–	–
Cyclophosphamide	++	++	+	+	+++	+	+
Methotrexate	+	++	++	++	+	–	+
5-Fluorouracil	+	+	+	+++	++	–	–
Capecitabine	+	+	+	++	+	–	–
Paclitaxel	++	+	+	+	+++	+++	–
Docetaxel	+++	++	+	+	+++	+	–
Vinorelbine	++	+	+	+	++	+++	–

[a] –, rare; +, mild; ++, moderate; +++, severe/frequent.

reduce the chemotherapy if the hematologic parameters have not recovered to acceptable levels by the next scheduled chemotherapy administration.

4.1.2. ACUTE GASTROINTESTINAL TOXICITY

Nausea and vomiting are the toxicities most feared by patients. A multitude of supportive medicines are now available that have made nausea and vomiting less troublesome. The development of $5\text{-}HT_3$ antagonists has revolutionized the field of supportive oncology. Other adjunctive antiemetic agents commonly used include prochlorperazine, metoclopramide, haloperidol, lorazepam, and dexamethasone.

Stomatitis and diarrhea can occur when chemotherapy causes damage to the gastrointestinal mucosa. These toxicities can significantly inhibit the ability to maintain proper hydration and nutrition. Aggressive supportive measures should be instituted at the first signs of these complications. Patients may require significant analgesia to maintain adequate levels of oral intake if stomatitis becomes severe. If these measures fail, the patient should be hospitalized for pain control and intravenous hydration. If the patient is having frequent liquid stools, antidiarrheals may be used to decrease the number of stools and therefore help to maintain the proper hydration status.

4.1.3. ACUTE NEUROLOGIC TOXICITY

Neurologic toxicity is often in the form of sensory peripheral neuropathy. Of the newer chemotherapeutic agents, paclitaxel has the most troublesome neuropathy. This problem is often dose- and schedule-dependent. It may become quite severe and is the dose-limiting toxicity for this agent. Often the neuropathy is reversible with discontinuation of the drug, but it may become permanent if not recognized early. The vinca alkaloids can also cause peripheral neuropathy but are also associated with autonomic dysfunction, which may produce constipation or ileus.

4.1.4. ACUTE DERMATOLOGIC TOXICITY

Dermatologic toxicity can present in various forms. Many chemotherapeutic agents can cause rashes or photosensitivity. Capecitabine, an oral 5-fluorouracil (5-FU) derivative, is taken for 21 consecutive days followed by 7 days without drug administration, mimicking protracted infusions of 5-FU. Like infusional 5-FU, capecitabine has been associated with a dermatologic complication known as palmar-plantar erythrodysesthesia or hand-foot syndrome. Pain and erythema of the hands and feet characterize this syndrome. It can be severe and is often a dose-limiting toxicity for the drug. Symptoms usually resolve with discontinuation or decrease in the dose.

Alopecia, although not physically harmful, can be psychologically damaging for patients receiving chemotherapy. Hair loss usually begins 2–3 weeks after the initiation of chemotherapy. Hair generally begins to regrow approximately 1 month after the discontinuation of chemotherapy treatment. Unfortunately, no preventive measures have proved to decrease this side effect. Patients should be reminded that hair growth will resume after chemotherapy and should be offered a wig to be worn during the treatment period.

4.1.5. ACUTE GENITOURINARY TOXICITY

Many chemotherapeutic agents are excreted by the kidney and may cause significant renal damage. Cyclophosphamide can cause hemorrhagic cystitis with prolonged exposure to the urothelium. This is usually of concern when cyclophosphamide is given in high doses. Hemorrhagic cystitis can occur, however, during the administration of CMF if proper hydration is not maintained while the patient is taking the oral cyclophosphamide. There is no specific therapy to reverse the cystitis once it has developed. Patients should be encouraged and reminded to maintain aggressive oral hydration and to void frequently throughout their chemotherapy treatment period.

4.1.6 ACUTE HYPERSENSITIVITY REACTIONS

Many chemotherapy drugs are associated with acute hypersensitivity reactions. Of those utilized in the treatment of breast cancer, the taxanes have the highest incidence. Paclitaxel must be administered in polyoxyethylated castor oil (Cremophor EL) to permit water solubility. Most hypersensitivity reactions are believed to be related to the Cremophor. Premedication with corticosteriods, diphenhydramine, and histamine H_2-antagonists such as cimetidine has greatly reduced the incidence of these adverse reactions. Docetaxel, although not prepared with Cremophor, has also been associated with acute hypersensitivity reactions. As with paclitaxel, premedication with corticosteroids has decreased the frequency of these reactions.

4.2. Long-Term Toxicity

Although many of the toxicities associated with the administration of chemotherapy are acute and reversible, serious complications may develop months to years after treatment with chemotherapy and can be permanent or fatal. This is particularly important when considering the administration of adjuvant therapy. These long-term toxicities tend to be rare, but even a low incidence can eliminate the potential benefits of adjuvant therapy in low-risk women. The three most significant long-term complications are premature menopause, cardiomyopathy, and the development of a second malignancy.

4.2.1. PREMATURE MENOPAUSE

Chemotherapy has long been known to cause ovarian oblation. This may in fact be beneficial during adjuvant therapy. Many women, however, never regain ovarian function once treatment has been completed. Although early-onset menopause is not a potentially fatal complication, it can be quite devastating to women. Patients often experience significant hot flashes and some dyspareunia. They are also prone to all the health issues associated with lack of estrogen including osteoporosis and the risk of cardiac disease. From a psychological standpoint, the loss of reproductive abilities can be very damaging not only to the patient but also her family, and they may require significant psychosocial support.

4.2.2. CARDIOMYOPATHY

Several drugs used in the treatment of breast cancer have the potential for significant and long-lasting cardiac toxicity. Anthracyclines have a well-established association with the development of cardiomyopathy. The incidence of cardiac dysfunction increases dramatically when the cumulative dose of doxorubicin, the most common anthracycline utilized for breast cancer treatment in the United States, exceeds 450 mg/m^2. This threshold dose may be less in patients with preexisting cardiac disease. All patients should have a baseline assessment of cardiac function prior to the institution of doxorubicin-based therapy. Recent trials have also shown an unacceptably high incidence of cardiomyopathy when doxorubicin was combined with trastuzamab *(35)*. This is of great importance as trastuzamab is now being tested in the adjuvant setting. Dexrazoxane is an iron chelator shown to decrease the cardiotoxic effects of doxorubicin *(37)*. This may be used in conjunction with chemotherapy in patients with prior anthracycline exposure or preexisting cardiac dysfunction if doxorubicin therapy is being considered.

4.2.3 SECOND MALIGNANCIES

Many cytotoxic chemotherapeutic agents are known carcinogens. Alkylating agents (i.e., cyclophosphamide), in particular, are associated with an increased risk of acute myelogenous leukemia (AML) and myelodysplastic syndrome (MDS). The greatest risk of developing chemotherapy-induced AML or MDS is within 2–3 years immediately following treatment; a slightly increased risk may continue, however, for 7–10 years after therapy. In a large case-controlled study, an increased risk of AML was observed in patients treated with regional radiotherapy, alkylating agents alone, or combination chemotherapy and radiotherapy. The risk was particularly high for patients treated with melphalan (a drug no longer used for the treatment of breast cancer). In patients treated with cyclophosphamide for less than 12 months or who received less than 20 g total, the risk was almost zero *(38)*. No significant increase in acute leukemia or solid tumors was noted in a long-term follow-up study of women treated with CMF *(39)*. Although these data are encouraging, the number of patients may not have been sufficiently large to detect small increases in risk. In general, the risk of recurrent breast cancer outweighs a small risk of secondary malignancy. In patients with a low risk of recurrent breast cancer, however, these issues become quite important and should be seriously considered before administering chemotherapy.

5. CONCLUSIONS

Chemotherapy for both early and advanced stage breast cancers has evolved greatly over the past 20 years. Significant improvements in overall survival, time to progression, and quality of life have been achieved. The 1990s have seen the development of several new chemotherapeutic agents with significant activity in metastatic breast cancer. The role of these agents in early-stage disease is currently under investigation. Despite these advances, breast cancer continues to claim the lives of thousands of women each year. Research involving optimal administration of the currently available agents and the development of new cytotoxic drugs continues. In addition, investigation of novel targeted therapies to be used in conjunction with traditional chemotherapy is ongoing. The combination of these modalities may continue to improve the outcomes for women with all stages of breast cancer.

REFERENCES

1. Fisher B, Carbone P, Economou SG, et al. (1975) L-phenyalanine mustard (L-PAM) in the management of primary breast cancer: a report of early findings. *N. Engl. J. Med.* **292,** 117–122.
2. Bonadonna G, Brusamolino E, Valagussa P, et al. (1976) Combination chemotherapy as an adjuvant treatment in operable breast cancer. *N. Engl. J. Med.* **294,** 405–410.
3. Early Breast Cancer Trialists' Collaborative Group (1998) Polychemotherapy for early breast cancer: an overview of the randomised trials. *Lancet* **352,** 930–942.
4. Fisher B, Redmond C, Legault-Poisson S, et al. (1990) Postoperative chemotherapy and tamoxifen compared with tamoxifen alone in the treatment of positive-node breast cancer patients age 50 years and older with tumors responsive to tamoxifen: results from the National Surgical Adjuvant Breast and Bowel Project B-16. *J. Clin. Oncol.* **8,** 1005–1018.
5. Mansour EG, Gray R, Shatila A, et al. (1989) Efficacy of adjuvant chemotherapy in high-risk node-negative breast cancer: an Intergroup Study. *N. Engl. J. Med.* **320,** 485–490.
6. Ludwig Breast Cancer Study Group (1989) Prolonged disease-free survival after one course of perioperative adjuvant chemotherapy for node negative breast cancer. *N. Engl. J. Med.* **320,** 491–496.
7. Fisher B, Redmond C, Dimitrov N, et al. (1989) A randomized clinical trial evaluating sequential methotrexate and fluorouracil in the treatment of patients with node-negative breast cancer who have estrogen-receptor-negative tumors. *N. Engl. J. Med.* **320,** 473–478.

8. Fisher B, Costantino J, Redmond C, et al. (1989) A randomized trial evaluating tamoxifen in the treatment of patients with node-negative breast cancer who have estrogen-receptor-positive tumors. *N. Engl. J. Med.* **320,** 473–478.

9. Fisher B, Dignam J, Wolmark N, et al. (1997) Tamoxifen and chemotherapy for lymph node-negative, estrogen receptor-positive breast cancer. *J. Natl. Cancer Inst.* **89,** 1673–1682.

10. Hutchins L, Green S, Ravdin P, et al. (1998) CMF versus CAF with and without tamoxifen in high risk node-negative breast cancer patients and a natural history follow-up study in low-risk node-negative patients: first results of Intergroup trial INT0102. *Proc. Annu. Meet. Am. Soc. Clin. Oncol.* **17,** 1a.

11. Tancini G, Bonadonna G, Valagussa P, et al. (1983) Adjuvant CMF in breast cancer: comparative 5-year results of 12 versus 6 cycles. *J. Clin. Oncol.* **1,** 2–10.

12. Fisher B, Brown AM, Dimitrov NV, et al. (1990) Two months of doxorubicin-cyclophosphamide with and without interval reinduction therapy compared with 6 months of cyclophosphamide, methotrexate, and fluorouracil in positive-node breast cancer patients with tamoxifen-nonresponsive tumors: results from the National Surgical Adjuvant Breast and Bowel Project B-15. *J. Clin. Oncol.* **8,** 1483–1496.

13. Henderson IC, Berry D, Demetri G, et al. (1998) Improved disease free survival and overall survival from the addition of sequential paclitaxel but not from the escalation of doxorubicin dose level in the adjuvant chemotherapy of patients with node-positive primary breast cancer. *Proc. Annu. Meet. Am. Soc. Clin. Oncol.* **17,** 101a.

14. Carpenter JT, Velez-Garcia E, Aron BS, et al. (1994) Five year results of a randomized comparison of cyclophosphamide, doxorubicin and fluorouracil (CAF) versus cyclophophamide, methotrexate and fluorouracil (CMF) for node positive breast cancer: a Southeastern Cancer Group Study. *Proc. Annu. Meet. Am. Soc. Clin. Oncol.* **13,** 66.

15. Levine MN, Bramwell VH, Pritchard KI, et al. (1998) Randomized trial of intensive cyclophosphamide, epirubicin, and fluorouracil compared with cyclophosphamide, methotrexate, and fluorouracil in premenopausal women with node-positive breast cancer. *J. Clin. Oncol.* **16,** 2651–2658.

16. Wood W, Budman D, Korzun A, et al. (1994) Dose and dose intensity of adjuvant chemotherapy for stage II, node-positive breast carcinoma. *N. Engl. J. Med.* **330,** 1253–1259.

17. Fisher B, Anderson S, Wickerham DL, et al. (1997) Increased intensification and total dose of cyclophosphamide in a doxorubicin-cyclophosphamide regimen for the treatment of primary breast cancer: findings from National Surgical Adjuvant Breast and Bowel Project B-22. *J. Clin. Oncol.* **15,** 1858–1869.

18. Peters W, Rosner G, Vredenburgh J, et al. (1999) A prospective, randomized comparison of two doses of combination alkylating agents as consolidation after CAF in high-risk primary breast cancer involving ten or more axillary lymph nodes: preliminary results of CALGB 9082/SWOG 9114/NCIC MA-13. *Proc. Annu. Meet. Am. Soc. Clin. Oncol.* **18,** 1a.

19. The Scandinavian Breast Cancer Study Group 9401 (1999) Results from a randomized adjuvant breast cancer study with high dose chemotherapy with CTCb supported by autologous bone marrow stem cells versus dose escalation and tailored FEC therapy. *Proc. Annu. Meet. Am. Soc. Clin. Oncol.* **18,** 2a.

20. Bezwoda WR (1999) Randomized, controlled trial of high dose chemotherapy (HD-CNVp) versus standard CAF chemotherapy for high risk, surgically treated primary breast cancer. *Proc. Annu. Meet. Am. Soc. Clin. Oncol.* **18,** 2a.

21. Carlson RW, Goldstein LJ, Gradishar WJ, et al. (1997) Update of the NCCN guidelines for the treatment of breast cancer. *Oncology* **11,** 199–220.

22. Sledge GW, Neuberg D, Ingle J, et al. (1997) Phase III trial of doxorubicin versus paclitaxel versus doxorubicin plus paclitaxel as first line therapy for metastatic breast cancer: an Intergroup trial. *Proc. Annu. Meet. Am. Soc. Clin. Oncol.* **16,** 2.

23. Winer E, Berry D, Duggan D, et al. (1998) Failure of higher dose paclitaxel to improve outcome in patients with metastatic breast cancer—results from CALGB 9342. *Proc. Annu. Meet. Am. Soc. Clin. Oncol.* **17,** 101a.

24. Stadtmauer EA, O'Neill A, Goldstein LJ, et al. (1999) Phase III randomized trial of high-dose chemotherapy and stem cell support shows no difference in overall survival or severe toxicity compared to maintenance chemotherapy with cyclophosphamide, methotrexate and 5-fluorouracil for women with metastatic breast cancer who are responding to conventional induction chemotherapy: the 'Philadelphia' Intergroup Study (PBT-1). *Proc. Am. Soc. Clin. Oncol.* **18,** 1a.

25. Mamousnas E, Brown A, Smith R, et al. (1998) Effect of Taxol duration of infusion in advanced breast cancer (ABC): results from NSABP B-26 trial comparing 3- to 24-hr infusion of high-dose Taxol. *Proc. Annu. Meet. Am. Soc. Clin. Oncol.* **17,** 101a.

26. Löffler TM, Freund W, Dröge C, et al. (1998) Activity of weekly Taxotere (TXT) in patients with metastatic breast cancer. *Proc. Annu. Meet. Am. Soc. Clin. Oncol.* **17,** 113a.

27. Seidmon AD, Hudis CA, Albanel J, et al. (1998) Dose-dense therapy with weekly 1-hour paclitaxel infusions in the treatment of metastatic breast cancer. *J. Clin. Oncol.* **16,** 3353–3361.

28. Gianni L, Capri G, Munzone E, et al. (1994) Paclitaxel efficacy in patients with advanced breast cancer resistant to anthracyclines. *Semin. Oncol.* **21,** 29–33.

29. Nabholtz JM, Thuerlimann B, Beswoda WR, et al. (1998) Taxotere improves survival over mitomycin C/vinblastine in patients with metastatic breast cancer who have failed an anthracycline containing regimen: final results of a phase III randomized trial. *Proc. Am. Soc. Clin. Oncol.* **17,** 101a.

30. Weber B, Vogel C, Jones S, et al. (1995) Intravenous vinorelbine as first-line and second-line therapy in advanced breast cancer. *J. Clin. Oncol.* **13,** 2722–2730.

31. Gammucci T, Piccart M, Brüning P, et al. (1998) Single agent Taxol (T) versus doxorubicin as first-line chemotherapy in advanced breast cancer. Final results of an EORTC randomized study with crossover. *Proc. Am. Soc. Clin. Oncol.* **17,** 111a.

32. Muss H, Case LD, Richards F, et al. (1991) Interrupted versus continuous chemotherapy in patients with metastatic breast cancer. *N. Engl. J. Med.* **325,** 1342–1348.

33. Coates A, Gebski V, Bishop JF, et al. (1987) Improving the quality of life during chemotherapy for advanced breast cancer. A comparison of intermittent and continuous treatment strategies. *N. Engl. J. Med.* **317,** 1490–1495.

34. Cobleigh MA, Vogel CL, Tripathy D, et al. (1998) Efficacy and safety of Herceptin (humanized anti-HER-2 antibody) as a single agent in 222 women with HER2 overexpression who relapsed following chemotherapy for metastatic breast cancer. *Proc. Am. Soc. Clin. Oncol.* **17,** 97a.

35. Slamon D, Leyland-Jones B, Shak S, et al. (1998) Addition of Herceptin (humanized anti-HER-2 antibody) to first line chemotherapy for HER2 overexpressing metastatic breast cancer markedly increases anticancer activity: a randomized, multinational controlled phase III trial. *Proc. Am. Soc. Clin. Oncol.* **17,** 98a.

36. Hortobagyi G, Theriault R, Porter L, et al. (1996) Efficacy of pamidronate in reducing skeletal complications in patient with breast cancer and lytic bone metastases. *N. Engl. J. Med.* **335,** 1785–1791.

37. Speyer J, Green M, Kramer E, et al. (1988) Protective effect of the bispiperazinedione ICRF-187 against doxorubicin-induced cardiac toxicity in women with advanced breast cancer. *N. Engl. J. Med.* **319,** 745–752.

38. Curtis RE, Boice JD, Stovall M, et al. (1992) Risk of leukemia after chemotherapy and radiation treatment for breast cancer. *N. Engl. J. Med.* **326,** 1745–1751.

39. Valagussa P, Tancini G, Bonadonna G (1987) Second malignancies after CMF for resectable breast cancer. *J. Clin. Oncol.* **5,** 1138–1142.

40. Goldhirsch A, Glick JH, Gelber RD, Senn HJ (1998) Meeting highlights; International Consensus Panel on the Treatment of Primary Breast Cancer. *J. Natl. Cancer Inst.* **90,** 1601–1608.

10 Hormonal Therapy of Breast Cancer

Halle C. F. Moore, MD and Kevin R. Fox, MD

CONTENTS

INTRODUCTION
HORMONAL THERAPY FOR METASTATIC DISEASE
HORMONAL THERAPY AS ADJUVANT TREATMENT
    FOR EARLY-STAGE DISEASE
BREAST CANCER PREVENTION
FUTURE DIRECTIONS
REFERENCES

1. INTRODUCTION

Studies of breast cancer epidemiology suggest an important role of hormonal factors in the development of breast cancer. An individual's risk of developing breast cancer is clearly correlated with the timing of menarche and menopause, parity, age of first pregnancy, use of exogenous estrogens, and female gender. Given the importance of the endocrine environment in the establishment of breast cancer, it is not surprising that hormonal manipulations have become a crucial aspect of therapy for this disease.

The responsiveness of breast cancer to endocrine therapy has been evident for over a century. The earliest successful treatment of advanced breast cancer consisted of surgical oophorectomy. Additional early treatments for metastatic breast cancer included adrenalectomy, hypophysectomy, and the

administration of synthetic androgens or estrogens (1). In the past several decades, newer drug therapies have come into use including competitive inhibitors of the estrogen receptor, inhibitors of adrenal aromatase activity, and other additive hormonal therapies such as synthetic progesterones. In addition to their role in the palliation of metastatic disease, hormonal therapies can decrease the risk of breast cancer recurrence and death when used in the adjuvant setting for early-stage disease. Recently, interest has developed in the use of hormonal agents to prevent breast cancer in healthy individuals at high risk of developing the disease.

2. HORMONAL THERAPY FOR METASTATIC DISEASE

Despite efforts at early detection and the reduction in the risk of death from breast cancer through the application of adjuvant therapy, approximately 40% of patients with early-stage breast cancer will develop metastatic disease, usually within 10 years of the diagnosis. In

From: *Current Clinical Oncology:*
Breast Cancer: A Guide to Detection and Multidisciplinary Therapy
Edited by: M. H. Torosian © Humana Press Inc., Totowa, NJ

Table 1
The Optimum Candidate for Hormonal Therapy of Metastatic Breast Cancer

Tumor rich in estrogen and/or progesterone receptor
No prior exposure to hormonal therapy or prior response to hormonal therapy
Greater than 2 years from diagnosis of breast cancer until recurrence
Metastatic involvement of bone and/or soft tissue predominantly
If visceral involvement, evidence of indolent disease behavior

general, metastatic breast cancer is incurable and therapy is directed at palliation of symptoms and prolongation of life. The median survival for patients with metastatic breast cancer is approximately 3 years. Patients with hormone-sensitive advanced disease, however, have been known to survive for 10–20 years or more. Because prolonged treatment may thus be required, therapy for advanced breast cancer should be effective but with modest and acceptable toxicity. In general, hormonal agents are easily administered, and side effects are tolerable, particularly in comparison with the effects of systemic chemotherapy. Hormonal therapy should be strongly considered for patients with hormone receptor-positive tumors confined to the soft tissues and/or bone and those with an indolent disease course as these patients are most likely to benefit from hormonal therapy (Table 1).

Most patients with breast cancer will have detectable amounts of estrogen or progesterone receptor in their tumor tissue. Approximately two-thirds of patients with such positive hormone receptors will respond to endocrine therapy. Response likelihood is related to the level of hormone receptor positivity and to the interval to development of progressive disease from the time of diagnosis. Patients who progress after initial response to one hormonal agent have a good chance of responding to subsequent hormonal treatments, although the likelihood of response diminishes following each progression. Although endocrine therapy can be safely combined with chemotherapy, such combined modality therapy is generally not recommended for metastatic disease. Although initial response rates are generally superior with chemohormonal therapy over endocrine therapy alone, sequential use of each modality results in equivalent survival (2,3). Similarly, combining more than one hormonal agent may increase response rates at the expense of increased toxicity with no impact on survival (4,5). The means of hormonal intervention is influenced by the menopausal status of the patient as well as by anticipated toxicity profiles of the various options. A list of commonly applied hormonal therapies is given in Table 2.

2.1. Therapy in Postmenopausal Patients

Breast cancer in postmenopausal women is frequently estrogen-dependent. Despite cessation of ovarian estrogen production in postmenopausal women, continued estrogen production occurs, predominantly through conversion of adrenal steroids into estrone and estradiol via aromatase activity (6).

Tamoxifen, a mixed estrogen agonist/antagonist, is generally considered standard first-line treatment for postmenopausal women with metastatic breast cancer who are candidates for endocrine therapy. Tamoxifen was approved for the treatment of advanced breast cancer in the United States in 1978. Subsets of postmenopausal women with strongly positive estrogen receptors have been identified with response rates to tamoxifen as high as 86% when tamoxifen was used as first line therapy for metastatic disease (7). In patients unselected by hormone receptor status, responses occur in approximately one-third of patients, which is

Table 2
Types of Hormonal Therapy for Metastatic Breast Cancer in Clinical Use

Antiestrogens (tamoxifen, toremifene)
Selective aromatase inhibitors (anastrazole, letrozole, exemestane,
　postmenopausal patients only)
Progestational agents (megesterol acetate)
Oophorectomy (premenopausal patients only)
Gonadotropin-releasing hormone agonists (premenopausal
　patients only)
Nonselective aromatase inhibitors (aminoglutethimide)
Androgens

similar to response rates seen with most other forms of hormonal therapy for breast cancer. The very favorable side effect profile of tamoxifen has led to its widespread acceptance as first-line hormonal therapy for postmenopausal advanced breast cancer. Most clinical trials of tamoxifen in breast cancer have used a dose of 10 mg twice daily; however, a single daily 20-mg dose appears to be equally effective and biologically equivalent (8).

An alternative is toremifine. This drug, like tamoxifen, has mixed estrogenic and antie-strogenic effects and appears to be similar in to tamoxifen both activity and toxicities (9). The two drugs have significant crossresistance, and patients who are refractory to tamoxifen are unlikely to respond to toremifene (10).

For many years, the most commonly applied second-line hormonal therapy in patients whose metastatic disease progressed on tamoxifen therapy was high-dose progesterone, usu-ally in the form of the synthetic progestational agent megesterol acetate. The undesirable toxicities of megesterol acetate (primarily weight gain and a tendency toward thromboem-bolic events) led to a search for less toxic agents to replace progesterone. The new selective aromatase inhibitors anastrozole and letrozole are appropriate second-line hormonal therapy choices for postmenopausal women who have disease progression following adjuvant tamoxifen (see Adjuvant Hormonal Therapy) or following an initial response to tamoxifen for metastatic disease. For several decades it has been known that "medical adrenalectomy" with the nonselective aromatase inhibitor aminoglutethimide could result in objective regression of advanced breast cancer (11). Aminoglutethimide has frequent side effects and requires hydrocortisone supplementation, given its nonselective interference with adrenal steroid hormone production. The recent development of selective aromatase inhibitors, which specifically inhibit the conversion of adrenal androgens into estrogens, has made this class of drug much easier to use, with less toxicity and potentially greater efficacy.

Clinical trials of anastrozole, the first selective aromatase inhibitor to be approved for use in this country, have demonstrated activity in tamoxifen-resistant, predominantly hormone receptor-positive metastatic breast cancer. In a randomized clinical trial comparing two doses of anastrozole with 40 mg of megesterol acetate four times a day, approximately 10% of patients had objective responses, with disease stability for more than 6 months in an addi-tional 25% of patients (12,13,23). Response rates were similar among the three arms of the trial; however, a modest survival advantage has emerged for patients randomized to anastro-zole 1 mg compared with megesterol acetate. This group also experienced the least amount of toxicity compared with patients randomized to megesterol acetate or the 10-mg dose of anastrozole. The most common side effects specifically associated with anastrozole are gas-trointestinal complaints.

Letrozole, another selective aromatase inhibitor recently approved for use in post-menopausal women with metastatic breast cancer has also been compared directly with megesterol acetate 160 mg daily *(14)*. The overall response rate to a 2.5-mg dose of letrozole was 24% compared with 16% for megesterol acetate, with no significant difference in survival. Like anastrozole, letrozole was found to be better tolerated than megesterol acetate, with predominant adverse effects associated with letrozole consisting of musculoskeletal pain and gastrointestinal complaints. Letrozole 2.5 mg has also been compared with aminoglutethimide 250 mg twice a day. Patients randomized to letrozole experienced a superior response rate, longer time to progression, and improved survival.

The third aromatase inhibitor approved for use in the United States, exemestane, differs from anstrazole and letrozole in several ways. Exemestane is a steroidal aromatase inhibitor and inhibits the aromatase enzyme via a noncompetitive mechanism. The clinical relevance of this difference remains to be determined. Like anastrazole and letrozole, exemestane, at a dose of 25 mg per day, has also been compared to megesterol acetate and proved superior with respect to response rate and time to progression, and showed an improvement in survival of borderline statistical significance *(15)*. Preliminary evidence also suggests that exemestane may be effective in patients who have failed prior aromatase inhibitors of the nonsteroidal type (anastrazole and letrozole) or aminoglutethimide. One phase II trial reported a response rate of 6.6% and an overall success rate (complete reponse, partial response, and stable disease for more than six months) of 24.3% in a cohort of 241 patients who had failed prior aromatase inhibitor therapy *(16)*.

For patients who remain candidates for hormonal therapy after progression on first-and second-line therapy, megesterol acetate remains an important therapeutic option. Megesterol acetate is a synthetic derivative of progesterone. When tested in hormone therapy-naïve metastatic breast cancer, the activity is comparable to that of tamoxifen *(17,18)*. Megesterol acetate can be difficult to tolerate, however, and commonly results in significant weight gain. Over 30% of patients may experience a $\geq 5\%$ weight gain with 10% of patients experiencing a $\geq 10\%$ weight gain. Peripheral edema is another side effect commonly associated with megesterol acetate. Because of the somewhat poorer tolerability of this drug, relative to tamoxifen and the selective aromatase inhibitors, megesterol acetate is generally considered as a third-line option. Other additive therapies that can be considered in patients who have progressed after initial responses to multiple hormonal manipulations include androgens and high-dose estrogens. These drugs, too, are associated with additional toxicities that affect tolerability of therapy.

2.2. Aromatase Inhibitors as First Line Treatment

The success of aromatase inhibitors in supplanting megesterol acetate as second-line therapy led naturally to a series of randomized trials in which the aromatase inhibitors were compared directly to tamoxifen as first-line therapy in the treatment of metastatic breast cancer. In these clinical trials, patients with no prior exposure to hormonal therapy for metastatic disease were eligible, and patients who had taken tamoxifen therapy as adjuvant treatment were also eligible, providing that tamoxifen had been discontinued at least 12 months before study entry. The first of these trials to be published compared anstrazole to tamoxifen in two separate trials of similar design *(19,20)*. These two studies, involving over 1000 patients, demonstrated clinical effectiveness for anastrazole that was at least equivalent to tamoxifen, with a suggestion of superiority for patients who were hormone-receptor positive as opposed to those whose hormone receptor status was unknown *(20)*. Letrozole has also been compared to tamoxifen in a single clinical trial of similar design to the tamoxifen/anastrazole trials above. In 907 patients studied, letrozole was superior to tamoxifen for most of the endpoints studied, including time to progression, overall response, and time to treatment failure *(21)*. Survival benefits were not described in the most recent report of this study, which included a voluntary crossover design, in which patients progressing on either therapy were permitted to take the opposite drug, and did so in approximately 50% of cases *(22)*. In all of these trials, the toxicity of the aromatase inhibitors was comparable to that of tamoxifen, with some suggestion that the number of thromboembolic events associated with the aromatase inhibitors might be smaller than the number observed with tamoxifen. Both anastrazole and letrozole have now been approved as first-line therapy for postmenopausal patients with hormone-responsive metastatic breast cancer.

2.3. Therapy in Premenopausal Patients

Approximately half of breast cancers in premenopausal women are hormone-receptor positive. As with postmenopausal women, the patients most likely to respond to hormonal therapy are those with strongly positive estrogen and progesterone receptors, whose disease is limited to the soft tissue and/or bones, and those with minimal prior therapy. The ovaries are the predominant source of estrogen production in premenopausal women, although additional estrogen production occurs via aromatization of adrenal androgens to estrogens.

Ovarian ablation, through either surgical, radiologic, or medical means, is an effective first-line therapy for premenopausal women with advanced breast cancer. In premenopausal patients unselected with respect to hormone receptor status, the objective response rate to oophorectomy is approximately 30%, whereas up to 75% of hormone receptor-positive premenopausal women may respond to this treatment. Patients under age 35 years are somewhat less likely to respond to this therapy. Surgical oophorectomy is associated with a more rapid response than ovarian radioablation; however, both procedures are effective. Recently, the use of synthetic gonadotropin releasing hormone (GnRH) analogs as a means of performing medical ovarian ablation has come into favor *(24)*. These agents essentially induce a postmenopausal state through downregulating receptors for pituitary luteinizing hormone releasing factor, resulting in inhibition of gonadotropin synthesis and subsequent inhibition of ovarian estrogen secretion. Serum estradiol levels reach the postmenopausal range within approximately 3 weeks of therapy. Advantages to medical ovarian ablation include avoidance of an operative procedure and the reversibility of treatment should the patient fail to benefit or experience excessive side effects. Activity of GnRH analogs in phase II trials and in one small phase III trial has demonstrated efficacy comparable to that of oophorectomy *(24,25)*.

Tamoxifen is also an effective agent in premenopausal women and is an appropriate second-line hormonal therapy, as well as an accepted alternative to oophorectomy as first line hormonal therapy, for metastatic breast cancer in this population. One small randomized comparison trial of oophorectomy versus tamoxifen has been conducted in premenopausal women with advanced breast cancer. Both treatments were well tolerated, with no significant difference in response rate, response duration, or survival identified between the two treatment arms *(26)*.

As in postmenopausal women, megesterol acetate is a potentially effective third line hormonal option in premenopausal women. One small randomized trial of high-dose megesterol acetate versus oophorectomy in previously untreated premenopausal women with metastatic breast cancer found the two therapies to be similar in terms of response rates and survival *(27)*. Furthermore, it was found that patients with disease progression after oophorectomy had a reasonable likelihood of subsequent response to megesterol acetate. In contrast to megesterol acetate, aromatase inhibitors are not felt to be effective in premenopausal women. This class of drug should be avoided in premenopausal patients, as inhibition of aromatase activity in women with functioning ovaries may lead to virilization and a polycystic ovary syndrome. Aromatase inhibitors could be considered for use in premenopausal women who have been treated with GnRH agonists, whose disease is progressing after initial response to such therapy, and in whom GnRH treatment will be continued to maintain its menopausal effect.

The value of combination hormonal therapy in premenopausal women is an interesting research question. Although tamoxifen is an active agent in both premenopausal and postmenopausal women, it is known to result in stimulation of estrogen production in functioning ovaries. It is possible that the high plasma estradiol levels result in competition with tamoxifen for binding to estrogen receptors, thereby hampering its efficacy in younger women. Because of this theoretical concern, the effect of combing tamoxifen with a GnRH agonist to prevent compensatory increases in estrogen production has been addressed. In a recent three-arm trial of first line therapy for advanced breast cancer in premenopausal patients, a combination of a luteinizing hormone releasing hormone (LHRH) agonist and tamoxifen therapy was compared with each drug as a single agent. Time to progression and survival were superior in patients randomized to combined treatment compared with LHRH agonist or tamoxifen alone. Because this trial did not include a crossover design, it is difficult to know whether sequential use of each therapy would result in equivalent survival *(28)*.

2.4. Conclusions

All patients with hormone receptor-positive metastatic breast cancer are theoretical candidates for endocrine therapy. Patients with rapidly progressive disease or extensive involvement of viscera, such as the liver, are suboptimal candidates for hormonal intervention and should be considered preferably for systemic cytotoxic chemotherapy. When choosing hormonal therapies, the menopausal status of the patient should be considered, as should the toxicity of the treatment chosen. Patients who respond to hormonal intervention have a respectable chance of responding to second- and even third-line hormonal therapies, and thus the sequential use of such therapies may potentially provide the patient with years of effective palliation with minimal toxicity. Patients who fail to respond at all to hormonal therapy or who have exhausted all legitimate hormonal therapies should be considered candidates for systemic chemotherapy. Tamoxifen should be considered the standard treatment of care for postmenopausal patients, although many of these patients will be taking or will already have taken tamoxifen as adjuvant treatment. For these patients, the aromatase inhibitors represent a new care standard for endocrine therapy of metastatic disease. Premenopausal patients should be considered for oophorectomy by whatever means the patient finds most acceptable, with tamoxifen standing as an acceptable alternative to oophorectomy in patients not currently taking the drug for adjuvant therapy purposes.

3. HORMONAL THERAPY AS ADJUVANT TREATMENT FOR EARLY-STAGE DISEASE

Insofar as most of patients with breast cancer will, at the time of initial diagnosis, have their disease confined to the breast with or without axillary nodal involvement, their disease will theoretically be curable by local measures, such as surgery with or without radiation therapy. In contrast to its palliative role in advanced disease, the purpose of systemic therapy for localized disease is to decrease the risk of cancer recurrence and death when it is at a potentially curable stage after appropriate surgery. As early as the 1950s prophylactic oophorectomy and adrenalectomy were performed in attempt to prevent breast cancer recurrence before the development of metastatic disease in patients who were felt to be at extremely high risk for relapse. The outcome of patients with this form of adjuvant endocrine therapy appeared to be better than was expected given the extent of their disease at presentation *(29)*. Patients appeared to have relatively little interference with quality of life as a result of the surgical procedures; however, potential operative morbidity as well as the permanent nature of such interventions limited the appeal of such therapy.

Over more recent decades, a series of clinical trials has assessed the value of adjuvant hormonal therapy, predominantly using the drug tamoxifen. Many of these trials were included in a large metaanalysis of adjuvant therapy trials in breast cancer conducted by the Early Breast Cancer Trialists Collaborative Group (EBCTCG). The 1992 Overview Analysis included data from 30,000 women with early-stage breast cancer randomized to receive or not receive tamoxifen on various trials *(30)*. In this analysis, a significant reduction in mortality was observed in patients who received up to 5 years of tamoxifen. The benefit continued even at 10 years of follow-up. Patients who were over 50 years appeared to benefit the most from adjuvant tamoxifen; however, all patient groups, regardless of age, nodal status, and hormone receptor levels experienced a benefit from tamoxifen.

The 1992 Overview also addressed the value of ovarian ablation in early breast cancer. Patients under 50 years of age with early breast cancer experienced a significant survival advantage when randomized to receive ovarian ablation versus no ovarian ablation. As with tamoxifen, the benefits of oophorectomy were sustained and persisted for 15 years of follow-up. Tamoxifen and oophorectomy have not been directly compared in any large randomized trial in the adjuvant setting, but tamoxifen has generally been favored, given its low toxicity and its reversibility. Tamoxifen also appears to have beneficial effects on bone density and cardiovascular events.

In 1998, the EBCTG published an updated version of the tamoxifen overview using data from approximately 37,000 women in 55 randomized trials of adjuvant tamoxifen *(31)*. Again, patients receiving tamoxifen experienced a survival advantage at 10 years compared with patients not receiving adjuvant tamoxifen. The beneficial effect was greatest in patients with hormone receptor-positive tumors, whereas the value of adjuvant tamoxifen in patients with tumors that are truly estrogen receptor-negative remains uncertain. In trials of roughly 5 years of tamoxifen, patients benefited from therapy regardless of age or menopausal status.

In the EBCTG overview, longer duration of therapy appeared to be associated with a more pronounced benefit to tamoxifen. Patients receiving approximately 5 years of tamoxifen had a greater benefit than did patients in trials of 1 or 2 years of tamoxifen. Prolonging tamoxifen therapy beyond 5 years, however, does not appear to be beneficial. The National Surgical Adjuvant Breast and Bowel Project (NSABP) trial B-14 addressed the issue of optimal tamoxifen duration by randomizing those patients getting tamoxifen to receive 5 years versus 10 years of therapy *(32)*. No advantage was seen to continuing tamoxifen beyond 5 years, and, in fact, there was a suggestion of a decrease in relapse-free and overall survival in those patients receiving the longer duration of therapy. Five years of therapy has, therefore, become the standard duration of tamoxifen in the adjuvant setting (Table 3).

Although tamoxifen alone may be effective adjuvant therapy for some patients with hormone receptor-positive early-stage breast cancer, several studies have addressed the value of adding chemotherapy to tamoxifen. NSABP trial B-16 randomized women over age 50 years with node-positive breast cancer, who were either progesterone-positive or over age 60 years regardless of receptor status, to receive tamoxifen alone versus tamox-

Table 3
The Role of Tamoxifen as Adjuvant Therapy in Early-Stage Breast Cancer

Tamoxifen reduces the risk of recurrence and death by 30–45%.
Both premenopausal and postmenopausal patients derive benefit.
The optimum duration of therapy is 5 years.
The benefit of tamoxifen is uncertain in estrogen and progesterone
  receptor-negative patients.
The benefit of tamoxifen continues to be realized after more than 10
  years of follow-up

ifen plus a 12 week course of doxorubicin-based chemotherapy. A significant advantage in disease-free survival was seen in patients receiving combination therapy, with 84% of patients alive and disease-free at 3 years compared with 67% of patients randomized to tamoxifen alone *(33)*. Additional reports have confirmed the utility of combination chemohormonal therapy in node-positive patients, and one trial, NSABP trial B-20, has found that node-negative patients also benefit from combined therapy. In the latter trial, premenopausal and postmenopausal patients with node-negative, receptor-positive tumors were randomized to tamoxifen alone versus tamoxifen plus non-doxorubicin-containing chemotherapy. A reduction of one-third in treatment failure was observed with addition of chemotherapy to tamoxifen *(34)*. The absolute improvement in survival at 5 years was a modest 3–4% reflecting the generally favorable prognosis of the patient population included in this study. Similar benefits relative to chemotherapy were observed regardless of tumor size or level of hormone receptor positivity. The importance of adding chemotherapy to adjuvant hormonal therapy, however, is likely to be greatest in patients whose risk for disease recurrence is high, including younger patients, and those with large tumors or lymph node involvement.

The presence of *HER2neu* oncogene overexpression in tumor tissue is a widely recognized prognostic factor that, if present, predicts for poorer disease-free and overall survival in patients with early-stage breast cancer. *HER2neu* has also emerged as a factor that may identify patients for whom hormonal therapy alone may be inadequate. *HER2neu* overexpression is more commonly associated with hormone receptor negativity, and 25% or fewer of tumors with positive hormone receptors will also overexpress *HER2neu*. In the Naples Gruppo Universitario Napoletan (GUN) trial of adjuvant tamoxifen in node-negative breast cancer, a retrospective analysis of the interaction between *HER2neu* expression status and outcome was performed. Overexpression of *HER2neu* was found to be a strong predictor for failure of tamoxifen, independent of estrogen receptor status *(35)*. Similarly, in a correlative study by the Southwest Oncology Group of *HER2neu* as a predictor of adjuvant therapy outcome, patients with *HER2neu* overexpression had a greater benefit to the addition of doxorubicin-based chemotherapy to tamoxifen over tamoxifen alone as adjuvant therapy *(36)*. These findings may indicate a particular sensitivity of *HER2neu*-overexpressing tumors to doxorubicin-containing chemotherapy or may reflect the inadequacy of tamoxifen alone in such tumors. The interaction of *HER2neu* status and response to tamoxifen remains a matter of ongoing clinical investigation. At the present time, the overexpression of *HER2neu* by hormone receptor-positive breast cancers should not influence the decision to employ tamoxifen in the adjuvant treatment of early-stage invasive breast cancer.

Table 4
Toxicities of Tamoxifen Therapy

Vasomotor symptoms (hot flashes)
Fluid retention
Weight gain
Vaginal dryness with or without atrophic vaginitis
Thromboembolic phenomena (uncommon)
Endometrial carcinoma (uncommon)

3.1. Tamoxifen in the Treatment of Ductal Carcinoma In Situ

Another recent development in adjuvant therapy for breast cancer has been the evaluation of tamoxifen in patients with ductal carcinoma *in situ* (DCIS). Patients with DCIS, or noninvasive breast cancer, are felt to be at essentially no risk for systemic spread of their disease. These patients remain at higher than average risk, however, for the development of new breast cancers, both invasive and noninvasive, in the contralateral breast. Patients with DCIS treated with breast-conserving surgery, with or without radiation to the breast, are also at risk for ipsilateral in-breast recurrences, which may be *in situ* or invasive. NSABP trial B24 evaluated the value of tamoxifen following lumpectomy and radiotherapy in women with DCIS. In this randomized, placebo-controlled trial, patients not receiving tamoxifen had a cumulative 5 year risk of a new breast cancer event (invasive or noninvasive breast cancer in either breast) of 13%. Patients randomized to tamoxifen had an 8.8% cumulative 5-year rate of new breast cancer events (p = 0.007), representing about a one-third reduction or an absolute benefit of approximately 4% reduction in new breast cancer events. Survival data from this cohort are not yet available *(37)*.

The benefits of tamoxifen need to be considered in relationship to potential risks and toxicities of therapy (Table 4). This is particularly true when treatment is considered for patients in whom the absolute benefit of tamoxifen is likely to be low. Tamoxifen has been associated with the development of endometrial cancer, with a yearly rate of approximately 1.6 cases per 1000 women taking tamoxifen. The incidence of endometrial cancer appears to be higher with prolonged tamoxifen use. The risk of thromboembolic phenomena is also increased with tamoxifen, with relative risks of this complication ranging from 1.3 to 7 in various studies. Other side effects of tamoxifen include menopausal symptoms such as hot flashes, mood disturbances, weight gain, and atrophic vaginitis. Such symptoms may be more pronounced in younger women.

3.2. Conclusions

Virtually all patients with hormone receptor-positive early-stage invasive breast cancer are legitimate candidates for tamoxifen therapy for the prevention of metastatic disease and death. There are, however, some patients whose breast cancers pose so little risk of systemic spread that tamoxifen may be considered unnecessary. These patients are considered in Table 5. The emergence of data from appropriately controlled clinical trials has raised the legitimate issue that perhaps all patients with hormone-receptor positive early-stage breast cancer should receive both chemotherapy and tamoxifen. This issue remains an ongoing matter of debate and will probably not be clarified by further clinical trials. The optimum therapy for each patient must be considered on an individual basis and must take into account the patient's perceived risk of recurrence and death, the relative benefit she will

Table 5
Features of the Patient Who May Be Able to Avoid Adjuvant Tamoxifen

Estrogen and progesterone receptor-negative breast cancer
Estrogen receptor-positive breast cancer of low histologic grade
    and measuring less than 1 cm, providing axillary nodes are negative
Microinvasive ductal carcinoma *in situ,* providing axillary nodes
    are negative
Colloid or mucinous histologies of invasive ductal cancers, providing
    axillary nodes are negative

probably derive from tamoxifen or from the combination of chemotherapy and tamoxifen, the anticipated toxicities of each, the patient's motivation to receive therapy, and their general medical condition.

4. BREAST CANCER PREVENTION

Similar to the investigation of the use of tamoxifen in noninvasive breast cancer is the recent interest in the drugs use to prevent breast cancer in healthy women who are perceived to be at increased risk for the development of breast cancer. It has been observed for some time that patients receiving tamoxifen have fewer in-breast recurrences after breast-conserving therapy, as well as a lower than expected incidence of new contralateral breast cancers (38). In a combined analysis of nine NSABP trials of early-stage breast cancer, the 5-year cumulative rate of contralateral breast cancer was 29.3 per 1000 women not receiving adjuvant hormonal therapy. Patients who received tamoxifen in these trials experienced a significantly lower 5-year cumulative rate of new contralateral primary breast cancer, 16.9 per 1000 women (39). In NSABP trial B-14, in which patients were randomized to either placebo or tamoxifen, the 5-year cumulative rate of contralateral breast cancer was 36.9 per 1000 women in patients receiving placebo, versus a rate of 20.8 per 1000 women randomized to tamoxifen. This translates into a 37% reduction in the annual incidence of contralateral breast cancer. Similarly, in the 1998 EBCTCG overview, a 47% reduction in contralateral breast cancers was seen in patients randomized to tamoxifen for about 5 years.

The first NSABP breast cancer prevention trial, NSABP P-1, was published in 1998 (40). This randomized, placebo-controlled trial assessed the effect of a 5-year course of tamoxifen on the incidence of breast cancer in 13,388 previously healthy women who were identified to be at high risk for breast cancer. Patients included in the study were either 60 years of age or older, had a history of lobular carcinoma in situ, or were over 35 years with a predicted 5-year risk for developing breast cancer of at least 1.66%, based on the Gail risk model, a model for the development of breast cancer based on clinical data derived from healthy women during the 1970s. The 5-year cumulative rate of invasive breast cancer in the control population was 6.67 per 1000 women, whereas the rate in patients randomized to tamoxifen was 3.43 per 1000 women. Tamoxifen was, therefore, associated with a 49% reduction in the risk of invasive breast cancer in this population (p < 0.00001). In this study, the reduction in new breast cancers was primarily a reduction in estrogen receptor-positive tumors. Whether tamoxifen truly prevents the development of malignancy or represents early treatment of occult breast cancers is unclear, but regardless of the mechanism, therapy appears to allow more patients to live free of breast cancer. Unfortunately, survival data are yet available from

NSABP trial P1, making it difficult to advise healthy patients of the relative risks and ulti-mate benefits of tamoxifen as preventive therapy.

Adding to the difficulty of determining whether healthy patients should receive tamox-ifen for the prevention of breast cancer are two additional randomized studies that failed to demonstrate a benefit for tamoxifen in the prevention of breast cancer (41,42). The first of these trials, conducted at the Royal Marsden hospital in the United Kingdom, random-ized 2471 healthy women ages 30–70 years who had a family history of breast cancer to receive tamoxifen or placebo (41). With a median follow-up period of 70 months, no sig-nificant difference in breast cancer incidence was observed between the two groups. Sim-ilarly, an Italian trial of 5408 healthy women with a prior hysterectomy failed to demonstrate a significant difference in breast cancer incidence between patients random-ized to tamoxifen versus placebo (42). In the latter trial, patients were not required to have a higher than average risk of developing breast cancer, and a low number of breast cancer events in this study resulted in poor statistical power to detect a difference between the two study arms. In addition to differences in patient populations and statistical power, the Royal Marsden and Italian trials differed from NSABP trial P1 in that the European trials allowed the use of exogenous estrogens.

In considering the use of tamoxifen in healthy individuals, it is important to understand the potential risks of this therapy. Patients with invasive breast cancer may experience a sur-vival benefit with tamoxifen despite a small increase in the risk of thromboembolic events or endometrial cancer. Although tamoxifen may be an effective agent for reducing the inci-dence of breast cancer in certain populations of individuals at risk for breast cancer, the sur-vival benefit has not yet been quantified. Healthy patients considering this preventive therapy should be informed of the potential risks of treatment, and patients should be carefully selected with attention to the criteria used in NSABP trial P1, as this is the only study in which tamoxifen has clearly shown efficacy as a preventive agent.

Another potentially effective agent for the prevention of breast cancer is the selective estrogen receptor modulator raloxifene. This drug, which, like tamoxifen, has both estro-gen agonist and antagonist activity, was developed for the treatment of osteoporosis with the hope of avoiding undesirable effects of estrogen including stimulatory effects on endometrial and breast tissue. In a trial of 7704 postmenopausal women with osteoporo-sis, patients were randomized to one of two doses of Raloxifene or to placebo. Although the primary end point of the study was to evaluate whether raloxifene decreased the risk of bone fractures, the rates of breast and endometrial cancers on each arm of the study were recorded as part of the safety database. In this population of postmenopausal women, a significantly lower incidence of breast cancer was observed in patients assigned to raloxifene than in patients receiving placebo, with a relative risk of 0.26 after a median follow-up period of 28.9 months (43). There was also a trend toward a reduction in the risk of endometrial cancer with raloxifene.

The potential role of raloxifene as a preventive agent for breast cancer in healthy post-menopausal women is encouraging and is currently under investigation in NSABP trial P2, which will directly compare raloxifene and tamoxifen for the prevention of breast cancer in postmenopausal women at risk for breast cancer. The current indication for raloxifene is in the treatment of osteoporosis, and it should not be prescribed solely as a breast cancer preventive agent outside the context of the P2 trial. Furthermore, this agent is not known to be effective in the treatment of metastatic breast cancer or in the adjuvant therapy of early-stage disease. It is also unclear how breast cancer recurrence will be affected if raloxifene is given to treat osteoporosis in patients who have completed 5 years of adjuvant tamoxifen, given the aforementioned finding that prolonged exposure to tamoxifen beyond 5 years may be harmful.

5. FUTURE DIRECTIONS

Ongoing research in breast cancer involves the development of new generations of selective estrogen receptor modulators. A search is under way for the ideal drug that has antiestrogenic activity in breast and endometrial tissues but estrogenic activity in bone, the cardiovascular system and central nervous system. Early clinical trials of pure selective estrogen receptor modulators, or SERMs, are underway. Prospects for advances in adjuvant endocrine therapy and therapy of metastatic breast cancer are also encouraging. Currently, the value of aromatase inhibitors in early breast cancer is being addressed in clinical trials in which these agents are being evaluated as alternatives to or as additions to tamoxifen. One study, by the Eastern Cooperative Oncology Group, is testing the value of adding letrozole after the completion of 5 years of adjuvant tamoxifen in a placebo-controlled trial in postmenopausal women. Clinical trials of the aromatase inhibitors as alternatives to tamoxifen in the first-line therapy of metastatic breast cancer are under way as well, and some have completed enrollment.

REFERENCES

1. Atkins H, Falconer MA, Hayward JL, et al (1966) The timing of adrenalectomy and of hypophysectomy in the treatment of advanced breast cancer. *Lancet:* **1,** 827–830.
2. The Australian and New Zealand Breast Cancer Trials Group (1986) A randomized trial in postmenopausal patients with advanced breast cancer comparing endocrine and cytotoxic therapy geven sequentially or in combination. *J. Clin. Oncol.* **4,** 186–193.
3. Cocconi G, De Lisi V, Boni C, et al (1983) Chemotherapy versus combination of chemotherapy and endocrine therapy in advanced breast cancer. *Cancer* **51,** 581–588.
4. Ingle JN, Twito DI, Schaid DJ, et al (1988) Randomized clinical trial of tamoxifen alone or combined with fluoxymesterone in postmenopausal women with metastatic breast cancer. *J. Clin. Oncol.* **6,** 825–831.
5. Ingle JN, Green SJ, Ahmann DL, et al (1986) Randomized trial of tamoxifen alone or combined with aminoglutethimide and hydrocortisone in women with metastatic breast cancer. *J. Clin. Oncol.* **4,** 958–964.
6. Ellis M, (1998) Selective aromatase inhibitos: current indication and future perspectives. *Dis. Breast Upd.* **2,** 1–11.
7. Ravdin PM, Green S, Dorr TM, et al (1992) Prognostic significance of progesterone receptor levels in estrogen receptor-positive patients with metastatic breast cancer treated with tamoxifen: results of a prospective southwest oncology group study. *J. Clin. Oncol.* **10,** 1284–1291.
8. Buzdar AU, Hortobagyi GN, Frye D, et al (1994) Bioequivalence of 10-mg once-daily tamoxifen relative to 10-mg twice-daily tamoxifen regimens for breast cancer. *J. Clin. Oncol.* **12,** 50–54.
9. Hayes DF, Van Zyl JA, Hacking A, et al (1995) Randomized comparison of tamoxifen and two separate doses of toremifine in postmenopausal patients with metastatic breast cancer. *J. Clin. Oncol.* **13,** 2556–2566.
10. Vogel CL, Shemano I, Schoenfelder J, et al (1993) Multicenter phase II efficacy trial of toremifine in tamoxifen-refractory patients with advanced breast cancer. *J. Clin. Oncol.* **11,** 345–350.
11. Lipton A, Santen RJ, (1973) Medical adrenalectomy using aminoglutethamide and dexamethasone in advanced breast cancer. *Cancer* **33,** 503–512.
12. Jonat W, Howell A, Blomqvist C, et al (1996) A randomized trial comparing two doses of the new selective aromatase inhibitor anastrozole (Arimidex) with megestrol acetate in postmenopausal patients with advanced breast cancer. *Eur. J. Cancer* **32A,** 404–412.
13. Howell A, Buzdar A, Jonat W, et al (1997) Significantly improved survival with 'Arimidex' (anastrozole (AN)) compared with megestrol acetate (MA) in postmenopausal women with advanced breast cancer (ABC): updated results of two randomixed trials. *Breast Cancer Res. Treat.* **46,** 27.
14. Dombernowsky P, Smith I, Falkson G, et al (1998) Letrozole, a new oral aromatase inhibitor for advanced breast cancer: double-blind randomized trial showing a dose effect and improved efficacy and tolerability compared with megestrol acetate. *J. Clin. Oncol.* **16,** 453–461.

15. Kaufman M, Bajetta L, Fein L, et al (2000) Exemestane is superior to megestrol acetate after tamoxifen failure in postmenopausal women with advanced breast cancer: results of a phase III randomized double-blind trial. *J. Clin. Oncol.* **18,** 1399–1411.

16. Lonning P, Bajetta E, Murray R, et al (2000) Activity of exemestane in metastatic breast cancer after failure of nonsteroidal aromatase inhibitors: a phase III trial. *J. Clin. Oncol.* **18,** 2234–2244.

17. Muss HB, Paschold EH, Black WR, et al (1985) Megestrol acetate v tamoxifen in advanced breast cancer: a phase III trial of the Piedmont Oncology Association (POA). *Sem. Oncol.* **XII,** 55–61.

18. Muss HB, Case DL, Atkins JN, et al (1994) Tamoxifen versus high-dose oral medroxyprogesterone acetate as initial endocrine therapy for patients with metastatic breast cancer. *J. Clin. Oncol.* **12,** 1630–1638.

19. Bonneterre J, Thurliman B, Robertson J, et al (2000) Anastrozole versus tamoxifen as first-line therapy for advanced breast cancer in 668 postmenopausal women: results of the tamoxifen or arimidex randomized group efficacy and tolerability study. *J. Clin. Oncol.* **18,** 3748–3757.

20. Nabholz J, Buzdar A, Pollak M, et al (2000) Anastrozole is superior to tamoxifen as first-line therapy for advanced breast cancer in postmenopausal women: results of a North American multicenter randomized trial. *J. Clin. Oncol.* **18,** 3758–3767.

21. Mourisden H, Gershanovich M, Sun Y, et al (2001) Superior efficacy of letrozole versus tamoxifen as first-line therapy for postmenopausal women with advanced breast cancer: results of a phase III study of the international letrozole breast cancer group. *J. Clin. Oncol.* **19,** 2596–2606.

22. Mourisden H, Sun Y, Gershanovich M, et al (2001) Final survival analysis of the double-blind, randomized multinational phase III trial of letrozole (Femara) compared to tamoxifen as first-line therapy for advanced breast cancer. *Breast Cancer Res Treat* **69,** 211.

23. Buzdar A, Jonat W, Howell A, et al (1996) Anastrozole, a potent and selective aromatase inhibitor, versus megestrol acetate in postmenopausal women with advanced breast cancer: results of overview analysis of two phase III trials. *J. Clin. Oncol.* **14,** 2000–2011.

24. Kaufmann M, Jonat W, Kleeberg U, et al (1989) Goserelin, a depot gonadotrophin-releasing hormone agonist in the treatment of premenopausal patients with metastatic breast cancer. *J. Clin. Oncol.* **7,** 1113–1119.

25. Taylor CW, Green S, Dalton WS, et al (1998) Multicenter randomized clinical trial of goserelin versus surgical ovariectomy in premenopausal patients with receptor-positive metastatic breast cancer: an intergroup study. *J. Clin. Oncol.* **16,** 994–999.

26. Buchanan RB, Blamey RW, Durrant KR, et al (1986) A randomized comparison of tamoxifen with surgical oophorectomy in premenopausal patients with advanced breast cancer. *J. Clin. Oncol.* **4,** 1326–1330.

27. Martoni A, Longhi A, Canova N, et al (1991) High-dose medroxyprogesterone acetate versus oophorectomy as first-line therapy of advanced breast cancer in premenopausal patients. *Oncol.* **48,** 1–6.

28. Klijn JG, Beex LV, Mauriac L, et al (2000) Combined treatment with buserelin and tamoxifen in premenepausal metastatic breast cancer: a randomized study. *J. Nat. Cancer Inst.* **92,** 903–911.

29. Patey DH, Nabarro JDN, (1970) Early ("prophylactic") oophorectomy and adrenalectomy in carcinoma of the breast: a ten-year follow-up. *Br. J. Cancer* **24,** 16–21.

30. Early Breast Cancer Trialists' Collaborative Group (1992) Systemic treatment of early breast cancer by hormonal, cytotoxic, or immune therapy. *Lancet* **339,** 1–15,71–85.

31. Early Breast Cancer Trialists' Collaborative Group (1998) Tamoxifen for early breast cancer: an overview of the randomixed trials. *Lancet* **351,** 1451–1467.

32. Fisher B, Dignam J, Bryant J, et al (1996) Five versus more than five years of tamoxifen therapy for breast cancer patients with negative lymph nodes and estrogen receptor-positive tumors. *J. Nat. Cancer Inst.* **88,** 1529–1541.

33. Fisher B, Redmond C, Legault-Poisson S, et al (1990) Postoperative chemotherapy and tamoxifen compared with tamoxifen alone in the treatment of positive-node breast cancer patients aged 50 years and older with tumors responsive to tamoxifen: results from the National Surgical Adjuvant Breast and Bowel Project B-16. *J. Clin. Oncol.* **8,** 1005–1018.

34. Fisher B, Dignam J, Wolmark N, et al (1997) Tamoxifen and chemotherapy for lymph node-negative, estrogen receptor-positive breast cancer. *J. Nat Can. Inst.* **89,** 1673–1682.

35. Carlomagno C, Perrone F, Gallo C, et al (1996) c-erbB2 overexpression decreases the beneifit of adjuvant tamoxifen in early-stage breast cancer without axillary lymph node metastases. *J. Clin. Oncol.* **14,** 2702–2708.

36. Ravdin PM, Green S, Albain KS, et al (1998) Initial report of the SWOG biological correlative study of c-erb-2 expression as a predictor of outcome in a trial comparing adjuvant CAF T with tamoxifen (T) alone. *Proc. ASCO* **17,** 97a.

37. Wolmark N, Dignam J, Fisher B, (1990) The addition of tamoxifen to lumpectomy and radiotherapy in the treatment of ductal carcinoma in situ (DCIS): preliminary results of NSABP protocol B-24. *Breast Cancer Research and Treatment* **50,** 227 (abst).

38. Ragaz J, Coldman A, (1998) Survival impact of adjuvant tamoxifen on competing causes of mortality in breast cancer survivaors, with analysis of mortality from contralateral breast cancer, cardiovascular events, endometrial cancer, and thromboembolic episodes. *J. Clin. Oncol.* **16,** 2018–29024.

39. Mamounas EP, Bryant J, Fisher B, et al (1998) Primary breast cancer (PBC) as a risk factor for subsequent contralateral breast cancer (CBC): NSABP experience from nine randomized adjuvant trials. *Breast Cancer Res. Treat.* **50,** 230 (abst).

40. Fisher B, Costantino JP, Wickerham DL, et al (1998) Tamoxifen for prevention of breast cancer: report of the National Surgical Adjvuant Breast and Bowel Project P-1 Study. *J. Natl. Cancer Inst.* **90,** 1371–1388.

41. Veronesi U, Maisonneuve P, Costa A, et al (1998) Prevention of breast cancer with tamoxifen: preliminary findings from the italian randomised trial among hysterectomised women. *Lancet* **352,** 93–97.

42. Powles T, Eeles R, Ashley S, et al (1998) Interim analysis of the incidence of breast cancer in the royal marsden hospital tamoxifen randomised chemoprevention trial. *Lancet* **352,** 98–101.

43. Cummings SR, Norton L, Eckert S, et al (1998) Raloxifene reduces the risk of breast cancer and may decrease the risk of endometrial cancer in post-menopausal women. Two-year findings from the Multiple Outcomes of Raloxifene Evaluation (MORE) Trial. *Proc. Am. Soc. Hematol.* **17,** 2a.

11 The Role of Surgery for Metastatic Breast Cancer

Lori Jardines, MD

x

CONTENTS

INTRODUCTION
MANAGEMENT OF PULMONARY METASTASES
MANAGEMENT OF DISCRETE LIVER METASTASES
MANAGEMENT OF BRAIN METASTASES
CONCLUSIONS
REFERENCES

1. INTRODUCTION

Breast cancer affects approximately 180,000 women annually in the United States. Despite advances in therapy, 20–30% of women who have been treated for localized breast cancer will develop metastatic disease, for which there is little chance for cure. However, a small, select group of patients with breast cancer who have isolated, distant disease are candidates for surgical resection and potential cure. In addition, surgery for palliation may also be indicated when a patient has metastatic breast cancer and symptoms that cannot be managed by other modalities. The role of surgery for breast cancer metastases to the lung, liver, and brain is discussed here in detail.

2. MANAGEMENT OF PULMONARY METASTASES

In 15–25% of patients with metastatic breast cancer, the lung is the first site of recurrence *(1)*. When a patient presents with a pulmonary nodule and a history of breast cancer, the differential diagnosis includes metastatic breast cancer, primary lung cancer, and benign causes of pulmonary nodules such as granulomas or hamartomas *(2,3)*. A single pulmonary nodule in a woman with a history of breast cancer is most likely secondary to a primary lung cancer. In a study by Cahan et al. *(4)*, 78 women with a diagnosis of breast cancer were evaluated for a solitary lung mass; over half were found to have lung cancer, and six were found to have benign disease.

Between 75 and 90% of patients presenting with pulmonary metastases are asymptomatic *(2)*. Therefore, the diagnosis is most often made on a routine imaging study. In most instances, the metastatic foci are peripheral in the lung *(2)*. When pulmonary metastatic disease is symptomatic, it may present as cough, shortness of breath, wheezing, or chest pain.

From: *Current Clinical Oncology:*
Breast Cancer: A Guide to Detection and Multidisciplinary Therapy
Edited by: M. H. Torosian © Humana Press Inc., Totowa, NJ

Therefore, a patient presenting with a history of breast cancer and a solitary lung nodule should first be evaluated with a chest computed tomography (CT) scan. If the mass has benign features on CT scan that suggest a granuloma, it requires no further intervention *(3)*. Positron emission tomography may be helpful in distinguishing metastatic disease from a primary lung neoplasm *(2)*. However, when the CT scan suggests a malignant process, the study can evaluate the extent of disease and can identify other small pulmonary nodules that were not visible on the chest radiograph, the presence of pleural disease or pleural effusions, and the status of the mediastinal lymph nodes. High-resolution CT scanning can identify lesions as small as 1–2 mm *(2)*. The patient should also undergo a complete metastatic evaluation including a CT scan of the abdomen to evaluate the liver and adrenal glands as well as a bone scan.

For patients with a suspicious solitary pulmonary nodule or an indeterminate nodule, surgery is the most reliable approach for making a diagnosis *(3)*. With the advent of video-assisted thoracoscopic surgery (VATS), the surgery is much less invasive than a formal thoracotomy *(5)*. This procedure can provide a significant amount of information since the pleural surfaces can be evaluated, small amounts of pleural fluid can be obtained for cytology, and mediastinal lymph nodes can be evaluated at the same time the lung nodule is resected. A transthoracic needle biopsy is another option whereby cytology material is obtained percutaneously under fluoroscopic or CT scan guidance *(2,3)*. This technique is limited since the false-negative rate is significant and needle aspiration cytology results can differ from the surgical specimen in over 30% of cases *(3)*. The major complication is pnemothorax, occurring in 10% of cases *(3)*.

When a patient with breast cancer is found to have a primary lung cancer and there is no other evidence of disease, the lung cancer should be treated aggressively. If the patient is found to have a solitary focus of metastatic breast cancer, some data suggest that surgical resection may improve survival. Lanza et al. *(6)* reported on 44 patients with breast cancer who underwent thoractomy and resection of pulmonary nodules. Three patients were found to have benign disease. Thirty seven patients with metastatic breast cancer underwent complete resection of all clinically evident disease. Most of the patients were treated by wedge resection. Thirty percent of those who underwent complete resection were disease-free at a mean of 49.2 months after resection. When disease recurred, it was most often disseminated or in locations not amenable to resection. Factors associated with improved outcome after thoracotomy were an initial disease-free interval of 1 year or longer and the presence of estrogen receptor-positive disease. Patients who underwent resection of a single pulmonary nodule had a survival advantage over patients who had two or more nodules resected, but this difference was not statistically significant. There were no operative deaths and minimal morbidity.

Staren et al. *(7)* compared outcome in patients with pulmonary metastases who were treated surgically verses medically. Some of the patients treated by surgery were also given adjuvant systemic therapy. Single nodules were diagnosed in 27 patients in the surgical group and in 20 patients in the medical group. Multiple nodules were seen in 6 patients in the surgical group and 10 patients in the medical group. Patients in the surgery group were treated by either surgery alone, surgery and adjuvant systemic therapy, or surgery and adjuvant radiotherapy. Outcome was not related to the number of nodules resected, the extent of the resection, estrogen receptor (ER) status, or disease-free interval. Patients in the medical group received systemic hormonal therapy and/or chemotherapy with or without radiation therapy. The 5-year survival was significantly longer in the group treated by surgery compared with the medically treated group (36 verses 11%). Many of the patients in the medical group were diagnosed by cytology, which can have a higher error rate in diagnosis. This might adversely affect the ability to compare outcomes between the medical and surgical groups.

Freidel et al. *(8)* reported on a group of 91 patients with breast cancer and isolated pulmonary metastases who underwent resection. Approximately three-fourths of the patients underwent limited resections. There were no operative deaths, and morbidity was minimal. Factors associated with outcome were completeness of resection, disease-free interval, ER status of the primary tumor, and number of pulmonary metastases. Patients who underwent complete resection had a 5-year survival of 31%. Patients with an initial disease-free interval of 2 years of longer had a 33% 5-year survival. Patients who underwent resection of a single metastatic pulmonary nodule had a 5-year survival of 35%, and no patients with more than five metastatic foci were alive beyond 3 years. No benefit was seen with the administration of adjuvant systemic therapy; however, during the time of the study there was no standard regimen.

3. MANAGEMENT OF DISCRETE LIVER METASTASES

Liver metastases are eventually found in 55–75% of patients with metastatic breast cancer *(9)*. Approximately 20% of patients with breast cancer will succumb to liver failure associated with metastatic disease *(9,10)*. The liver is an uncommon site for solitary, initial metastatic disease, which is seen in only 3–9% of patients *(9,11)*. Cytotoxic chemotherapy for the control of hepatic metastases does not offer long-term survival. In addition, liver metastases are not responsive to hormonal therapy *(12)*. A small percentage of these patients have disease that is localized and amenable to resection, therefore possibly achieving long-term survival *(10)*.

Most patients with a history of breast cancer who present with isolated liver metastases are asymptomatic, and the disease is detected by elevation of liver enzymes on routine screening liver function tests. These findings then lead to either a CT scan or magnetic resonance imaging (MRI) of the abdomen to evaluate the liver further *(10)*. When minimal liver metastases are identified and the patient is a potential candidate for exploration and possible resection, a thorough evaluation is indicated to ensure there are no other sites of distant disease. The patient should undergo a CT scan of the chest, abdomen and pelvis along with a bone scan. If there is no evidence of pulmonary, pleural, or abdominal extrahepatic disease or bone disease, the patient may be a candidate for resection.

In 1991 Elias et al. *(13)* published their initial study including 12 patients who had undergone hepatic resection for metastases from breast cancer. The study was subsequently updated in 1995 when 32 patients underwent exploratory laparotomy for isolated liver metastases with a plan for resection *(14)*. Six of the patients were found to have diffuse metastatic disease at exploration and were not candidates for resection. In five patients, benign hepatic lesions were identified at laparotomy. The remaining 21 patients underwent liver resection and sampling of perihepatic lymph nodes. Nineteen patients undergoing resection received preoperative chemotherapy, and 12 received postoperative chemotherapy. Twelve patients underwent major liver resection. There were no operative deaths in the entire surgical group, and the morbidity was minimal. Thirteen patients had a single focus of disease, and eight patients had multiple sites within the liver. Twenty-four percent had positive hepatic lymph nodes. Two patients underwent a second liver resection at 16 and 12 months after the first resection for recurrent, isolated liver metastases. From the time of liver resection, median survival for the entire group was 26 months, with a 5-year survival rate of

9%. After resection, the site of first recurrence was in the liver for nine patients, with a mean time to recurrence of 15.9 months. For the other patients, the first site of recurrence was the brain ($n = 3$) or bone ($n = 1$) or disseminated at multiple sites ($n = 3$). The authors did not particularly recommend hepatic resection for liver metastases secondary to breast cancer since it serves mainly as a cytoreductive procedure and its efficacy is hampered by the limitations of available chemotherapy.

Raab et al. *(12)* reported on 34 patients with metastatic breast cancer confined to the liver. The median age at the time of surgery was 47 years, and the median time interval between primary breast surgery and liver resection was 27.3 months (range 8.5–197 months). Nearly 60% of the patients had a solitary metastatic focus within the liver. In 30 patients, the resection was felt to be curative. Two patients had undergone a prior resection at an outside institution and underwent a second resection with Raab's group. One of these patients underwent a third liver resection for recurrent isolated hepatic metastases. Surgical complications included bile leak (seven patients), postoperative bleeding (two patients), and infection (one patient). There was one death postoperatively. Two patients received adjuvant regional chemotherapy. The median survival for all patients was 27 months, and the 5-year survival was 18%. For those patients who underwent a potentially curative resection, the median survival was 41.5 months, and the 5-year survival was 22%. Patients who underwent palliative resection had a median survival of 5 months with a maximum survival of 20 months. The authors commented on two patients with extensive liver disease who underwent resection and survived for 5 years without evidence of recurrence.

Schneebaum et al. *(9)* compared systemic chemotherapy with regional therapy in the treatment of isolated liver metastases secondary to breast cancer. The median survival for patients treated with systemic chemotherapy was 5 months. Within the group receiving regional chemotherapy, 12 received regional chemotherapy alone since they were unresectable at the time of exploration, 5 underwent resection and regional chemotherapy, and 1 underwent resection alone. The median survival for patients treated regionally by surgery was 42 months and by chemotherapy 25 months. There were no operative deaths, and the postoperative morbidity was minimal, primarily associated with catheter complications. This is a small, very select group of patients; however, resection and regional chemotherapy may improve survival in resectable patients with liver metastases secondary to breast cancer.

Recently, cryosurgery has been used to treat hepatic metastases from breast cancer in a small group of patients *(15)*. No deaths were associated with the procedure, and morbidity was minimal. Further research is necessary to determine whether this is a useful technique in the treatment of this uncommon problem.

4. MANAGEMENT OF BRAIN METASTASES

Breast cancer commonly metastasizes to the brain and is second only to lung cancer as the most common cause of metastatic disease to the brain *(16)*. The incidence of clinically apparent brain metastasis ranges from approximately 6 to 16% (17–19). In autopsy series, this range increases to 18–30% *(16,20)*. Infiltrating ductal carcinoma is more likely to metastasize to the brain than infiltrating lobular cancer *(21)*. In addition, brain metastases are more commonly seen in women with premenopausal breast cancer *(22,23),* and in patients whose tumors are ER-negative *(24)*.

Brain metastases secondary to breast cancer are frequently solitary *(23,25)*. However, with the more widespread use of MRI, small additional foci of brain metastases are being identified *(16)*. Brain metastases are commonly seen in patients with widespread disease;

however, up to 30% will have no other site of disease *(23)*. It is important to distinguish patients with single brain metastasis regardless of the presence of extracranial disease and patients with solitary brain metastases who have no other sites of metastatic disease *(16)*.

The most common signs and symptoms of brain metastases are headache, weakness, mental status changes, seizures, ataxia, sensory disturbance, papilledema, and speech problems. Rarely, brain metastases are detected in an asymptomatic patient who is undergoing a routine screening study *(25)*. Patients with breast cancer who present with neurologic symptoms should be evaluated with contrast-enhanced MRI scan. The most common location for brain metastases is below the junction of the gray and white matter *(26)*.

A dural-based mass in a patient with breast cancer could be secondary to either a metastasis to the brain or a meningioma *(26)*. When a patient with breast cancer has multiple brain lesions, the diagnosis is most consistent with metastatic disease. When only one brain lesion is visualized, other causes, such as a primary brain tumor or infectious etiologies, must be ruled out *(27)*. Such patients will often require biopsy to establish the diagnosis. A study by Patchell et al. *(27)* revealed that 11% of patients with a history of cancer who presented with a single brain mass did not have metastatic disease but instead had a primary brain tumor.

Without treatment, patients with untreated brain metastases have a median survival of 2–8 weeks *(28,29)*. Patients with breast cancer who have brain metastases treated with whole brain irradiation have a median survival of 12–16 weeks *(17,30–33)*. Treatment has been directed toward the relief of symptoms and the prevention of progressive disease. Whole brain irradiation combined with chemotherapy or hormonal therapy has traditionally been used to treat patients with brain metastases secondary to breast cancer. There is some evidence that chemotherapeutic agents cross the blood-brain barrier and are useful in controlling intracranial disease *(34)*. With improvements in surgical technique, there may be a role for surgery in the management of brain metastases secondary to breast cancer to relieve neurologic symptoms and prolong life *(23,25,27,35)*.

Patchell et al. *(27)* reported on a group of 48 patients who had a prior history of cancer and presented with solitary metastases to the brain. Most of these patients had nonbreast primary lesions. All patients underwent brain biopsy to establish the diagnosis of metastatic cancer. Twenty-five patients were randomized to surgery followed by radiation therapy, and 23 were randomized to receive radiation alone. Patients who had undergone radiation therapy alone had a median survival of 15 weeks, whereas patients treated by surgery and radiotherapy had a median survival of 40 weeks. In addition, the patients treated by both modalities remained functionally independent and had an improved quality of life for a significantly longer period. The local control rate was improved in patients who had undergone surgical resection and radiotherapy. Operative mortality and morbidity rates were 4 and 8%, respectively. In patients treated with radiation therapy, the 30-day mortality rate was 4%, and the 30-day morbidity rate was 17%.

Wronski et al. *(25)* reported on a group of 70 patients with primary breast cancer and metastatic disease to the brain who were treated by surgical resection. The median age at diagnosis of breast cancer was 46 years, and the median age at diagnosis of brain metastasis was 50 years. Ninety-seven percent of patients presented with metachronous brain metastases, and 3% had a synchronous presentation of their breast primary and brain lesions. Four patients presented with stage IV disease, and two were inoperable at the time of presentation of the primary tumor. Multiple brain metastases were identified in 23% of patients. Nearly 90% of patients received postoperative radiotherapy. There were four postoperative deaths, and morbidity was minimal. Over half of the patients died from neurologic causes, and 30% died from systemic disease. The median survival was approximately 14 months.

Fifteen patients received whole brain irradiation preoperatively and were referred for surgery owing to lack of response or recurrence. These patients had a median survival of 6.3 months compared with a median survival of 15.8 months for patients who received radiation therapy postoperatively. There was no statistical difference in survival for patients who underwent resection of a single versus multiple metastatic foci. By the end of the study, five patients were alive at 32, 55, 73, 101, and 120 months after craniotomy, respectively.

Pieper et al. *(23)* retrospectively reported on a group of 63 patients with breast cancer who underwent resection of nonrecurrent brain metastases. None of the patients were treated with preoperative radiation therapy. The median age at presentation of the brain metastases was 50 years. In nearly 30% of the patients, the brain was the first site of relapse. Eighty-seven percent of patients presented with a single metastatic site of disease in the brain. In 85% of the patients, a complete resection was accomplished. Fifty-four patients were treated with postoperative whole brain irradiation, and 21 of these patients did not receive chemotherapy. Thirty-five patients received postoperative chemotherapy. There were 3 deaths within the first 30 days after surgery; however, these patients died from progressive systemic disease. Twenty-four patients died from systemic disease, 20 died from neurologic causes, and 4 died from both systemic and neurologic disease. Patients with multiple brain metastases had a diminished survival compared with patients who had a single focus of disease. The use of postoperative radiation therapy was associated with an improved survival. The overall median survival was 16 months, and 3- and 5-year survival rates were 22 and 17%, respectively.

A report from Salvati et al. *(36)* identified 34 patients with breast cancer who developed a single brain metastasis. Nine underwent resection alone, and the remainder were treated by surgery and radiation therapy. All patients underwent gross removal of the brain lesion. The mean survival for patients treated by both modalities was 28 months, whereas the mean survival for patients treated by surgery alone was 15 months.

There are conflicting reports as to whether patients with multiple brain metastases benefit from surgical resection. Hazuka et al. *(37)* reported on a group of 18 patients with multiple brain metastases and a group of 28 patients with a single brain metastasis who underwent resection and radiation therapy. The median survival for the patients with multiple metastases was 5 months, whereas the median survival for patients with a single metastasis was 12 months. Bindal et al. *(38)* and Wronski et al. *(25)* reported on surgical resection in patients with multiple brain metastases. Both groups found no significant difference in outcome in patients with single versus multiple brain metastases treated by resection. These results are conflicting, and it is not clear whether patients with multiple brain metastases benefit from resection. The morbidity and mortality observed for patients in both studies was low; therefore, from a technical standpoint, it is possible to resect multiple brain metastases. Patients who present with multiple brain metastases with a large symptomatic lesion should be considered for surgical resection followed by whole brain irradiation.

5. CONCLUSIONS

The role of surgery for patients with metastatic breast cancer is limited. However, there is clearly a role for surgical intervention in a select patient population. Resection of limited metastatic disease can prolong duration of life and improve quality of life. In some instances, patients have sustained significant disease-free intervals.

Patients who have isolated, minimal pulmonary metastatic disease are a select patient population. Based on data from retrospective studies, these patients may achieve long disease-free intervals and possible cure with aggressive treatment. With the advent of VATS, there is a minimally invasive method to perform wedge and segmental resections, although lobectomies can also be performed using this technology. Patients who benefit the most from metastasectomy are those with a prolonged initial disease-free interval, minimal metastatic pulmonary nodules, and ER-positive disease. There may be a role for adjuvant systemic therapy and radiotherapy post resection.

Isolated liver metastases secondary to breast cancer are uncommon. The presence of multiple liver metastases precludes aggressive surgical therapy such as hepatic resection, and these are best treated with systemic or regional cytotoxic chemotherapy. Patients who might benefit from liver resection are those with a solitary hepatic metastasis and a long disease-free interval between the time of initial diagnosis and the identification of metastatic disease. The addition of systemic and/or regional chemotherapy to resection may improve outcome and potentially cure some patients of their disease. The role of cryosurgery for the treatment of hepatic metastases requires further study.

Patients with solitary brain metastases secondary to breast cancer appear to benefit from resection followed by whole brain irradiation. The addition of systemic therapy to local treatment to improve survival is not well defined and deserves further investigation. Patients with multiple brain metastases and a large symptomatic lesion should be considered for resection of the symptomatic metastatic site followed by whole brain radiation. The role of surgery for patients with multiple brain lesions is controversial.

REFERENCES

1. Friedel G, Linder A, Toomes H (1994) The significance of prognostic factors for the resection of pulmonary metastases of breast cancer. *Thorac. Cardiovasc. Surg.* **42,** 71–75.
2. Greelish JP, Freidberg JS (2000) Secondary pulmonary malignancy. *Surgi. Clin. North Am.* **80,** 633–657.
3. Mentzer SJ, Sugarbaker DJ (2000) Management of discrete pulmonary nodules. In: Harris J (ed.), *Disease of the Breast.* Lippincott Williams and Wilkins, Philadelphia, PA, pp. 901–905.
4. Cahan WG, Castro EB, Huvos AG (1974) Primary breast cancer and lung carcinoma in the same patient. *J. Thorac. Cardiovasc. Surg.* **68,** 546–550.
5. DeCamp M Jr, Jaklitsch M, Mentzer SJ, et al. (1995) The safety and versatility of video-thoracoscopy: a prospective analysis of 895 consecutive cases. *J. Am. Coll. Surg.* **181,** 113–120.
6. Lanza L, Natarajan G, Roth JA, Putnam JB (1992) Long-term survival after resection of pulmonary metastases from carcinoma of the breast. *Ann. Thorac. Surg.* **54,** 244–248.
7. Staren E, Salerno C, Rongione A, et al. (1992) Pulmonary resection for metastatic breast cancer. *Arch. Surg.* **127,** 1282–1284.
8. Freidel G, Toomes H (1994) The significance of prognostic factors for the resection of pulmonary metastases from breast cancer. *Thorac. Cardiovasc. Surg.* **42,** 71–75.
9. Schneebaum S, Walker MJ, Young D, et al. (1994) The regional treatment of liver metastases from breast cancer. *J. Surg. Oncol.* **55,** 26–32.
10. Talamonti MS (2000) Management of discrete liver metastasis. In: Harris J (ed.), *Diseases of the Breast.* Lippincott Williams and Wilkins, Philadelphia, PA, pp. 907–910.
11. Jardines L, Callans LS, Torosian M (1993) Recurrent breast cancer: presentation, diagnosis, and treatment. *Semin. Oncol.* **20,** 538–547.
12. Raab R, Nussbaum K-T, Behend M, et al. (1998) Liver metastases of breast cancer: results of liver resection. *Anticancer Res.* **18,** 2231–2234.
13. Elias D, Lasser P, Spielman M, et al. (1991) Surgical and chemotherapeutic treatment of hepatic metastases from carcinoma of the breast. *Surg. Gynecol. Obstet.* **172,** 461–464.
14. Elias D, Lasser PH, Montrucolli D, et al. (1995) Hepatectomy for liver metastases from breast cancer. *Eur. J. Surg. Oncol.* **21,** 510–513.
15. Bilchik AJ, Sarantou T, Wardlaw JC, Ramming KP (1997) Cryosurgery causes a profound reduction in tumor markers in hepatoma and non-colorectal hepatic metastases. *Am. Surg.* **63,** 796–800.
16. Wen PY, Shafman TD (2000) Brain metastases. In: Harris J (ed.), *Diseases of the Breast.* Lippincott Williams and Wilkins, Philadelphia, PA, pp. 841–853.

17. DiStefano A, Yap HY, Hortobgyi GN, et al. (1979) The natural history of breast cancer patients: with brain metastasis. *Cancer* **44,** 1913–1918.

18. Lee Y-TN (1985) Patterns of metastasis and natural course of breast carcinoma. *Cancer Metastasis Rev.* **4,** 153–172.

19. Posner JB, Chernik NL (1978) Intracranial metastases from systemic cancer. *Adv. Neurol.* **19,** 579–592.

20. Tsukada Y, Fouad A, Pickren JW, et al. (1983) Central nervous system metastasis from breast carcinoma: autopsy study. *Cancer* **52,** 2349–2354.

21. Jain S, Fisher C, Smith P, et al. (1993) Patterns of metastatic breast cancer in relation to histological type. *Eur. J. Cancer* **29,** 2155–2157.

22. Sparrow GEA, Rubens RD (1981) Brain metastases from breast cancer: clinical course, prognosis, and influence on treatment. *Clin. Oncol.* **7,** 291–297.

23. Pieper DR, Hess KR, Sawaya RA (1997) Role of surgery in the treatment of brain metastases in patients with breast cancer. *Ann. Surg. Oncol.* **4,** 481–490.

24. Stewart JF, King RJ, Sexton SA, et al. (1981) Oestrogen receptors, sites of metastatic disease and survival in recurrent breast cancer. *Eur. J. Cancer Clin. Oncol.* **17,** 449–454.

25. Wronski M, Ehud A, McCormick B (1997) Surgical treatment of 70 patients with brain metastases from breast carcinoma. *Cancer* **80,** 1746–1754.

26. Wen PY, Loeffler JS (1999) Management of brain metastases. *Oncology* **13,** 941–966.

27. Patchell RA, Tibbs PA, Walsh JW, et al. (1990) A randomized trial of surgery in the treatment of single metastases to the brain. *N. Engl. J. Med.* **322,** 494–500.

28. Boogerd W, Vos VW, Hart AA, Baris G (1993) Brain metastases in breast cancer: natural history, prognostic factors and outcome. *J. Neurooncol.* **13,** 165–174.

29. Lang EF, Slater J (1964) Metastatic brain tumor: results of surgical and non surgical treatment. *Surg. Clin. North Am.* **44,** 865–872.

30. Cairncross JG, Kim J-H, Poner JB (1980) Radiation therapy for brain metastases. *Ann. Neurol.* **7,** 529–541.

31. Zinn S, Wampler GL, Stablein D, et al. (1981) Intracerebral metastases in solid tumor patients: natural history and results of treatment. *Cancer* **48,** 384–394.

32. Kamby C, Soerenson PS (1988) Characteristics of patients with short and long survivals after detection of intracranial metastases from breast cancer. *J. Neurooncol.* **6,** 37–45.

33. West J, Maor M (1980) Intracranial metastases: behavioral patterns related to primary site and results of treatment by whole brain irradiation. *Int. J. Radiat. Oncol. Biol. Phys.* **6,** 111–115.

34. Rosner D, Nemoto T, Lane WW (1986) Chemotherapy induces regression of brain metastases in breast cancer patients: update study. *Cancer* **58,** 832–840.

35. Sause WT, Crowley JJ, Morantz R, et al. (1990) Solitary brain metastasis: results of an RTOG/SWOG protocol evaluation of surgery + RT versus RT alone. *Am. J. Clin. Oncol.* **13,** 427–432.

36. Salvati M, Capoccia G, Orlando ER, et al. (1992) Single brain metastases from breast cancer: remarks on clinical pattern and treatment. *Tumori* **78,** 115–117.

37. Hazuka MB, Burlson W, Stroud DN, et al. (1993) Multiple brain metastases are associated with poor survival in patients treated with surgery and radiotherapy. *J. Clin. Oncol.* **11,** 369–375.

38. Bindal RK, Sawaya R, Leavens ME, et al. (1993) Surgical treatment of multiple brain metastases. *J. Neurosurg.* **79,** 210–215.

12 Male Breast Cancer

Mahmoud El-Tamer MD, FACS,
and Lucy J. Kim, MD

CONTENTS

INTRODUCTION
PREVALENCE
RISK FACTORS
PRESENTATION AND WORKUP
HISTOLOGY
TREATMENT
PROGNOSIS
CONCLUSIONS
BIBLIOGRAPHY

1. INTRODUCTION

Male breast cancer is an uncommon disease, and much of our knowledge has been gained through multiple retrospective studies. What is encouraging is that the conclusions drawn from these studies have been largely consistent. Breast cancer treatment in men has been mostly guided by studies in women. These guidelines have been established owing to the similarities of disease behavior between the two genders. Because of the consistency of conclusions and similarities in the disease process, a relative consensus on how to treat male breast cancer has been generated despite the absence of randomized prospective trials in men.

2. PREVALENCE

Breast cancer accounts for less than 1% of all cancers in men and is 100-fold less frequent than in women. Over the last 10 years, for unclear reasons, there has been a gradual increase in incidence of male breast cancer in the United States. Unlike in women, the incidence of breast cancer in men does not carry a bimodal distribution but increases exponentially throughout life. Also unlike in women, breast cancer affects a predominantly older population in men with a mean age at presentation in the mid-sixties. The epidemiology of breast cancer in men corresponds to that in women with respect to geographic distribution. North America and northern Europe carry the highest incidence and Japan the lowest.

From: *Current Clinical Oncology:*
Breast Cancer: A Guide to Detection and Multidisciplinary Therapy
Edited by: M. H. Torosian © Humana Press Inc., Totowa, NJ

3. RISK FACTORS

As in women, the hormonal milieu probably plays a role in the development of breast cancer in men. One of the largest risk factors is a rare genetic abnormality, Klinefelter's syndrome, which results from the inheritance of an extra X chromosome. The risk of breast cancer is approximately 20 times higher in men with this condition. Patients with Klinefelter's syndrome usually have atrophic testes with high levels of gonadotropins but low levels of androsterone and normal to low levels of estrogen, resulting in a high estrogen-to-androgen ratio. Supporting the theory that hormones play a risk factor, male breast cancer has also been reported in hermaphrodites, in men who underwent feminizing surgery, and in men who received exogenous estrogen for the treatment of prostate cancer. Both Klinefelter's syndrome and male breast cancer are rare diseases. Hence it is unusual, even for the busy general surgeon or health practitioner, to encounter a patient with both disease processes. However, a breast lesion in a patient with Klinefelter's syndrome ought to be considered with more suspicion than in other men. It has been reported that 4% of men with breast cancer have Klinefelter's syndrome, although in most recent large series this figure has been lower.

Gynecomastia has also been suggested to be a risk factor for male breast cancer. Clinically, gynecomastia has been noted in 4–23% of patients with breast cancer. However, microscopic evidence of gynecomastia has been reported to be higher, ranging from 26.5 to 88%. It has been implied that gynecomastia and breast cancer represent different ends of the spectrum of the same disease. It has also been suggested that gynecomastia may be a premalignant lesion, although no conclusive proof exists. It is unclear whether gynecomastia predisposes to the development of cancer or whether the two diseases, breast cancer and gynecomastia, are induced by the same hormonal imbalance (estrogen/androgen). Clearly, a causal relationship has never been documented.

Other risk factors debated in the literature are liver disorders (cirrhosis and bilharziasis), testicular injury, orchitis, history of head injury with ensuing hyperprolactinemia, prostate cancer, and chest irradiation. Exposure to electromagnetic fields or exposure of the testis to heat are considered to be occupational hazards.

As in women, there appears to be a genetic influence to the development of breast cancer in men. In as high as 30% of cases and particularly in younger patients, a positive family history can be elicited in one or more first-degree relatives. Furthermore, the relative risk of a man with an affected mother or sister, compared with the general population, is 2.33 and 2.23, respectively. That risk increases if the affected relative acquired the disease at an age younger than 45 years. In addition, there also exist clusters of male family members with breast cancer.

In the past decade, germline mutations in chromosomes 17q and 13q have been associated with a high risk of developing breast cancer in women. These genetic mutations in breast cancer genes 1 and 2 (*BRCA1* and *BRCA2*) account for 5–10% of breast cancer cases in women. Men who are carriers of the mutated genes not only transmit the disease to their progeny but are at a greater risk for developing breast cancer. Men carrying the *BRCA2* mutation have a 100-fold increase in risk of developing breast cancer, with an estimated lifetime risk reaching 6%. Men who are carriers of the *BRCA1* mutation are also at a higher risk than the general population but to a lesser degree than *BRCA2* carriers.

4. PRESENTATION AND WORKUP

Men with breast cancer usually present with a breast mass (75–95%). Clinically the mass is painless, eccentric, and ill defined. The mass may be preceded by or associated with nip-

Table 1
Clinical Features Suggestive of Gynecomastia or Carcinoma

Feature	Gynecomastia	Carcinoma
Age	Young	Old
Mass	Diffuse	Localized
	Rubbery	Hard
	Centered nipple/areola	Frequently eccentric
Skin fixation	Rare	Frequent
Ulceration	None	Frequent
Nipple discharge	Infrequent	Common
Bilateral	Common	Rare

ple discharge in up to 80% of cases. Serosanguineous discharge in a man represents an ominous sign because of its association with carcinoma in 75% of cases. Because the male breast is smaller, involvement of the skin and nipple-areola complex or the underlying chest wall is more frequent than in women with breast cancer. Skin fixation and ulceration can be found in up to 44 and 13% of cases, respectively.

Frequent breast complaints for which men may seek medical advice are gynecomastia, a palpable mass, or breast pain. It is crucial to identify patients with cancer in this clinical scenario. Medical history and physical exam may be helpful in separating benign from malignant disease. Age is important, as breast cancer in men rarely affects patients younger than 40 years of age. However, gynecomastia remains the most common cause of breast masses even in older men. In a review of more than 800 breast biopsies, 96% of the findings were benign, with gynecomastia as the most common benign pathology (91%). Other benign findings included lipoma, fibrosis, and inflammatory and normal breast tissue. Medication history is important to elicit. Anabolic steroids, marijuana, cimetidine, and antipsychotic as well as some antihypertensive drugs, among others, have been associated with gynecomastia.

Clinically, patients with gynecomastia present with a diffusely enlarged and frequently tender breast, and symptoms are commonly bilateral. In contrast, patients with carcinoma have a hard palpable mass that usually only involves one breast. The presence of nipple discharge is not physiologic and is usually associated with malignancy. Evidence of skin ulceration or fixation is also highly suggestive of malignancy and mandates a biopsy. The clinical findings listed in Table 1, although not diagnostic, may be helpful in the differential diagnosis.

Mammography may aid in the diagnosis of breast cancer. The malignant mammographic findings, in order of frequency, are mass, architectural deformity, or microcalcifications. However, a false-negative mammogram is more frequent in men than in women, with an incidence of 10–20%. There is currently an emerging role for sonography as an adjunct to mammography, particularly in patients with a breast mass and a negative mammogram. Sonography may be helpful in differentiating carcinomas from gynecomastia.

Needle sampling of a breast mass can be performed with fine needle aspiration (FNA) or a core needle biopsy (CNBx). Both techniques are accessible and easy to perform. Fine needle aspiration is a cytologic test and is usually performed with a 10-mL syringe and a 22-gage needle. The reliability of an FNA depends on the experience of the institution and particularly the cytopathologist. Core needle biopsy is a histologic test and is performed percutaneously or

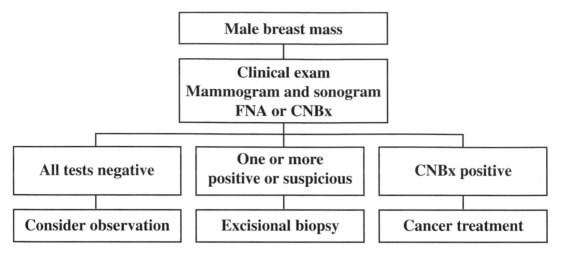

Fig. 1. Management of palpable lump in men. FNA, fine needle aspiration; CNBx, core needle biopsy.

through a 2-mm skin incision. It requires a dedicated needle and preferably a biopsy instrument. We prefer to use a 14-gage needle and usually retrieve an average of two to three cores of tissue. Both modalities are currently more utilized in the management of female breast lesions. If the pathologist reports a diagnosis of cancer by CNBx, the surgeon may proceed with definitive surgery. If the diagnosis is made by FNA, an open biopsy is advisable prior to proceeding with definitive surgery. The incidence of a false-negative test with either an FNA or CNBx varies from 3 to 10%. However, the rate of an equivocal, atypical, or inadequate specimen depends on the experience of the operator and/or cytopathologist.

The gold standard of managing a palpable breast mass in men is excisional biopsy. However, more recently, and in certain clinical situations, we have extrapolated from the management of women with breast masses by using the triple test. The triple test includes a clinical exam, a mammographic and/or sonographic evaluation, and a cytologic or histologic assessment. If all three tests are consistent with a benign process, we may observe the patient and avoid excisional biopsy, as outlined in Figure 1, particularly if the histologic and cytologic results are consistent with the clinical and radiologic findings.

5. HISTOLOGY

The male breast consists almost exclusively of ducts and has no lobular structures. The ductal cell lining is the most common source of malignant transformation in the male breast. Some experts have denied the existence of lobular carcinoma of the male breast, although rare cases have been reported. Infiltrating ductal carcinoma is the most common histology (80%). Ductal carcinoma *in situ* occurs in 5–15% of the cases. Other unusual subtypes include medullary, tubular, papillary, small cell, and mucinous carcinoma as well as Paget's disease. Medullary and papillary carcinomas appear to carry a better prognosis.

In comparison with women, malignant breast lesions in men may arise more frequently from cells other than the lining of the breast, i.e., sarcomas, lymphomas, overlying skin cancers, and metastatic prostate cancer. Therefore, it is important to rule out these lesions during the workup.

Breast cancer in men is more frequently positive for estrogen and progesterone receptors (ER and PR) than in women, with an incidence of 65–85% ER-positive and 70–80% PR-positive. This difference may be related to the older age at presentation in men. A proportion of male breast cancer seems to be associated with overexpression of *c-erbB-2* (Her-2/*neu* oncogene), which reflects an increase in proliferative activity. The importance of this is unclear, however. Male breast cancer is staged using the TNM staging system of the American Joint Committee on Cancer and the Union International Contre le Cancer. The staging system uses the same guidelines and recommendations as for women.

6. TREATMENT

6.1. Surgery

As in most solid tumors, surgical therapy is the mainstay of treatment. Classically the procedure of choice was a formal radical mastectomy. In the recent past the operative treatment has shifted to modified radical mastectomies. The shift away from radical mastectomy has not made a negative impact on prognosis. Studies have failed to detect any difference in disease recurrence or survival rates between patients treated with radical, modified radical, or simple mastectomies. Anatomically, the male breast is a small organ and usually underlies the nipple-areola complex. Malignant breast tumors in men tend to be palpable and in close proximity to the overlying skin and underlying muscle. We start the surgical resection with an elliptic skin incision that includes the skin overlying the tumor and nipple-areola complex. Flaps are raised in all directions to separate the breast from the skin and subcutaneous tissue. The specimen is usually resected *en bloc* with a segment of the pectoralis major muscle that only underlies the tumor. Resecting the pectoralis major muscle is particularly important when the tumor is invasive and in close proximity to the muscle as it allows the achievement of a widely negative surgical margin and may obviate the use of adjuvant radiation therapy. If invasion to the pectoralis muscle occurs, a radical mastectomy is strongly advised. Simple mastectomy is the procedure of choice for *in situ* breast cancer. Axillary lymph node dissection has been the standard of care in the management of male breast cancer. Level I and II axillary lymph nodes are routinely resected in continuity with the breast. Knowledge of nodal status is important in guiding further treatment. Recently sentinel lymph node biopsy has emerged as a reliable alternative to axillary node dissection in node negative patients.

The role and appropriateness of breast conservation in men is debatable. In small, uncontrolled series, favorable outcomes were reported for simple mastectomy or lumpectomy followed by radiation therapy with respect to local recurrence, survival, and morbidity. These findings were not confirmed by other studies. Many question the justification of radiation therapy for breast conservation, given that mastectomy in men does not carry the same implications as it would in women.

6.2. Radiation

The rationale for postoperative radiotherapy is based on data from female breast cancer. The use of radiation is generally reserved for locally advanced disease or tumors with extensive axillary metastasis. More recently, two prospective randomized studies from the Netherlands and Canada demonstrated a significant improvement in survival in women who received postmastectomy radiation to the chest wall. Men may benefit more from adjuvant radiation therapy, given the central topography of the tumor, the frequency of dermal and muscular involvement, and the high rate of axillary involvement. For these reasons, as well as to treat the internal mammary lymph nodes, some authors recommend the use of adjuvant radiation therapy in men. Adjuvant radiation therapy is strongly recommended for T3 and T4 lesions, for four or more positive axillary lymph nodes, and for close or involved surgical margins (<2 mm). Given the size of the male breast, margin status rather than size of the tumor is frequently the determining factor for adjuvant radiation therapy. Hence, some surgeons recommend routine resection of the pectoralis major muscle that underlies the tumor, as it allows a wider deep surgical margin and may obviate the need for postoperative radiation to the chest wall.

6.3. Hormonal Therapy

Although the role of hormonal therapy in male breast cancer has not been evaluated by prospective randomized trials, male breast cancers have a high incidence of ER and PR positivity, giving the rationale for hormonal manipulation. In the past, orchiectomy was used as the standard treatment, with a response rate close to 80%. Adrenalectomy and hypophysectomy have been long dropped from the surgical armamentarium. Tamoxifen, a selective estrogen receptor modulator, has replaced orchiectomy. This is secondary to the psychological impact and reluctance of men to accept orchiectomy. Response rates with tamoxifen have been as high as 80%. Although tamoxifen in men is generally well tolerated, it has been associated with treatment-limiting symptoms such as weight gain and loss of libido. The use of tamoxifen and orchiectomy are not exclusive of each other, and patients who fail tamoxifen may still respond to orchiectomy. Other hormonal agents are used as second- or third-line treatments and include androgens, estrogens, progestins, antiandrogens, aminoglutethimide, and luteinizing hormone-releasing hormone (LH-RH) analogs.

Adjuvant hormonal therapy has been recommended for locally advanced tumors, those with axillary involvement as well as metastatic disease. In the recent past, the use of tamoxifen, in the adjuvant setting, has expanded to include men with stage I and II breast cancer. In a nonrandomized trial, tamoxifen significantly improved the disease-free survival in this setting.

6.4. Chemotherapy

Adjuvant chemotherapy is controversial secondary to lack of prospective randomized trials and limited retrospective data. Many extrapolate from data available in women. Treatment was usually reserved for stage III and IV disease; however, recently adjuvant chemotherapy has been used in patients with node-positive stage II disease. Treatment consists of multiple courses of cyclophosphamide, methotrexate or doxorubicin, and 5-fluorourocil. For node-positive patients, adjuvant chemotherapy has resulted in 5-year survival rates in excess of 80%. However, in the metastatic setting, less than half of the patients who received chemotherapy responded, and, in those who did respond, median survival rates ranged from 4 to 23 months. Our approach to the management of breast cancer is outlined in Figure 2.

7. PROGNOSIS

It has been a common belief that men with breast cancer had a worse prognosis compared with women. Recent large series (matched for stage and number of positive nodes) have shown that men and women with breast cancer had similar survival rates. The most important prognostic factor in men with breast cancer is number of histologically positive nodes. Ten-year survival rates for patients with histologically negative nodes range from 51 to 77% whereas patients with more than four positive nodes had a 10-year survival rate ranging from 4 to 14%. The size of the primary tumor is also important. The ER and PR status of the tumor does not seem to be an important prognostic factor.

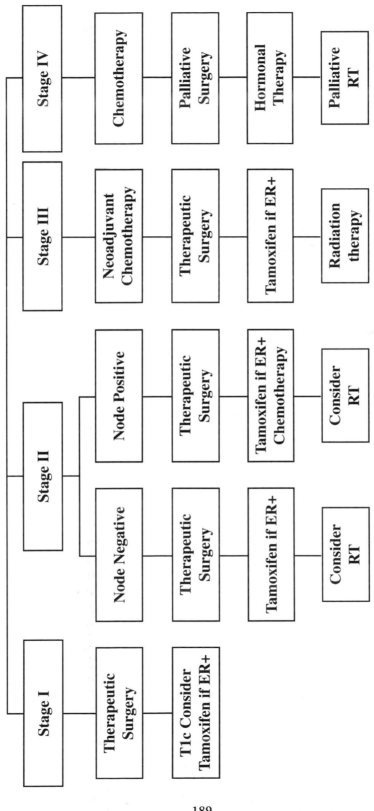

Fig. 2. Management of male breast cancer. ER, estrogen receptor; RT, radiation therapy.

Distant relapse in men seems to be similar to that in women, with bone, lung, liver, and brain as the most common sites. The incidences of systemic and locoregional failure were reported at 18–40% and 5–19%, respectively.

Because of the older age of presentation, comorbid disease frequently coexists, and often the patient dies of causes unrelated to breast cancer. In one series, 39.5% of deaths were unrelated to the cancer itself. At Columbia-Presbyterian Medical Center, 52 men were diagnosed with breast cancer over the past 18 years. Only 25% of the deaths in those men were related to breast cancer. The other causes of mortality were related to other cancers in 25% of the cases and to nonmalignant causes in the rest.

8. CONCLUSIONS

Breast cancer is an uncommon disease in men. Its diagnosis and management is influenced to a great extent by data available from the disease in women. Surgery is the mainstay of treatment, although hormonal manipulation, chemotherapy, and radiation are important adjuncts. The prognosis and outcome in men with breast cancer is similar to that in women. Hopefully, as we learn and understand more of female breast cancer, we will be able to improve survival in men with the disease.

BIBLIOGRAPHY

Anelli TFM, Anelli A, Tran KN, et al. (1994) Tamoxifen administration is associated with a high rate of treatment-limiting symptoms in male breast cancer patients. *Cancer* **74,** 74–77.

Appelqvist P, Salmo M (1982) Prognosis in carcinoma of the male breast. *Acta Chir. Scand.* **148,** 499–502.

Bagley CS, Wesley MN, Young RC, et al. (1987) Adjuvant chemotherapy in males with cancer of the breast. *Am. J. Clin. Oncol.* **10,** 55–60.

Bezwoda WR, Hesdorffer C, Dansey R, et al. (1987) Breast cancer in men: clinical features, hormone receptor status, and response to therapy. *Cancer* **60,** 1337–1340.

Borgen PI, Wong GY, Vlamis V (1992) Current management of male breast cancer. *Ann. Surg.* **215,** 451–457.

Crichlow RW (1972) Carcinoma of the male breast. *Surg. Gynecol. Obset.* **134,** 1011–1019.

Crichlow RW, Galt SW (1990) Male breast cancer. *Surg. Clin. North Am.* **70,** 1165–1177.

Cutuli B, Lacroze M, Dilhuydy JM, et al. (1995) Male breast cancer: results of the treatments and prognostic factors in 397 cases. *Eur. J. Cancer* **31A,** 1960–1964.

Gough DB, Donohue JH, Evans MM, et al. (1993) A 50-year experience of male breast cancer: is outcome changing? *Surg. Oncol.* **2,** 325–33.

Griffith H, Muggia FM (1989) Male breast cancer: update on systemic therapy. *Rev. Endocr. Rel. Cancer* **31,** 5–11.

Guinee VF, Olsson H, Moller T (1993) The prognosis of breast cancer in males: a report of 335 cases. *Cancer* **71,** 154–161.

Heller KS, Rosen PP, Schottenfeld D, et al. (1978) Male breast cancer: a clinicopathologic study of 97 cases. *Ann. Surg.* **188,** 60–65.

Hultborn R, Friberg S, Hultborn KA (1987) Male breast carcinoma: a study of the total material reported to the Swedish Cancer Registry 1958–1967 with respect to clinical and histopathologic parameters. *Acta Oncol.* **26,** 241–256.

Kinne D, Hakes T (1991) Male breast cancer. In: Harris J, Hellman S, Henderson C, et al. (eds.) *Breast Diseases.* JB Lippincott, Philadelphia, pp. 782–789.

Lilleng R, Paksoy N, Vural G, et al. (1995) Assessment of fine needle aspiration cytology and histopathology for the diagnosing male breast masses. *Acta Cytol.* **39,** 877–881.

Lipshy KA, Denning DA, Wheeler WE (1996) A statewide review of male breast carcinoma. *Contemp. Surg.* **49,** 71–75.

McLauchlan SA, Erlichman C, Liu FF, et al. (1996) Male breast cancer: an 11 year review of 66 patients. *Breast Cancer Res. Treat.* **40,** 225–230.

Memon MA, Donohue JH (1997) Male breast cancer. *Br. J. Surg.* **84,** 433–435.

Paatel HZ, Buzdar AV, Hortobagy GN (1989) Role of adjuvant chemotherapy in male breast cancer. *Cancer* **64,** 1583–1585.

Ribeiro GG (1977) Carcinoma of the male breast: a review of 200 cases. *Br. J. Surg.* **64,** 381–383.

Ribeiro GG (1983) Tamoxifen in the treatment of male breast carcinoma. *Clin. Radiol.* **34,** 625–628.

Robinson R, Montague ED (1982) Treatment results in males with breast cancer. *Cancer* **49,** 403–406.

Stierer M, Rosen H, Weitensfelder W, et al. (1995) Male breast cancer: the Austrian experience. *World J. Surg.* **19,** 687–693.

Thomas DB (1993) Breast cancer in men. *Epidemiol. Rev.* **15,** 220–231.

Tavtigian SV, Simard J, Rommens J, et al. (1996) The complete BRCA2 gene and mutation in chromosome 13q-linked kindreds. *Nat. Genet.* **12,** 333–337.

Williams WL, Powers M, Wagman LD (1996) Cancer of the male breast: a review. *J. Natl. Med. Assoc.* **88,** 439–443.

13 Oncogenes in the Development of Breast Cancer

Xiao Tan Qiao, MD, Kenneth L. van Golen, PhD, and Sofia D. Merajver, MD, PhD

CONTENTS

INTRODUCTION
HER-2/*NEU (C-ERB*B-2) ONCOGENE AND PROTEIN
BCL-2 GENE AND PROTEIN
THE *BRCA* AND *P53* TUMOR SUPPRESSOR GENES
APOPTOSIS AND ONCOGENESIS: *P53, BCL*-2,
  AND HER-2/*NEU* (C-ERBB-2)
ACKNOWLEDGMENTS
REFERENCES

1. INTRODUCTION

The diagnosis, treatment, and prevention of breast cancer are being influenced by recent advances in our understanding of the molecules implicated in tumor development and progression. The Human Genome Project will increase knowledge of the molecular determinants of breast cancer suddenly and drastically. The utilization of this knowledge in the clinic, however, will lag by a few years. It is thus important to consider the present state of knowledge of some of the key molecular markers that are presently used in the clinic to care for breast cancer patients and individuals at high risk for developing breast cancer. In this chapter, we summarize the main features of two oncogenes (*bcl2* and HER-2/*neu*) and three tumor suppressor genes (*BRCA1, BRCA2,* and *p53*). For each of these genes and gene products, we review the present knowledge of their function, with special emphasis on those aspects that have led to or supported their translation to the clinic.

2. HER-2/*neu (c-erbB-2)* ONCOGENE AND PROTEIN

The HER-1/*neu* gene's influence on cancer development was discovered in the process of researching what DNA changes were induced as normal cells were transformed into cancer cells by a carcinogen. HER-2 (*c-erbB-2* or *neu*), a protooncogene *(1)*, was identified because the DNA of rat tumor cells transformed by *N*-ethyl-*N*-nitrosourea induced transformation of mouse embryo fibroblast NIH3T3 cells *(2)*. Specifically, they induced fibrosarcomas when injected into nude mice. Working independently, researchers found

From: *Current Clinical Oncology:*
Breast Cancer: A Guide to Detection and Multidisciplinary Therapy
Edited by: M. H. Torosian © Humana Press Inc., Totowa, NJ

the *neu* gene to be homologous to the avian erythroblastosis virus (AEV) transforming gene *v-erbB*. Later, the human homolog of the rat *neu* gene was cloned and named *c-erbB-2*, HER-2, MAC117, and NGL.

2.1. Structure and Function

The human HER-2/*neu* gene was mapped to chromosome 17q21. It contains an open reading frame of 3765 nucleotides and has a major transcript of 4.8 kb, which translates into a 1255-amino acid protein. The functional gene product of the HER-2/*neu* gene was termed *p185* in accordance with its molecular weight (185,00 Daltons); the primary translation product has a relative molecular mass of 137,895 Daltons. This difference in apparent molecular masses is owing in part to *N*-linked glycosylation. Phosphorylation has also been found to be a key modification of HER-2/*neu*-encoded protein.

The HER-2/*neu* gene sequence and its protein product are closely related to the epidermal growth factor receptor (EGFR), with which it shares an overall homology of 50%. Similar to EGFR, HER-2/*neu* is a transmembrane glycoprotein having intrinsic tyrosine kinase activity and can be grouped as a member of the growth factor receptor tyrosine kinase (RTK) gene superfamily. HER-2/*neu* is comprised of the following domains: 1) a cleaveable signal peptide sequence; 2) the extracellular ligand-binding domain, containing two cysteine-rich regions, which are important for ligand binding; 3) a transmembrane domain; and 4) the intracellular/cytoplasmic domain.

The extracellular domain of *p185* shows 44% homology with the ligand-binding domain of the EGFR. The cytoplasmic and transmembrane portion of the EGFR shows 90% homology with the erbB protein. Within the ligand-binding domain lie two cysteine-rich regions that are completely conserved between these two RTK proteins. The cytoplasmic component of HER-2/*neu* contains the tyrosine kinase domain that lies immediately inside the plasma membrane and contains an ATP binding site. This is a key region to target for small molecule drug development. Another important residue is the threonine at position 954, the location for phosphorylation mediated by protein kinase C (PKC). All the autophosphorylation sites of HER-2/*neu* reside within the carboxy-terminal tail. The C-terminal portion contains the SH2 and SH3 domains, which are sites of interaction with other proteins, such as other members of the RTK family. HER-2/*neu* appears not to have a single specific ligand, but rather its growth modulation function depends on its ability to act as a co-receptor for multiple stroma-derived growth factors.

2.2. Oncogenic Features

In the rat a single-point mutation of a T to A at nucleotide position 2012 of the *c-neu* protooncogene results in the protooncogene being activated to the *neu* oncogene. This point mutation causes a change at amino acid residue 664 from valine to glutaminc acid in the transmembrane domain of the protein product and was shown to activate constitutively the intrinsic tyrosine kinase activity. In human breast cancer cells, amino acid 664 is a "hot spot" for activation of increased tyrosine kinase activity in vitro.

Increased expression of the HER-2/*neu* protooncogene has been observed in human breast cancer *(3)*. The HER-2/*neu* gene was found to be amplified or rearranged in many primary breast cancers, in breast cancer cell lines, and in metastatic breast cancer lesions *(4–6)*. One of the early reports described a 2- to 20-fold amplification of the HER-2/*neu* gene in about 30% of primary human breast cancer in a study of 189 cases. In addition, there is a significant direct correlation between the level of HER/*neu* gene amplification and its protein overexpression *(7)*.

Animal mammary tumor models that overexpress *neu* or *neu* homologs have been developed. These animal models have been used to identify genetic and somatic events that appear to cooperate with the *c-erbB-2/neu* oncogene in carcinogenesis and progression.

2.3. Implications of HER-2/neu Status on Breast Cancer Management

During the 1990s, HER-2/*neu*-related research has resulted in distinct contributions to breast cancer treatment. The HER-2/*neu* gene has been reported to be amplified or overexpressed in many different cancers including breast cancer, ovarian cancer, gastric tumors, colon cancer, lung cancer, oral cancer, kidney and salivary gland adenocarcinoma, gastric cancer *(8),* and cervical cancer. In contrast to gene amplification, mutation occurs at a very low frequency.

First found to be amplified in a human mammary tumor, HER-2/*neu* has been the focus of extensive studies on archival and fresh tumor biopsies. Approximately 20% of primary breast cancers exhibit either HER-2/*neu* gene amplification and/or overexpression by membrane protein staining *(9–23).* HER-2/*neu* expression varies in different breast lesions.

In benign tumors, overexpression is very rare, approximately 3 of 149. In contrast, over 90% of noninvasive ductal carcinomas *in situ* of comedo type tumors overexpressed HER-2/*neu,* whereas cribriform, solid, or papillary histologies rarely do. Overexpression of HER-2/*neu* was found in 4 of 10 cases of extramammary Paget's disease (and in none of 9 cases of mammary Paget's disease.) This evidence supports the hypothesis that mammary disease and extramammary disease follow different pathways of growth. Among different types of invasive breast cancer, invasive ductal carcinoma has demonstrated HER-2/*neu* protein overexpression in 30% of cases, whereas activation or overexpression is generally not observed in invasive lobular carcinoma.

An established marker for poor prognosis in breast cancer, HER-2/*neu* oncoprotein may also be predictive of response to treatment in some subpopulations. The level of HER-2/*neu* expression correlated with the number of lymph node metastases in primary and recurring breast cancers. The correlations found from clinical data are strong but not yet sufficient to define fully the role of HER-2/*neu* expression in aggressive breast cancer *(9,24–27).* Nevertheless, HER/*neu* gene amplification or overexpression in human primary breast cancers was shown to be a powerful predictor of the risk of recurrence *(28),* and thus this information is routinely used in breast cancer treatment to tailor the number of cycles and the type of chemotherapy given.

The $p185^{neu}$ on the cell surface of HER-2/*neu* overexpressing tumor cells is a good target for receptor-directed immunotherapies. Using the anti-human *p185* monoclonal antibody 4D5 together with chemotherapy may increase the chemosensitivity of the *p185*-overexpressing breast cancer cells to paclitaxel and docetaxel *(29,30).* In conclusion, HER-2/*neu* antibody-based cancer therapy is promising *(31–33),* and further studies are needed to define better the potential benefits to cancer patients.

3. bcl-2 GENE AND PROTEIN

The contribution of *bcl-2* to oncogenesis rests mainly on its role in extending cell survival by blocking or impairing the onset of apoptotic cell death. Normal development and maintenance of normal breast tissue is dependent on a balance between cell proliferation and cell death. Apoptosis or programmed cell death plays an important role in mammary gland development and involution after pregnancy and lactation. Aberrant, permanent perturbation in the balance between mitosis and apoptosis, a relative decrease in cell death, appears to contribute to neoplastic development. In rodent models of mammary tumorigenesis, it has been shown that constitutively active *bcl-2,* acting in concert with conditions that promote excessive cell proliferation and permit the accumulation of mutation, contributes to mammary tumorigenesis *(34,35).* Prolonged dysregulated cell survival allows the accumulation of possible deletions and mutations that are necessary for neoplastic transformation. It has been demonstrated that inhibition of apoptosis, which prolongs the cell life span, can contribute to breast neoplastic development and progression and can modulate response to treatment *(36,37).* There are hormonal and nonhormonal factors that regulate apoptosis of mammary epithelial cells. More recently, hormone-independent factors participating in the regulation of mammary epithelial cell apoptosis have been studied widely, including the *bcl-2* family.

bcl-2 was first isolated in 1984 from the breakpoint of the t(14:18) translocation that occurs frequently in B-cell leukemia and non-Hodgkin's follicular lymphoma. In 1988, it was shown that introduction of the gene into interleukin-3 (IL-3)-dependent myeloid and lymphoid cell lines promoted survival of these cells after withdrawal of IL-3 but did not stimulate their proliferation. Subsequently, the *bcl-2* gene was shown specifically to inhibit apoptosis as the mechanism of increased survival *(38). bcl-2* is the prototype member of a large gene family encoding proteins that can either inhibit *(bcl-2, bcl-x$_L$)* or promote *(bax, bcl-x$_S$,* bak) apoptosis. The balance in expression of these factors is the major determinant of whether or not a cell undergoes apoptosis. For instance, if *bcl-2* expression is higher than that of *bax,* apoptosis is generally suppressed; if the opposite is true, apoptosis is promoted. Most structure and function studies of *bcl-2* involve systems based on reagents devised from lymphoma and leukemia. Study of the characteristics of *bcl-2* in breast cancer is in its initial stages.

3.1. Structure, Function, and Oncogenesis

The wild-type *bcl-2* gene was cloned as a novel gene located at chromosome 18q21; it has a three-exon structure with an enormous 370-kb intron 2. *bcl-2* is 717 nucleotides long and codes for a *bcl-2* α-protein with molecular mass of 26 kDa. It is a membrane-associated protein containing a hydrophobic carboxyl terminus located in the inner mitochondria membrane; its lipophilic character suggests that it may be a membrane-spanning protein.

bcl-2's location suggests a possible role in the metabolic functions of the inner mitochondria membrane, i.e., oxidative phosphorylation and electron transport. It has been noted that decreasing cytosolic Ca^{2+} and increasing mitochondrial Ca^{2+} are correlated with *bcl-2* overexpression, suggesting that *bcl-2* may be involved in the regulation of intracellular Ca^{2+} distribution. However, *bcl-2* protects against apoptosis even in cells without mitochondria. *bcl-2* has also been localized to the nuclear membrane and to the mitotic nuclei in epithelial cell lines, suggesting that it may protect DNA from damage caused by nuclease activation. *bcl-2* may also act as an antioxidant, and *bcl-2* was able to block cell death induced by γ-irradiation, which produces reactive oxygen species (ROS). In addition, H_2O_2- and dexamethasone-induced apoptosis can be overcome by *bcl-2* expression. It has been noted that the death-suppressive effect of antioxidants such as *N*-acetyl-L-cysteine (NAC) and glutathione peroxidase was mediated through inhibition of lipid peroxidation, a mechanism similar to the one ascribed to *bcl-2* in its antioxidant function. It is known that *bcl-2* expression can occur at any stage of the cell cycle, but the mechanism by which *bcl-2* inhibits apoptosis is still under investigation.

The function of *bcl-2* as a cell death suppressor provided the first clue that altered gene expression could enhance cell survival without affecting cell proliferation. In the *bcl-2* gene family, a group of genes with a sequence homology to *bcl-2* produce proteins that share two highly conserved domains, *bcl-2* homologs 1 and 2 *(BH1, BH2)*. They are divided functionally into two groups: 1) cell death suppressors such as *bcl-2* and *bcl-X1,* and MCL-1; and 2) cell death promoters such as *bax, bcl-x$_S$,* bak, and *bad* cell death promoters. The *BH1* and *BH2* domains regulate heterodimerization; regulation of cell death by members of this gene family may be achieved through competing dimerization.

Normal *bcl-2* expression is associated with proliferating cells and cells that have a need for longevity. *bcl-2* is often demonstrated in breast glandular epithelial cells where regulation of hyperplasia and involution is controlled by hormones and growth factors, during the normal life cycle in complex differentiating epithelium with long-lived stem cells (skin, intestine, memory B cells), and in fully differentiated long-lived stem cells and noncycling cells (neurons).

The protein product of the *bcl-2* gene that acts to inhibit apoptosis is maximally expressed in the normal fetal breast where there is immunohistochemical localization in the basal epithelium of the developing breast bud and in the surrounding stroma; similar patterns of staining have been reported in male and female tissues. *bcl-2* reactivity is lost soon after birth and it is also expressed in hormonally regulated epithelium of the normal adult breast. These observations suggest that upregulation of *bcl-2* contributes to morphogenesis of the fetal breast by its inhibitory effect on apoptosis.

The *bcl-2* protooncogene actively blocks apoptosis and is triggered or regulated by several factors and events such as withdrawal growth factor, wild-type p53 protein, X-irradiation, IL-2, IL-3, IL-4, IL-6, IL-10, interferon-γ (INF-γ), transforming growth factor-β (TGF-β), and telomerase. Roles for *bcl-2* in epithelial differentiation, morphogenesis, and tumorigenesis and its response to hormone regulation have been reported from different groups; it seems to be an important factor in regulating complex pathways.

In vitro, breast cancer cell growth is influenced by *bcl-2* expression that prolongs the cell cycle and decreases tumor proliferation. These results may be the basis for *bcl-2* expression to be associated with a favorable outcome in breast cancer *(39)*. The mechanism by which *bcl-2* promotes tumorigenesis appears to be by conferring survival advantage to a variety of cell types by inhibiting apoptosis, an important feature in many normal biologic processes.

3.2. Implications in Clinical Breast Cancer

A number of investigators have studied *bcl-2* expression in breast tumor tissues and revealed highly heterogeneous staining patterns throughout the tumors. In general, *bcl-2* expression is present with decreasing frequency as tumors progress. It is expressed in over 95% of normal breast epithelium specimens, 79–91% of *in situ* cancer samples, and 45–79% of invasive breast carcinomas. *bcl-2* expression correlates with other favorable features of breast cancer: hormone receptor positivity, small tumor size, low tumor grade, greater disease-free survival, and decreased metastatic progression in T1 breast cancer *(40)*. In estrogen receptor-positive tumors, *bcl-2* expression inversely correlates with expression of EGFR, *c-myc,* and *p53.*

Loss of *bcl-2* expression is generally regarded as a relatively late event in the progression of the disease. In breast cancer, its expression is associated with favorable clinicopathologic features, whereas loss of *bcl-2* gene expression is linked to poor prognosis *(41,41)*. However, in T1 breast cancers, *bcl-2* expression was strongly associated with both apoptosis loss and presence of lymph node metastases *(42)*.

One study suggests that *bcl-2* cooperates with *c-myc* in vitro to promote proliferation and sometimes to induce tumors in nude mice. Because *bcl-2* expression prolongs the life span of cells, it increases the risk for those cells to acquire other changes, such as chromosomal abnormalities and small deletions, which may result in malignant progression.

The association of *bcl-2* expression with the sensitivity of epithelial cells to drugs, radiation, and hormone therapy very much depends on the type of malignancy. Its effect on therapeutic response and hence on prognosis is not clear-cut, and additional studies are needed. Berchem et al. *(43)* reported that phosphorylation of *bcl-2* may be responsible for sensitivity of docetaxel. Patients with elevated *bcl-2* immunostaining, especially those who coexpressed high levels of estrogen receptors, appeared to derive the greatest benefit from endocrine therapy *(44)* and had better response to tamoxifen treatment in metastatic breast cancer *(45)*. *bcl-2*-negative breast tumors over 1 cm in size are more likely to be treated with chemotherapy *(46)*. Recently preclinical studies of the combination therapy of *bcl-2* antisense oligonucleotide plus chemotherapeutic drugs showed efficacy in inhibiting breast tumor growth *(47)*, suggesting that *bcl-2* may be a useful target for anti-tumor therapy.

4. THE *BRCA* AND *p53* TUMOR SUPPRESSOR GENES

The *BRCA* (*BRCA1* and *BRCA2*) and *TP53* genes fit the traditional description of tumor suppressor genes, according to Knudson's classic "two-hit" model *(48)*. In familial cancers, an individual inherits a germline mutation; thus this "first hit" is present in all cells of the body. A somatic mutation represents the "second hit" on a given cell, resulting in loss of the wild-type allele, thus rendering both copies of the gene inactive. In sporadic cancers, loss of function of a tumor suppressor gene is accomplished by two somatic alterations that affect the corresponding alleles on both chromosomes. Knudson's model accurately accounts for the early onset of familial cancers owing to a preexisting germline mutation, whereas the accumulation of two somatic mutations in a single cell, a much less likely event, may occur once in several decades, giving rise to a sporadic cancer, typically of late onset.

It is estimated that mutations in *BRCA1* alone account for 50% of all familial early-onset female breast cancers *(49)*, whereas mutations in *BRCA2* may be responsible for up to 35% of the remaining hereditary breast cancers *(50,51)*. The *p53* gene is the most commonly somatically mutated gene in human cancer, with mutations occurring in approximately 50% of all cancers; depending on the study, it is found to be altered in 15–60% of all breast cancers. Several methods have been employed to screen for mutations in both the *BRCA* and *TP53* genes. These include direct sequencing of anomalous single-strand conformational polymorphism products (SSCP), heteroduplex analysis (HA), constant denaturant gradient gel electrophoresis, protein truncation test (PTT), and hydrazine-osmium-tetroxide (HOT) chemical cleavage.

During mutation screening, a host of polymorphisms have been identified for the *BRCA1, BRCA2,* and the *TP53* genes. Polymorphisms can be missense or other alterations that cause either no change, or a 1-amino acid substitution in the protein sequence, or another change that appears not to be associated with disease. By definition, polymorphisms do not significantly modify the protein's function but may actually significantly alter the protein's primary structure; a salient example is the case of a polymorphic stop codon in *BRCA2* (which truncates the last 98 amino acids). Polymorphisms are found to varying degrees in the general population and are typically not associated with obvious disease. It is possible, however, that certain missense alterations cause subtle modifications of protein structure or expression, which may impact on function without causing overt clinical disease.

4.1. BRCA Gene Structure

It has long been recognized that a family history of breast cancer is a contributing factor to the risk of developing breast cancer. In 1990, a breast cancer susceptibility gene responsible for early-onset breast cancer was localized to chromosome 17q21 *(52)*. A subsequent study confirmed this finding and also implicated this hereditary breast cancer gene in familial breast and ovarian cancer *(53)*. This gene, now known as *BRCA1,* was identified in 1994 by a combination of classical positional cloning with candidate gene strategies. *BRCA1* is a large, well-characterized gene contained in an 81-kb segment of genomic DNA that is rich in Alu-like repetitive sequences. The intron lengths range in size from 403 bp to 9.2 kb and contain a ribosomal protein pseudogene within intron 13. Three polymorphic intragenic microsatellite markers (D17S1323, D17S1322, and D17S855) localize to introns 12, 19, and 20, respectively.

The transcribed region of the *BRCA1* gene itself has 5,651 nucleotides in 24 exons, 22 of which are coding exons; almost half of the coding sequence is contained within exon 11. *BRCA1* encodes a 204-kDa cell cycle-regulated nuclear phosphoprotein composed of 1,863 amino acids, with a zinc finger domain near the N terminus, typical of nucleic acid binding proteins *(54)*. The BRCA1 protein also has two functional nuclear localization motifs, located at amino acids 503 and 607; interestingly, in spite of its nuclear localization, BRCA1 may also exhibit growth-inhibitory granin-like properties, although this function is considered controversial.

Splice variants of *BRCA1* mRNA present in normal breast cells have been identified. These alternatively spliced mRNAs code for truncated proteins; however, it is unknown whether these truncated proteins exhibit tumor suppressor function or dominant negative interactions. In breast cancer-prone families, truncations of the BRCA1 protein owing to inherited mutations are correlated with a high mitotic index of breast tumor cells in the affected carriers *(55)*. One naturally occurring splice variant of BRCA1 was isolated from breast tumor and colon epithelial cDNA libraries and has been useful in BRCA1 localization studies. BRCA1-Δ11b, which is missing exon 4 and most of exon 11, has been shown to lose its ability to localize to the nucleus and is consequently confined to the cytoplasm. This variant of BRCA1 is expressed at similar levels in tissues, tumors, and cell lines. Unlike the full-length BRCA1 protein, BRCA1-Δ11b protein overexpression is not toxic to the cell, suggesting that this isoform has a role in cellular proliferation and differentiation. Two other naturally occurring splice variants, BRCA1a and BRCA1b, have been identified and code for 110- and 100-kDa proteins, respectively. The 110-kDa protein retains the amino-terminal region and appears to function as a transcriptional activator, whereas BRCA1b only retains the C-terminal end of the full-length protein, possibly acting as a negative regulator of transcriptional activity.

The *BRCA2* gene is notably similar to the *BRCA1* gene in its tissue and phylogenetic expression, as well as structure. *BRCA2* was localized to chromosome 13q12–13 using linkage analysis of cancer-prone kindreds. Utilizing the lessons learned in cloning *BRCA1,* a partial sequence for *BRCA2* was reported less than a year and a half later *(56)*, almost simultaneously with the complete coding sequence of *BRCA2 (57)*. The *BRCA2* gene has 10,254 nucleotides in 27 exons, with a very large exon 11 containing almost half of the coding sequence. Like *BRCA1, BRCA2* codes for a large, negatively charged protein with a putative granin domain.

4.2. BRCA Gene and Protein Function

A variety of experiments using animal models have aided in the understanding of *BRCA1* and *BRCA2* function. *Brca1* expression is increased in the rapidly dividing cells of the murine mammary gland during ductal morphogeneis and pregnancy and in the rapidly dividing cells of the mouse embryo. Introduction of wild-type *BRCA1* into a variety of tumor cell lines, including breast and ovarian tumor lines, results in growth inhibition; introduction of antisense BRCA1 nucleotides into primary mammary epithelial cells increases cell proliferation.

Several transgenic mouse models have confirmed the role of *Brca1* in cell proliferation and differentiation. Homozygotes, with mutations in exons 5 and 6 *(Brca1$^{5-6}$)* died *in utero* 4.5–6.5 days after gestation with poorly differentiated embryonic tissues. Similar embryonic lethality and differentiation results were observed in embryos carrying homozygous deletion in the 5′-end of exon 11 of *BRCA1*. However, in both cases, the heterozygotes were developed normally, indicating that at least one normal *Brca1* allele is required for normal embryonic development and is essential for cellular proliferation. In contrast, homozygous *Brca1* exon 11 knockout embryos *(Brca1^{11-})* died at 9.5–13.5 days post gestation owing to severe neurologic defects. These data implicate *Brca1* in murine neurologic development and suggest that alternate forms of the Brca1 protein may have distinct functions on differentiating cells during embryogenesis.

Brca1$^{5-6}$ mutants showed a decrease in expression of the *p53* inhibitor mdm2 and an increase in the G1 cell cycle inhibitor *p21*. To test whether embryonic lethality brought about by the *Brca1$^{5-6}$* mutation could be circumvented, double-mutant mice (which were *Brca1$^{5-6}$* null) on either a *p53* null *(p53$^-$)* or *p21* null *(p21$^-$)* background were produced. Survival was prolonged in the *Brca1$^{5-6}$/p53$^-$* embryos from 7.5 to 9.5 days after gestation. Although none of the Brca1$^{5-6}$/p21$^-$ embryos survived past 10.5 days post gestation, they were developmentally similar to their wild-type littermates. Therefore, since deletion of *p53* or *p21* was unable to rescue the *Brca1$^{5-6}$* embryos completely, a complex process of embryo development involving interactions between several molecules is postulated.

A recent study demonstrated that mice heterozygous for *Brca1 (Brca1$^{+/-}$)* and deficient for *p53 (p53$^{-/-}$)* had the same survival rate as mice that were *Brca1$^{+/+}$/p53$^{-/-}$*. However, mammary tumors developed in 4 of 23 *Brca1$^{+/-}$/p53$^{-/-}$* mice compared with only 1 *Brca1$^{+/+}$/p53$^{-/-}$* mouse. Although these data are suggestive of a trend of increased incidence of mammary tumors in *Brca1$^{+/-}$/p53$^{-/-}$* mice, statistical significance was not reached.

Three potential nuclear localization motifs were identified in *BRCA1* at amino acids 503, 606, and 651. Mutation of each of these individual motifs determined that the nuclear localization signals at amino acid 503 and 607 were needed for transporting *BRCA1* to the nucleus while the nuclear localization motif at 651 was nonfunctional. The putative role of BRCA1 protein in DNA repair is supported by these data coupled, with independent in vitro studies demonstrating that *Brca1* coprecipitates with *Rad51,* the human homolog of the *E. coli* RecA DNA repair protein. More recently, Cortez et al. *(58)* demonstrated that the BRCA1 protein is phosphorylated by the checkpoint kinase ATM (mutated in ataxia telangiectasia) in response to ionizing radiation. It is thought that phosphorylation of wild-type BRCA1 modulates the interaction of BRCA1 with other proteins such as Rad51, thereby mediating DNA repair. It is reasonable to speculate that in normal developing embryos, Brca1, acting in concert with Rad51, is able to repair DNA damage effectively, but in homozygous *Brca1^{11-}* mutant embryos the repair machinery is lost or defective, and a *p53* cell cycle checkpoint is induced. In the *Brca1^{11}/p53$^{-/-}$* mouse the checkpoint is lost, and severe chromosomal abnormalities can accumulate. Paralleling the experiments on *Brca1* knockouts, *Brca2* knockout mice demonstrate that at least one normal copy of the *Brca2* gene is required for normal embryogenesis. Mouse experiments have helped to correlate findings derived from human normal and tumor breast cells, which show cell cycle regulation of *BRCA2* corresponding to a general upregulation of mRNA during S-phase and mitosis.

BRCA2 is also implicated in DNA repair *(59)*, as shown in experiments that introduced various mutations in the mouse *BRCA2* gene by homologous recombination. Mice were developed that had a disruption in exon 11 of the *Brca2* gene *(Brca2^11^)*. Some of the mice that were homozygous for this *Brca2* mutation were viable and lived to adulthood, but not beyond 5.5 months of age. Fibroblasts cultured from the embryos of *Brca2^11^* mutant mice overexpressed p21 and p53, which is reminiscent of the observation in the *Brca1^5–6^* mice. When the *Brca2^11^* mutant fibroblasts were exposed to X-rays, the cells repaired double-stranded DNA breaks at a considerable slower rate than fibroblasts from wild type *Brca2* mice or from mice that were heterozygous for the exon 11 deletion mutation.

4.2.1. THE ROLE OF BRCA1 AND BRCA2 IN DNA REPAIR

The *Brca1* knockout mouse data described above provide strong evidence that Brca1 has a role in double-stranded DNA repair. This is further supported by the data indicating that Brca1 is phosphorylated by ATM in response to double-stranded DNA breaks *(58)*. BRCA1 and the human homolog of the bacterial RecA protein, Rad51, have been found to be associated by both in vivo and in vitro experiments *(60)*. Immunostaining of both meiotic and mitotic cells in S-phase demonstrated that BRCA1 and Rad51 were colocalized in nuclear foci. Furthermore, the two proteins were coimmunoprecipitated from cells in S-phase. In vitro, BRCA1 and Rad51 formed complexes, and BRCA1 residues 768–1064 were identified to be key in the formation of these complexes with Rad51. Tissue culture experiments that analyzed murine cells containing targeted truncated Brca2 demonstrated increased chromosomal abnormalities and had increased sensitivity to genotoxic agents, further implicating Brca2 in DNA repair *(61)*.

The human BRCA2 protein, like BRCA1, has been shown to associate with Rad51 and is therefore also involved in DNA repair. Murine embryonic fibroblasts containing a *Brca2* gene with a C-terminal deletion at exon 27 *(Brca2^27^)* were generated. These clones did not bind murine Rad51 and consequently were hypersensitive to γ-irradiation, suggesting a deficiency in DNA repair mechanisms. In addition, the *Brca2^27^* mutant cells had a decreased proliferation rate and were prematurely senescent, presumably owing to inefficient DNA repair. These data seem to indicate that the farthest portion of Brca2 downstream of the Rad51 binding element is functionally important in DNA repair mediated by the Brca2/Rad51 complex. Multiple sites in BRCA2, termed BRC repeat motifs, interact with Rad51. The BRC repeat motifs are comprised of 59 amino acid residues that are conserved in evolution and are required for Rad51 interaction with BRCA2. In vitro experiments have demonstrated that interaction of Rad51 with these BRC repeat motifs of BRCA2 are critical for cellular response to DNA damage caused by genotoxic agents *(62)*. The identification of the specific regions of BRCA2 involved with binding to RAD51 and effecting the DNA repair action of the complex will assist in providing useful end points for functional assays. This experimental evidence will need to be reconciled with the possibility that truncation of the last 90–100 amino acids of the C-terminus of BRCA2 appears not to be associated with disease in humans. In spite of mounting evidence for a role of BRCA1 in DNA repair, all clinical evidence so far suggests that there are no clinical implications for irradiation of the breast during local-regional therapy for stage I or II breast cancer.

4.2.2. *BRCA* MUTATIONS IN BREAST AND OVARIAN CANCERS

Since its isolation in 1994, more than 100 mutations have been described in the *BRCA1* gene alone. Most of these mutations were identified in individuals who belong to families with several generations affected by either breast or breast and ovarian cancer *(63–65)*. Founder-effect mutations, common mutations presumably originating from a single ancestor within a historically isolated ethnic group, have been identified in several populations such as Ashkenazi Jews, French Canadians, Japanese, Italians, Swedes, Finns, Icelanders, Belgians, and Dutch. Salient examples of these are the *BRCA1* 185delAG, *BRCA1* 5382insC mutations, and *BRCA2* 6174delA in Ashkenazi Jewry.

The *BRCA1* 185delAG frameshift mutation is a 2-bp deletion at base 185 in exon 2, which causes a premature truncation of the protein by producing a premature stop at codon 39 *(66)*. Other types of frameshift mutations, caused either by deletions of 1–40 bp or insertions of up to 11 bp, have been identified that also result in premature stop codons. Additionally, single-base pair substitutions resulting in missense, nonsense, or splicing mutations have been described. Nearly 80% of mutations found so far in the *BRCA1* gene would produce a truncated protein. In many cases, however, it is not known whether the shorter or aberrant BRCA1 proteins are indeed expressed. A somewhat different set of mutations occurs in the regulatory regions of the *BRCA1* gene, such as methylatable CpG islands in promoters, enhancers, and repressors. These mutations cause an alteration in the level of gene transcription and are generally characterized by the absence of mRNA. Research is under way to define the clinical significance of these mutations better.

The role of *BRCA1* has been extensively investigated in sporadic breast and ovarian cancer. Several somatic mutations have been identified in the coding regions of *BRCA1* in sporadic ovarian tumors; however, until recently, none had been found in sporadic breast cancers *(67)*. Indications of involvement of the *BRCA1* gene in the formation of sporadic breast carcinomas derive from loss of heterozygosity experiments, putative loss of protein through unknown mechanisms, and the observation that the promoter region of *BRCA1* was hypermethylated in some invasive tumors *(68)*. Although loss of *BRCA1* function occurs in sporadic breast cancers, neither the mechanism involved in this phenomenon nor its implications are known at the present time.

Germline mutations in *BRCA2* predispose female carriers to breast and ovarian cancer and male carriers to breast cancer and possibly prostate cancer. The most common disease-associated mutations detected in the *BRCA2* gene of breast and ovarian patients have been microdeletions resulting in a frameshift, with notably few point mutations, compared with *BRCA1*. Founder mutations have also been identified in the *BRCA2* gene in members of defined ethnic groups. This is once again well illustrated in the Ashkenazi Jewish population. A recurrent germline mutation, 6147delT, was detected in 8% of Ashkenazi Jewish women between the ages of 42 and 50 who were diagnosed with early-onset breast cancer *(69)*. The 6147delT mutation is present in 1.5% of Ashkenazi Jews *(69)*.

Unlike *BRCA1,* loss of heterozygosity at the *BRCA2* locus has been observed in 30–40% of sporadic breast and ovarian cancers *(70);* however, very few somatic mutations or deletions have been found in the remaining allele *(71, 72)*. This suggests that either *BRCA2* may be an infrequent target for somatic inactivation or intron or regulatory sequences may be the primary targets of somatic mutation. In a study of 45 unselected grade 3 sporadic infiltrating ductal carcinomas, 21 cases demonstrated a concurrent loss of heterozygosity in the *BRCA1* and *BRCA2* loci. This suggests a common pathway of tumorigenesis in familial and sporadic breast cancers that involves these two *BRCA* genes.

In addition to an increase in the risk of familial female breast and ovarian cancer, mutations in the *BRCA2* gene are also associated with an increased risk of sporadic and familial forms of pancreatic, hepatic, prostate, and particularly male breast cancers. Mutations in the *BRCA* genes, which are found in these types of cancers, are similar to those of breast and ovarian carcinomas, so no phenotype-genotype correlations have been established. In one study, mutations in the central region of the *BRCA2* gene appear to carry higher risk of ovarian cancer than mutations at either the 5′- or 3′-ends of the gene. This observation needs to be confirmed in studies of large numbers of *BRCA2* carriers. Specific studies exploring the functional consequences of different mutations will be required before the phenotype-genotype correlations can be fully validated and applied in the clinic. With increasing numbers of individuals being tested for the *BRCA* genes, it has become crucial to be able to define what constitutes a true deleterious mutation in these genes; this key information is at present lacking, but several groups are working on this problem.

4.3. p53 Structure and Function

The p53 protein was first described in 1979 as an abundant transformation-related antigen in chemically and virally transformed murine cells *(73)*. Two years later, p53 was found to be expressed in several human cell lines and was thought to be a transformation-related antigen *(74)*. Not until several years later did researchers realize that the protein they had been studying was the mutant form of a tumor suppressor protein, which, when expressed in the wild-type form, exists in low levels transiently during the cell cycle *(75–79)*. The *TP53* gene spans a 20-kb area of human chromosome 17p13.1 and is composed of 11 exons. Exons 2–11 code for the full-length and processed mRNA, which is 2.2–2.5 kb in size. This message is found in all cells of the body, with the highest mRNA levels being found in the spleen and thymus.

The p53 protein is a 393-amino acid nuclear phosphoprotein. The p53 protein contains essentially four functional domains. Amino acids 1–100 compose the transactivational domain, responsible for the transcriptional effect *p53* has on other genes. Amino acids 100–300 comprise the core DNA binding domain. The next 60 amino acids make up the oligomerization domain; active wild-type *p53* tetramers are able to recognize the DNA binding consensus sequence, 5′-Pu, Pu, Pu, C, A/T, T/A, G, Py, Py, Py-3′, allowing transcription of specific p53-regulated genes. The final 33 amino acids comprise the negative regulatory domain that controls wild-type p53 activity and longevity *(80)*.

Most mutations in the *TP53* gene that occur in human cancers are located in the evolutionarily conserved regions of exons 6–11 *(81)*. Most of these mutations (75–80%) are missense mutations, producing a faulty p53 protein *(81,82)*. Commonly, the shape of the protein is altered, consequently increasing the stability and half-life of the mutant protein (the wild-type p53 protein has a half-life of approximately 20 minutes) *(75)*. More than 60% of the time, alterations in the shape of the p53 protein result in localization in the cytoplasm instead of the nucleus *(83,84)*. Phenotypically, three distinct properties are observed when a mutant p53 is present in a cell: 1) loss of function, which can be reversed with the introduction of wild-type p53; 2) gain of a new function, such as enhancement of tumorigenesis; and 3) dominant loss of function, which when introduced into cells with wild-type p53 sequesters by oligomerization and abrogates wild-type p53 function.

Over the years a picture has emerged of how wild-type p53 performs its tumor suppressor functions through regulation of apoptosis and cellular immortalization. In brief, loss of wild-type p53 function leads to loss of important G1 and/or G2 cell cycle checkpoints that occur in response to DNA damage and double-strand breaks. In the presence of mitogenic stimulation, uncontrolled and aberrant cellular proliferation occurs. Cells that lack wild-type p53 (either through mutation or through sequestration of the wild-type protein by a dominant mutant protein) bypass a G1/S-phase delay in response to DNA damage from a variety of agents Normally, it is at the checkpoint that a cell "decides" to repair the damaged DNA, or if the damage is too extensive, p53 begins a signaling cascade leading to apoptosis *(85)*. Abrogation of this checkpoint leads to uncontrolled replication of damaged DNA, resulting in amplifications, deletions, or mutations of other genes with an overall result of genomic instability of the cell leading to tumor cell development and progression. Jerry et al. demonstrated that almost 50% of cells within hyperplastic alveolar nodules, the most common pre-neoplastic lesions in mouse mammary glands, contained p53 mutations. As the lesions progressed to form tumors, almost 100% of the cells contained mutant p53, with the protein localizing in the nucleus. This study suggests that inactivation of the wild-type p53 pathway is a common and early event in mammary tumor development.

4.3.1. *P53* IN BREAST AND OVARIAN CANCER

In addition to germline mutations in the *BRCA1* and *BRCA2* genes, mutations in the *p53* gene are responsible for a rare hereditary predisposition to breast and ovarian cancers. The role of *p53* in hereditary breast cancer is observed in patients with Li-Fraumeni syndrome, who carry germline mutations in the *p53* gene. Most commonly, early-onset breast cancer affects women of these families, who often have a relative suffering from a childhood cancer, such as leukemia, brain tumor, or sarcoma. Very early onset of cancers, within the second or third decade of life, in a family with several cases of childhood malignancies suggests the presence of *p53* germline mutations.

Loss of wild-type p53 function, which leads to an increase in genomic instability, has also been demonstrated in sporadic cases of breast cancer *(86)*. Missense mutations account for 80% of all observed mutations in breast cancer *(87)*. Analysis of the *p53* gene in breast cancer has demonstrated that most mutations, over 90%, occur in exons 5–9. A small percentage of breast tumors have mutations in exons 4, 9, and 10 and in the flanking splice junctions of exons 1,2,3, and 11. Of these mutations, over 50% are GC to AT transitions, with a large number of these affecting CpG dinucleotides that are methylated.

Owing to its short half-life (approx 20 minutes) and modest expression level, the wild-type p53 protein is virtually undetectable in the nucleus of cells by immunohistochemical (IHC) staining. In contrast, mutant forms of p53 within tumors are readily detectable by IHC owing to a 10–20-fold increase in their half-life. IHC staining of human breast tumors has led to a variety of useful conclusions. Studies have demonstrated that anywhere from 20 to 55% of breast tumors stain positive for mutant p53 protein. Furthermore, this pattern of staining ranges from strictly nuclear staining to staining within the cytoplasm *(88)*.

Results from IHC studies appear to be influenced by several factors such as the type of antibody used, frozen versus paraffin-embedded tissues, time of fixation, and type of fixative. Generally, the most consistent results are derived from studies using tissues that have been fixed rapidly (within 15 minutes of removal) and have employed antigen retrieval in conjunction with the monoclonal antibody Pab 1801 or the polyclonal antibody CM1 *(87)*.

4.4. BRCA1 and p53 Tumor Suppressor Interactions

In vitro and in vivo experiments have shown that *BRCA1* associates with another tumor suppressor gene, *p53,* and regulates *p53*-responsive gene transcription. Coactivation of *p53*-dependent genes by *BRCA1* has been shown to be dependent on the presence of wild-type *p53* and wild-type *BRCA1,* suggesting a possible synergistic regulation of downstream genes by these two tumor suppressors. Investigation of the status of *p53* in breast tumors arising in *BRCA1* and *BRCA2* mutation carriers indicated that *p53* was mutant in 66% of the *BRCA*-related tumors compared with only 35% of grade-matched non-*BRCA*-associated tumors *(89)*.

It has been suggested that the CDK-inhibitor p21 is transactivated by *BRCA1* in a *p53*-dependent manner, therefore arresting cells before S-phase. S-phase progression was inhibited by *BRCA1* in cells that had wild-type *p21* but not in either *p21* null or *BRCA1* transactivation-deficient mutant cells. Taken together, this evidence suggests that the tumor suppressor action of *BRCA1* with *p53* may be mediated via cooperative *BRCA1* regulation of wild-type *p21*.

5. APOPTOSIS AND ONCOGENESIS: *p53, bcl-2,* AND HER-2/*neu (c-erbB-2)*

It has been suggested that exposure to environmental DNA-damaging agents contributes to the development of the vast majority of human tumors *(90)*. Therefore, an understanding of the molecular events involved in the cellular responses to such exposures should provide insights into mechanisms of human carcinogenesis. There are many interrelating effector events in apoptosis, and the malignant phenotype *p53,* as well as HER-2/*neu (c-erbB-2)* and *bcl-2* mutations in breast cancer, has attracted the attention of those studying this phenomenon.

The *p53* tumor suppressor gene is involved in genetic regulation of apoptosis. It acts as a direct "apoptogene," a gene that causes apoptosis, and it has been suggested that the product of the *p53* gene acts as a "molecular policeman" monitoring the integrity of the genome. If a cell's DNA is damaged, the *p53* gene product accumulates through a posttranslational stabilization mechanism and arrests the cell cycle at G1 to allow extra time for repair. If repair fails, *p53* may trigger deletion of the cell by apoptosis. To what extent *p53* is involved in regulating apoptosis under normal conditions is unknown. A major mechanism whereby abnormalities of *p53* contribute to the development and progression of tumors may be abrogation of the normal pathway that leads to the self-destruction of mutant cells.

bcl-2 is unique among oncogenes because it exerts its oncogenic effect via the inhibition of apoptosis and not via enhanced cell cycle progression. *bcl-2* is normally expressed in tissues characterized by extended viability or self-renewal that involves the process of apoptosis. In many malignancies, *bcl-2* overexpression confers an inhibition of programmed cell death upon malignant cells, even in the absence of gene arrangements *(91)*. *bcl-2* has been shown to inhibit apoptosis triggered by wild-type *p53,* and an inverse correlation between *bcl-2* expression and *p53* mutation has been observed in breast cancer and other malignant diseases.

The loss of function of *p53* in cells may effect the function of *bcl-2*. Tumor cell numbers would increase as a result of both unregulated proliferation and resistance to cell death. The study has suggested that *bcl-2* oncoprotein expression is frequently associated with an overexpression of *p53*. Loss of the *p53* tumor suppressor gene or overexpression of the apoptosis inhibitor protein *bcl-2* have been reported in oncogenically transformed cells that have lost their apoptotic potential. *p53* was also found to downregulate *bcl-2* and to regulate the *bcl-2/bax* balance. *bax* is a member of the *bcl-2* family that acts as a apoptosis promoter; wild-type *p53* function may be required for optimal expression of *bcl-2* since *p53* mutation in some cell types results in a marked reduction in *bax* and an increase in *bcl-2* expression.

HER-2/*neu (c-erbB-2)* is known as an EGFR protooncogene that plays an important role in the prognosis and transformation of neoplasms *(92);* its involvement in apoptosis is thought to be limited. One report, however, demonstrated that HER-2/*neu* overexpression in ovarian tumor cell lines transfected with an endoplasmic reticulum form of an anti-HER-2/*neu* single-chain antibody undergoes specific cytotoxicity through the induction of apoptosis *(93)*. Another study using anti-HER-2/*neu* monoclonal antibodies induced tyrosine phosphorylation of HER-2/*neu* proteins, causing cell morphology changes and apoptosis.

ACKNOWLEDGMENTS

This work was supported by the Susan G. Komen Breast Cancer Foundation, by the National Institutes of Health (grants 5T32 CA09537-16 and RO1-CA77612), the Venture Investment Fund of the University of Michigan Health System, and the Blodgett-Butterworth Research Foundation.

REFERENCES

1. Schubert D, Heinemann S, Carlisle W, et al. (1974) Clonal cell lines from the rat central nervous system. *Nature* **249,** 224–227.
2. Shih C, Padhy LC, Murray M, Weinberg RA (1981) Transforming genes of carcinomas and neuroblastomas introduced into mouse fibroblasts. *Nature* **290,** 261–264.
3. Yokota J, Yamamoto T, Miyajima N, et al. (1988) Genetic alterations of the c-erbB-2 oncogene occur frequently in tubular adenocarcinoma of the stomach and are often accompanied by amplification of the v-erbA homologue. *Oncogene* **2,** 283–287.
4. Kraus MH, Popescu NC, Amsbaugh SC, King CR (1987) Overexpression of the EGF receptor-related proto-oncogene erbB-2 in human mammary tumor cell lines by different molecular mechanisms. *EMBO J.* **6,** 605–610.
5. Slamon DJ, Godolphin W, Jones LA, et al. (1989) Studies of the *HER-2/neu* proto-oncogene in human breast and ovarian cancer. *Science* **244,** 707–712.
6. van de Vijver MJ, van de Bersselaar R, Devilee P, Cornelisse C, Peterse J, Nusse R (1987) Amplification of the neu (c-erbB-2) oncogene in human mammmary tumors is relatively frequent and is often accompanied by amplification of the linked c-erbA oncogene. *Mol. Cell Biol.* **7,** 2019–2023.
7. Slamon DJ, Clark GM, Wong SG, et al. (1987) Human breast cancer correlation of relapse and survival with amplification of the *HER-2/neu* oncogene. *Science* **235,** 177–182.
8. King CR, Kraus MH, Aaronson SA (1985) Amplification of a novel v-erbB-related gene in a human mammary carcinoma. *Science* **229,** 974–976.
9. Venter DJ, Tuzi NL, Kumar S, Gullick WJ (1987) Overexpression of the c-erbB-2 oncoprotein in human breast carcinomas: immunohistological assessment correlates with gene amplification. *Lancet* **2,** 69–72.
10. Ali IU, Campbell G, Lidereau R, Callahan R (1988) Lack of evidence for the prognostic significance of c-erbB-2 amplification in human breast carcinoma. *Oncogene Res.* **3,** 139–146.
11. Barnes DM, Lammie GA, Millis RR, Gullick WL, Allen DS, Altman DG (1988) An immunohistochemical evaluation of c-erbB-2 expression in human breast carcinoma. *Br. J. Cancer* **58,** 448–452.
12. Berger MS, Locher GW, Saurer S, et al. (1988) Correlation of c-*erbB*-2 gene amplification and protein expression in human breast carcinomas with nodal status and nuclear grading. *Cancer Res.* **48,** 1238–1243.
13. Guerin M, Gabillot M, Mathieu MC, et al. (1989) Structure and expression of c-erbB-2 and EGF receptor genes in inflammatory and non-inflammatory breast cancer: prognostic significance. *Int. J. Cancer* **43,** 201–208.
14. Thor AD, Schwartz LH, Koerner FC, et al. (1989) Analysis of c-erbB-2 expression in breast carcinomas with clinical follow-up. *Cancer Res.* **49,** 7147–7152.
15. Walker RA, Gullick WJ, Varley JM (1989) An evaluation of immunoreactivity for c-erbB-2 protein as a marker of poor short-term prognosis in breast cancer. *Br. J. Cancer* **60,** 426–429.
16. Borg A, Tandon AK, Sigurdsson H, et al. (1990) HER-2/neu amplification predicts poor survival in node-positive breast cancer. *Cancer Res.* **50,** 4332–4337.
17. Baak JP, Chin D, van Diest PJ, Ortiz R, Matze–Cok P, Bacus SS (1991) Comparative long-term prognostic value of quantitative HER-2/neu protein expression, DNA ploidy, and morphometric and clinical features in paraffin-embedded invasive breast cancer. *Lab. Invest.* **64,** 215–223.
18. Clark GM, McGuire WL (1991) Follow-up study of HER-2/neu amplification in primary breast cancer. *Cancer Res.* **51,** 944–948.
19. McCann AH, Dervan PA, O'Regan M, et al. (1991) Prognostic significance of c-erbB-2 and estrogen receptor status in human breast cancer. *Cancer Res.* **51,** 3296–3303.
20. Allred DC, Clark GM, Molina R, et al. (1992) Overexpression of HER-2/neu and its relationship with other prognostic factors change during the progression of in situ to invasive breast cancer. *Hum. Pathol.* **23,** 974–979.

21. Ciocca DR, Fujimura FK, Tandon AK, et al. (1992) Correlation of HER-2/neu amplification with expression and with other prognostic factors in 1103 breast cancers [see comments]. *J. Natl. Cancer Inst.* **84,** 1279–1282.

22. Tiwari RK, Borgen PI, Wong GY, Cordon–Cardo C, Osborne MP (1992) HER-2/neu amplification and over-expression in primary human breast cancer is associated with early metastasis. *Anticancer Res.* **12,** 419–425.

23. Schonborn I, Zschiesche W, Spitzer E, et al. (1994) c-erbB-2 overexpression in primary breast cancer: independent prognostic factor in patients at high risk. *Breast Cancer Res. Treat.* **29,** 287–295.

24. Varley JM, Swallow JE, Brammar WJ, Whittaker JL, Walker RA (1987) Alterations to either c-erbB-2(neu) or c-myc proto-oncogenes in breast carcinomas correlate with poor short-term prognosis. *Oncogene* **1,** 423–430.

25. Adnane J, Gaudray P, Simon MP, Simony–Lafontaine J, Jeanteur P, Theillet C (1989) Protooncogene amplification and human breast tumor phenotype. *Oncogene* **4,** 1389–1395.

26. Garcia I, Dietrich PY, Aapro M, Vauthier G, Vadas L, Engel E (1989) Genetic alterations of c-myc, c-erbB-2, and c-IIa-ras protooncogenes and clinical associations in human breast carcinomas. *Cancer Res.* **49,** 6675–6679.

27. King CR, Swain SM, Porter L, Steinberg SM, Lippman ME, Gelmann EP (1989) Heterogeneous expression of erbB-2 messanger RNA in human breast cancer. *Cancer Res.* **49,** 4185–4191.

28. Nagai MA, Marques LA, Torloni H, Brentani MM (1993) Genetic alterations in c-erbB-2 protooncogene as prognostic markers in human primary breast tumors. *Oncology* **50,** 412–417.

29. Cole SP, Bhardwaj G, Gerlach JH, et al. (1992) Overexpression of a transporter gene in a multidrug-resistant human lung cancer cell line [see comments]. *Science* **258,** 1650–1654.

30. Moscow JA, Cowan KH (1988) Multidrug resistance. *J. Natl. Cancer Inst.* **80,** 14–20.

31. Hung MC, Matin A, Zhang Y, et al. (1995) HER-2/neu-targeting gene therapy—a review. *Gene* **159,** 65–71.

32. Wels W, Moritz D, Schmidt M, Jeschke M, Hynes NE, Groner B (1995) Biotechnological and gene therapeutic strategies in cancer treatment. *Gene* **159,** 73–80.

33. Dhingra K, Hittelman WN, Hortobagyi GN (1995) Genetic changes in breast cancer—consequences for therapy? *Gene* **159,** 59–63.

34. Barbacid M (1986) Oncogenes and human cancer: cause or consequence? *Carcinogenesis* **7,** 1037–1042.

35. Morris DW, Cardiff RD (1987) Multistep model of mouse mammary tumor development. *Adv. Viral Oncol.* **7,** 123–140.

36. Schedin PJ, Thackray LB, Malone P, Fontaine SC, Friis RR, Strange R (1996) Programmed cell death and mammary neoplasia. *Cancer Treat Res.* **83,** 3–22.

37. Wu J (1996) Apoptosis and angiogenesis: two promising tumor markers in breast cancer (review). *Anticancer Res.* **16,** 2233–2239.

38. Hockenbery D, Nunez G, Milliman C, Schreiber RD, Korsmeyer SJ (1990) Bcl-2 is an inner mitochondrial membrane protein that blocks programmed cell death. *Nature* **348,** 334–336.

39. Knowlton K, Mancini M, Creason S, Morales C, Hockenbery D, Anderson BO (1998) Bcl-2 slows in vitro breast cancer growth despite its antiapoptotic effect. *J. Surg. Res.* **76,** 22–26.

40. Sierra A, Castellsague X, Escobedo A, Moreno A, Drudis T, Fabra A (1999) Synergistic cooperation between c-Myc and Bcl-2 in lymph node progression of T1 human breast carcinomas. *Breast Cancer Res. Treat.* **54,** 39–45.

41. Leek RD, Kaklamanis L, Pezzella F, Gatter KC, Harris AL (1994) bcl-2 in normal human breast and carcinoma, association with oestrogen receptor-positive, epidermal growth factor receptor-negative tumours and in situ cancer. *Br. J. Cancer* **69,** 135–139.

42. Sierra A, Castellsague X, Tortola S, et al. (1996) Apoptosis loss and Bcl-2 expression: key determinants of lymph mode metastases in T_1 breast cancer. *Clin. Cancer Res.* **2,** 1887–1894.

43. Berchem GJ, Bosseler M, Mine N, Avalosse B (1999) Nanomolar range docetaxel treatment sensitizes MCF-7 cells to chemotherapy induced apoptosis, induces G2M arrest and phosphorylates bcl-2. *Anticancer Res.* **19,** 535–540.

44. Gee JM, Robertson JF, Ellis IO, et al. (1994) Immunocytochemical localization of BCL-2 protein in human breast cancers and its relationship to a series of prognostic markers and response to endocrine therapy. *Int. J. Cancer* **59,** 619–628.

45. Elledge RM, Green S, Howes L, et al. (1997) bcl-2, p53, and response to tamoxifen in estrogen receptor-positive metastatic breast cancer: a Southwest Oncology Group study. *J. Clin. Oncol.* **15,** 1916–1922.

46. Gasparini G, Barbareschi M, Doglioni C, et al. (1995) Expression of bcl-2 protein predicts efficacy of adjuvant treatments in operable node-positive breast cancer. *Clin. Cancer Res.* **1,** 189–198.

47. Yang D, Ling Y, Almazan M, et al. (1999) Tumor regression of human breast carcinomas by combination therapy of anti-bcl-2 antisense oligoneuleotide and chemotherapeutic drugs. American Association for Cancer Research 90th Annual Meeting, poster no.4814.

48. Rittling SR, Novick KE (1997) Osteopontin expression in mammary gland development and tumorigenesis. *Cell Growth Differ.* **8,** 1061–1069.

49. Ford D, Easton DF, Bishop DT, Narod SA, Goldgar DE (1994) Risks of cancer in *BRCA1*-mutation carriers. Breast Cancer Linkage Consortium. *Lancet* **343,** 692–695.

50. Rebbeck TR, Couch FJ, Kant J, et al. (1996) Genetic heterogeneity in hereditary breast cancer: role of *BRCA1* and *BRCA2*. *Am. J. Hum. Genet.* **59,** 547–553.

51. Krainer M, Silva-Arrieta S, Fitzgerlad MG, et al. (1997) Differential contributions of *BRCA1* and *BRCA2* to early-onset breast cancer. *N. Engl. J. Med.* **336,** 1416–1421.

52. Hall JM, Lee MK, Newman B, et al. (1990) Linkage of early-onset familial breast cancer to chromosome 17q21. *Science* **250,** 1684–1689.

53. Narod SA, Feunteun J, Lynch HT, et al. (1991) Familial breast-ovarian cancer locus on chromosome 17q12-q23. *Lancet* **338,** 82–83.

54. Chen Y, Farmer AA, Chi-Fen C, Jones DC, Chen PL, Lee WH (1996) BRCA1 is a 220-kDa nuclear phospho-protein that is expressed and phosphorylated in a cell cycle-dependent manner. *Cancer Res.* **56,** 3168–3172.

55. Sobol H, Stoppa-Lyonet D, Bressac-de-Paillerets B, et al. (1996) Truncation at conserved terminal regions of *BRCA1* protein is associated with highly proliferating hereditary breast cancers. *Cancer Res.* **56,** 3216–3219.

56. Wooster R, Bignell G, Lancaster J, et al. (1995) Identification of the breast cancer susceptibility gene BRCA2. *Nature* **378,** 789–792.

57. Tavtigian SV, Simard J, Rommens J, et al. (1996) The complete *BRCA2* gene and mutations in chromosome 13q-linked kindreds. *Nat. Genet.* **12,** 333–337.

58. Cortez D, Wang Y, Qin J, Elledge SJ (1999) Requirement of ATM-dependent phosphorylation of BRCA1 in the DNA damage response to double-strand breaks. *Science* **286,** 1162–1166.

59. Shen SX, Weaver Z, Xu X, et al. (1998) A targeted disruption of the murine BRCA1 gene causes gamma-irra-diation hypersensitivity and genetic instability. *Oncogene* **17,** 3115–3124.

60. Scully R, Chen J, Plug A, et al. (1997) Association of BRCA1 with Rad51 in mitotic and meiotic cells. *Cell* **88,** 265–275.

61. Patel KJ, Yu V, Lee H, et al. (1998) Involvement of BRCA2 in DNA repair. *Mol. Cell* **1,** 347–357.

62. Chen PL, Chen CF, Chen Y, Xiao J, Sharp ZD, Lee WH (1995) The BRC repeats in BRCA2 are critical for RAD51 binding and resistance to methyl methanesulfonate treatment. *Proc. Natl. Acad. Sci. USA.* **95,** 5287–5292.

63. Merajver SD, Frank TS, Xu J (1995) Germline *BRCA1* mutations and loss of the wild-type allele in tumors from families with early onset breast and ovarian cancer. *Clin. Cancer Res.* **1,** 1–6.

64. Serova O, Montagna M, Torchard D, et al. (1996) A high incidence of *BRCA1* mutations in 20 breast-ovarian cancer families. *Am. J. Hum. Genet.* **58,** 42–51.

65. Couch FJ, Weber BL (1996) Mutations and polymorphisms in the familial early-onset breast cancer (*BRCA1*) gene. Breast Cancer Information Core. *Hum. Mutat.* **8,** 8–18.

66. Berman DB, Wagner-Costalas J, Schultz DC, et al. (1996) Two distinct origins of a common *BRCA1* mutation in breast-ovarian cancer families: a genetic study of 15 185delAG-mutation kindreds. *Am. J. Hum. Genet.* **58,** 1166–1176.

67. Zittoun RA, Mandelli F, Willemze R, et al. (1995) Autologous or allogeneic bone marrow transplantation compared with intensive chemotherapy in acute myelogenous leukemia. European Organization for Research and Treatment of Cancer (EORTC) and the Gruppo Italiano Malattie Ematologiche Maligne dell'Adulto (GIMEMA) Leukemia Cooperative Groups [see comments]. *N. Engl. J. Med.* **332,** 217–223.

68. Dobrovic A, Simpfendorfer D (1997) Methylation of the BRCA1 gene in sporadic breast cancer. *Cancer Res.* **57,** 3347–3350.

69. Neuhausen S, Gilewski T, Norton L, et al. (1996) Recurrent *BRCA2* 6174delT mutations in Ashkenazi Jewish women affected by breast cancer. *Nat. Genet.* **13,** 126–128.

70. Cleton-Jansen A-M, Collins N, Lakhani SR, et al. (1995) Loss of heterozygosity in sporadic breast tumors at the BRCA2 locus on chromosome 13q12-q13. *Br. J. Cancer* **72,** 1241–1244.

71. Lancaster JM, Wooster R, Mangion J, et al. (1996) *BRCA2* mutations in primary breast and ovarian cancers. *Nat. Genet.* **13,** 238–240.

72. Foster KA, Harrington P, Kerr J, et al. (1996) Somatic and germline mutations of the *BRCA2* gene in sporadic ovarian cancer. *Cancer Res.* **56,** 3622–3625.

73. DeLeo AB, Jay G, Appella E, Dubois GC, Law LW, Old LJ (1979) Detection of a transformation-related anti-gen in chemically induced sarcomas and other transformed cells of the mouse. *Proc. Natl. Acad. Sci. USA* **76,** 2420–2424.

74. Crawford LV, Pim DC, Gurney EG, Goodfellow P, Taylor-Papadimitriou J (1981) Detection of a common feature in several human tumor cell lines—a 53,000-dalton protein. *Proc. Natl. Acad. Sci. USA* **78,** 41–45.

75. Oren M (1985) The p53 cellular tumor antigen: gene structure, expression and protein properties. *Biochem. Biophys. Acta* **823,** 67–78.

76. Eliyahu D, Michalovitz D, Eliyahu S, Pinhasi-Kimhi O, Oren M (1989) Wild-type p53 can inhibit oncogene-mediated focus formation. *Proc. Natl. Acad. Sci. USA* **86,** 8763–8767.

77. Eliyahu D, Goldfinger N, Pinhasi-Kimhi O, et al. (1988) Meth A fibrosarcoma cells express two transforming mutant p53 species. *Oncogene* **3,** 313–321.

78. Finlay CA, Hinds PW, Levine AJ (1989) The p53 proto-oncogene can act as a suppressor of transformation. *Cell* **57,** 1083–1093.

79. Kurose A, Sasaki K, Ishida Y, et al. (1995) Flow cytometric analysis of p53 expression during the cell cycle. *Oncology* **52,** 123–127.

80. Vogelstein B Kinzler KW (1992) p53 function and dysfunction. *Cell* **70,** 523–526.

81. Nigro JM, Baker SJ, Preisinger AC, et al. (1989) Mutations in the p53 gene occur in diverse human tumour types. *Nature* **342,** 705–708.

82. Blondal JA, Benchimol S (1994) The role of p53 in tumor progression. *Semin. Cancer Biol.* **5,** 177–186.

83. Martinez J, Georgoff I, Levine AJ (1991) Cellular localization and cell cycle regulation by a temperature-sensitive p53 protein. *Genes Dev.* **5,** 151–159.

84. Zerrahn J, Deppert W, Weidemann D, Patschinsky T, Richards F, Milner J (1992) Correlation between the conformational phenotype of p53 and its subcellular location. *Oncogene* **7,** 1371–1381.

85. Yonish-Rouach E, Resnitzky D, Lotem J, Sachs L, Kimchi A, Oren M (1991) Wild-type p53 induces apoptosis of myeloid leukaemic cells that is inhibited by interleukin-6. *Nature* **352,** 345–347.

85a. Jerry DJ, Ozbun MA, Kittrell FS, Lane DP, Medina D, Butel JS (1993) Mutations in p53 are frequent in the preneoplastic stage of mouse mammary tumor development. *Cancer Res.* **53,** 3374–3381.

86. Faille A, DeCremoux P, Extra JM, et al. (1994) p53 mutations and overexpression in locally advanced breast cancers. *Br. J. Cancer* **69,** 1145–1150.

87. Bautista S, Theillet C (1997) p53 mutations in breast cancer: incidence and relations to tumor aggressiveness and evolution of the disease. *Path. Biol.* **45,** 882–892.

88. Allred DC, Clark GM, Elledge R, et al. (1993) Association of p53 protein expression with tumor cell proliferation rate and clinical outcome in node-negative breast cancer. *J. Natl. Cancer Inst.* **85,** 200–206.

89. Crook T, Brooks LA, Crossland S, et al. (1998) p53 mutation with frequent novel codons but not a mutator phenotype in BRCA1 and BRCA2-associated breast tumours. *Oncogene* **17,** 1681–1689.

90. Doll R, Peto R (1981) The causes of cancer: quantitative estimates of avoidable risks of cancer in the United States today. *J. Natl. Cancer Inst.* **66,** 1191–1308.

91. Pezzella F, Tse AG, Cordell JL, Pulford KA, Gatter KC, Mason DY (1990) Expression of the bcl-2 oncogene protein is not specific for the 14;18 chromosomal translocation. *Am. J. Pathol.* **137,** 225–232.

92. Lupu R, Cardillo M, Cho C, et al. (1996) The significance of heregulin in breast cancer tumor progression and drug resistance. *Breast Cancer Res. Treat.* **38,** 57–66.

93. Grim J, Deshane J, Feng M, Lieber A, Kay M, Curiel DT (1996) erbB-2 knockout employing an intracellular single-chain antibody (sFv) accomplishes specific toxicity in erbB-2 expressing lung cancer cells. *Am. J. Respir. Cell Mol. Biol.* **15,** 348–354.

II   SPECIAL CLINICAL SITUATIONS

14 Primary Chemotherapy

Deborah L. Toppmeyer, MD

CONTENTS

INTRODUCTION
THEORETICAL ADVANTAGES OF PRIMARY CHEMOTHERAPY
POTENTIAL DISADVANTAGES TO PRIMARY CHEMOTHERAPY
REVIEW OF CURRENT STUDIES OF PRIMARY CHEMOTHERAPY
    IN OPERABLE BREAST CANCER
CURRENT AND FUTURE DIRECTIONS IN NEOADJUVANT THERAPY
CONCLUSIONS
REFERENCES

1. INTRODUCTION

Primary chemotherapy of breast cancer refers to the use of chemotherapy before definitive local treatment. Other synonymous terms include preoperative chemotherapy, neoadjuvant chemotherapy, induction chemotherapy, and upfront chemotherapy. Beginning in the early 1970s, primary chemotherapy has been explored to improve local control and survival in women with large breast tumors or inflammatory breast cancer. Primary chemotherapy produced regression of breast cancer in 60–90% of women *(1)* and made a significant impact on survival in inflammatory and locally advanced disease. Although primary chemotherapy was incorporated into standard treatment algorithms for select tumors such as Ewing's sarcoma, and carcinomas, and locally advanced and inflammatory breast cancer, its role in the treatment of resectable breast cancer is undefined. The rationale, benefits, and disadvantages of neoadjuvant chemotherapy in the treatment of operable breast cancer with a primary focus on the randomized clinical trials examining this modality are reviewed here. Recommendations on critical questions and potential future directions in this modality are addressed.

2. THEORETICAL ADVANTAGES OF PRIMARY CHEMOTHERAPY

The concept of primary chemotherapy is attractive for several reasons. It may potentially 1) downstage the primary tumor, leading to improved rates of breast conservation; 2) define the chemosensitivity of the tumor, resulting in the design of individualized chemotherapy regimens; and 3) help eliminate micrometastases and consequently improve overall survival.

From: *Current Clinical Oncology:*
Breast Cancer: A Guide to Detection and Multidisciplinary Therapy
Edited by: M. H. Torosian © Humana Press Inc., Totowa, NJ

2.1. Downstaging of the Primary Tumor

First, the ability to reduce the size of the primary tumor improves the likelihood of breast conservation and may decrease deaths from metastatic disease. Cytoreduction may also decrease the risk of local recurrence since larger tumors, despite adequate surgical margins, have a greater propensity for local failure. This principle was best demonstrated in patients with inoperable, locally advanced (LABC) or inflammatory breast cancer (IBC) *(2)*. The poor overall survival rate of patients with LABC is well documented. Bloom et al. followed 250 patients with LABC and observed a median survival of 2.7 years that was not affected by adjuvant radiation therapy to improve local control. In this study, 5-year survival rates with surgery alone, radiotherapy alone, or a combination of surgery and radiotherapy were 35, 29, or 33%, respectively.

The introduction of systemic chemotherapy had a significant impact on both local and distant disease. For example, chemotherapy increased survival, presumably owing to irradication of micrometastatic disease. Furthermore, systemic therapy converted patients with inoperable tumors to surgical candidates by cytoreduction of the primary tumor *(2,3)*.

The use of primary chemotherapy followed by surgery and radiation therapy is now the standard of care for LABC. A number of primary chemotherapy regimens and schedules have been studied in LABC. To date, no single regimen appears to be superior to another. The overall response rates range from 50 to 90% with clinical complete responses of 20% or less *(2)*. The controversial issue is whether or not the administration of primary therapy offers a benefit over adjuvant therapy in this population. Several studies found no overall survival benefit for primary chemotherapy compared with that of adjuvant chemotherapy in LABC. However, primary chemotherapy facilitates the surgical management of advanced tumors, limiting the need for complex reconstruction techniques. Furthermore, in highly selected patients breast conservation has been offered to patients with LABC with equivalent outcomes to modified radical mastectomy *(3)*. Therefore, the ability to downstage the primary tumor provides one of the rationales for administering primary chemotherapy in operable breast cancer.

2.2. Determining Chemosensitivity of the Tumor by Response and by Evaluation of Prognostic Molecular Markers

The initial responsiveness to primary chemotherapy can be used to select subsequent chemotherapy regimens. Patients with a poor initial response to chemotherapy may benefit from changing to a non-cross-resistant regimen, a novel schedule of established agents, or investigational therapies. In the future, chemotherapy may be selected based on molecular markers such as HER-2/*neu,* P-glycoprotein, bcl-2, and other drug-resistance mechanisms. As such markers may serve as surrogate markers for tumor response or chemosensitivity, neoadjuvant treatment of primary breast tumors allows sequential evaluation of proven and potential prognostic tumor markers (i.e., ploidy, S-phase, Ki67m HER-2/*neu,* mutant p53, or microtubule-associated protein 4 [MAP4] expression). Sequential analysis of these markers on tumor tissue obtained by core biopsies or fine needle aspiration (FNA) may provide insight into their significance. Indeed, Chang et al. *(4)* recently reported that expression and changes in expression of particular molecular markers predict for a good clinical response (GCR). GCR, in turn, appears to be a valid surrogate marker for survival *(4)*.

As a companion study to a primary chemotherapy plus endocrine therapy trial initiated by Powles et al. *(5)* in 1995, an evaluation of predictive molecular markers in primary operable breast cancer was performed. The predictive markers studied included estrogen receptors

(ERs), progesterone receptors (PRs), p53, bcl-2, Ki67, c-erbB-2, S-phase fraction, and ploidy. FNA of the primary breast tumor was performed twice before neoadjuvant chemotherapy and was repeated on day 10 or 21 of the first cycle of treatment. The results of this study demonstrated that a decrease in Ki67 expression, a measure of tumor proliferation, on day 10 or 21 of treatment significantly predicted for subsequent objective response *(4)*. Future studies may support the use of this biologic marker to guide treatment changes that would optimize GCR. Modern chemotherapy will probably be based on a predictive model to define the appropriate multimodality management strategy for individual breast cancer patients rather than a standardized approach based on histology alone.

2.3. Improved Treatment of Micrometastatic Disease

An extrapolation of the Goldie-Coldman hypothesis suggests that the potential for eradication of metastatic tumor clones is greater before surgery and that this approach should improve survival *(6)*. Accordingly, earlier introduction of non-cross-resistant chemotherapy would prevent the establishment of drug-resistant variants that arise from continued cell growth and somatic mutation. Thus, shortening the interval between diagnosis and the initiation of systemic therapy of breast cancer might lead to a better outcome. To date, this theoretical advantage has not been supported by clinical studies comparing perioperative chemotherapy with postoperative chemotherapy, and the value of earlier administration of chemotherapy in this setting has yet to be proved *(7–9)*.

A second hypothetical benefit, offered by Skipper, is that cytoreduction of the primary tumor mass may alter the growth characteristics of micrometastatic disease. This effect has been linked to the presence of a growth-stimulating factor in the serum *(10)*. Indeed, Fisher et al. *(11)* used an animal model to confirm this hypothesis, demonstrating improved tumor kinetics and survival when chemotherapy was administered before primary resection of the tumor. These provocative data provided the rationale for the design and conduct of primary chemotherapy trials in women with operable breast cancer.

3. POTENTIAL DISADVANTAGES TO PRIMARY CHEMOTHERAPY

Although primary chemotherapy offers some potential benefits, several disadvantages to this approach exist. The most significant disadvantage of primary chemotherapy is the loss of diagnostic and prognostic information gleaned from the initial examination of the lymph nodes and primary tumor specimen. Such information may help select certain subgroups that are at greater risk of recurrence and may therefore benefit from specific therapies or clinical research protocols.

3.1. Diagnostic Limitations

The appropriate use of primary chemotherapy rests on an accurate initial diagnosis of a palpable breast mass. The combination of physical examination, mammography, and FNA, the triple test, can enhance the accuracy of the diagnosis at the time of initial evaluation. When all three diagnostic evaluations suggested the lesion to be benign (3/457 cases), the false-negative rate was 0.7% *(12)*. However, if one component of the triple test is discordant, a surgical biopsy should be performed. Although both surgical and systemic treatments are initiated on the basis of an FNA alone, the potential for error remains. A review of the literature reveals a range of false-negative results from 1 to 35% as well as a range of false-positive results from 0.5 to 18%. The accuracy of the diagnosis is dependent on the experience of the surgeon and the expertise of the cytopathologist. A major limitation of the FNA is an inability to distinguish invasive from noninvasive carcinomas. Epithelial proliferations, duct papillomas, fibroadenomas, fat necrosis, mastitis, gynecomastia, and radiation changes may lead to false-positive diagnoses *(13)*. The most common reason for a false-negative FNA is an inadequate sample. Core biopsies are likely to result in better samples and may be performed on palpable lesions and also on nonpalpable lesions using mammographically guided stereotactic needle biopsy. The sensitivity of core biopsies increases with the size of the mass and ranges from 75 to 90% *(14)*. Compared with FNA, core needle biopsies are more likely to yield an accurate diagnosis, including additional histologic information such as histology, nuclear grade, and molecular markers such as HER-2/*neu* and ER and PR status. However, the reliability of the histologic information obtained from core needle biopsy remains inferior to that obtained by open biopsy. Furthermore, the ability to distinguish gross intraductal carcinoma from invasive carcinoma is limited. One to 2% of patients will be misdiagnosed with invasive disease and will receive unnecessary chemotherapy.

3.2. Loss of Preoperative Prognostic Information

Primary chemotherapy may interfere with the analysis of axillary lymph node metastases, the most important prognostic factor in breast cancer. Lymph node status is used to stratify patients according to risk of recurrence. This information is also used to recommend adjuvant treatment and to identify individuals for participation in appropriate clinical trials. Failure to determine the lymph node status can result in overtreatment of patients with an excellent prognosis and undertreatment of patients with a poor prognosis.

Compartmentalizing patients according to risk of recurrence is less important today than in the past since the indications for chemotherapy have broadened for breast cancer as a whole. The importance of axillary node dissection in guiding adjuvant treatment recommendations rests on whether the information gained will affect decisions regarding 1) the need for adjuvant treatment; 2) the chemotherapy regimen selected; or 3) the dose intensity of the selected regimen.

The primary prognostic factor in determining the need for adjuvant chemotherapy has become tumor size rather than lymph node status. In general, premenopausal and postmenopausal patients with hormone receptor negative tumors 1 cm or larger receive adjuvant chemotherapy regardless of lymph node status. Although adjuvant therapy recommendations may be influenced by molecular markers such as HER-2/*neu* expression as well as ER and PR status, the guidelines for the adjuvant administration of chemotherapy or chemoendocrine therapy have been liberalized, with a greater number of patients receiving treatment. Thus, determining the lymph node status in patients with tumors measuring 1 cm or larger may have less importance since most patients in this group will receive adjuvant therapy based on tumor size alone *(15)*.

Second, the choice of chemotherapy may be less dependent on lymph node status than on the presence of molecular markers expressed by the tumor. For example, overexpression of HER-2/*neu* (an oncogene overexpressed in 25–30% of breast tumors) in the primary breast tumor may be predictive of response to anthracyline-based chemotherapy (e.g., 60 mg/m^2 of doxorubicin q 3–4 weeks) and resistance to standard cyclophosphamide, methotrexate, and 5-fluorouracil (CMF) *(16–18)*. However, the use of HER-2/*neu* expression to predict for response to specific chemotherapy regimens remains controversial *(19)* and complicated by the lack of standardization of HER-2/*neu* assays. Nonetheless, based on these data, there is an increasing trend to recommend an anthracyline-based regimen over CMF in patients diagnosed with HER-2/*neu*-positive tumors regardless of lymph node status.

More recently, lymph node status has been an important factor for determining whether or not to add paclitaxel to the standard adjuvant regimen. Taxanes have demonstrated a benefit in the adjuvant setting in patients with node-positive breast cancer. For example, an interim analysis of an adjuvant intergroup trial led by the Cancer and Leukemia Groups B suggested an increased recurrence-free and overall survival when paclitaxel was added to the standard adjuvant regimen of doxorubicin and cyclophosphamide (AC). Women with operable node-positive breast cancer ($n = 3,170$) were randomly assigned to receive one of three doses of doxorubicin (60, 75, or 90 mg/m^2) in combination with cyclophosphamide (600 mg/m^2). In a second randomization, women received four cycles of paclitaxel at 175 mg/m^2 after CA or they received no further therapy. The addition of paclitaxel to CA reduced the annual odds of recurrence and death by 22%. This translated into an absolute improvement in overall survival of 2% and a 4% improvement in disease-free survival *(20)*.

Based on these provocative preliminary data, CA plus paclitaxel has supplanted CA alone as the new standard adjuvant regimen in high-risk, node-positive disease. Most patients in this study had four or more positive nodes. Whether a taxane can improve the results in patients with three or fewer positive nodes is the subject of active clinical investigation. The administration of primary chemotherapy not only precludes identifying patients for enrollment in these clinical trials but also raises the question of the optimal ncoadjuvant regimen to select for women whose nodal status is unknown. This very question, however, forms the basis of the ongoing National Surgical Adjuvant Breast and Bowel Project (NSABP) B-27 trial described later in this chapter *(21)*.

Third, the use of high-dose chemotherapy for high-risk breast cancer remains controversial. Therefore, the need for preoperative lymph node dissection to determine eligibility for this type of therapy may be a moot point. The interim analyses of two out of three randomized trials addressing the benefit of high-dose chemotherapy with autologous bone marrow or stem cell support did not favor the high-dose approach *(22–24)*. The Cancer and Leukemia Group B/Southwest Oncology Group (CALGB/SWOG) intergroup trial randomized women with 10 or more positive lymph nodes to high-dose chemotherapy with cyclophosphamide, cisplatin, and BCNU as well as bone marrow or peripheral blood stem cell support compared with intermediate-dose chemotherapy using the same agents with granulocyte colony-stimulating factor (G-CSF) support. No difference in overall survival was observed (78% versus 80% in the high-dose and intermediate-dose arms, respectively) after a median follow-up of 37 months. Notably, a significantly higher treatment-associated mortality rate was seen in the high-dose arm (7.4%) compared with the intermediate-dose arm (0%). Despite a trend toward an improved relapse-free survival in the high-dose arm (68% versus 64%), this difference between the two arms did not reach statistical significance *(22)*.

These data were consistent with the Scandanavian group's study of 5-fluororacil/epirubicin/cyclophosphamide (FEC) followed by high-dose chemotherapy versus tailored FEC, i.e., the escalated dose to myelosuppression. After a median follow-up of 5 years, there was no survival advantage found for the high-dose chemotherapy arm *(23)*. The only study that suggested an advantage to dose intensification was reported by Bezwoda et al. *(24)*. Patients were randomized to standard CAF versus cyclophosphamide, mitoxantrone, and etoposide for two high-dose cycles with stem cell support. Interim analyses demonstrated an improved overall- and relapse-free survival in the high-dose arm *(24)*. Although additional follow-up is needed to define the role of high-dose chemotherapy accurately in breast cancer, the administration of high-dose therapy to patients with 10 or more positive nodes should be done only in the context of well-designed clinical trials.

Despite the potential loss of prognostic information with neoadjuvant therapy, residual tumor size and lymph node status following primary chemotherapy may also be of significance. Both clinical and pathologic complete responses predicted an improved overall and disease-free survival rate (25,26) in patients receiving neoadjuvant chemotherapy. Thus, despite concerns regarding neoadjuvant chemotherapy, loss of prognostic information alone is not enough to discourage exploration of this approach through well-designed clinical trials.

4. REVIEW OF CURRENT STUDIES OF PRIMARY CHEMOTHERAPY IN OPERABLE BREAST CANCER

Several studies using neoadjuvant chemotherapy were designed to test the hypothetical advantages of this approach over adjuvant therapy. Unfortunately, the significant heterogeneity among clinical trials in terms of patient selection, local-regional and systemic treatments, primary and secondary end points, and definition of tumor response make it difficult to draw firm conclusions. Furthermore, few trials have examined the effect of primary chemotherapy on systemic control of disease or overall survival. We will review both the randomized and nonrandomized studies addressing neoadjuvant chemotherapy in operable breast cancer.

4.1. Randomized Clinical Trials of Primary Chemotherapy in Operable Breast Cancer

The initial randomized phase III trials of primary chemotherapy compared with adjuvant therapy asked the question whether or not primary chemotherapy could improve disease-free and overall survival in patients with high-risk early, operable breast cancer. A second objective was to determine whether neoadjuvant chemotherapy could increase the number of patients eligible for breast-conserving therapy.

Five prospective randomized trials have addressed the use of primary chemotherapy in the management of operable breast cancer (Tables 1 and 2). The largest is the NSABBP B-18. Patients ($n = 1523$) who had primary palpable, operable breast cancer (T1–3, N0–1, M0) were randomized to standard doxorubicin and cyclophosphamide (60 mg/m^2 and 600 mg/m^2, respectively) for four 3-week cycles before or after definitive surgery. The primary end points were disease-free and overall survival. Secondary end points included the effects of chemotherapy on 1) the clinical and pathologic response of primary breast cancer to preoperative chemotherapy; 2) the effect of preoperative chemotherapy on axillary lymph node status; and 3) the rate of breast-conserving therapy following preoperative chemotherapy. The response rate in the group receiving primary chemotherapy was 79% (35% complete response and 44% partial response). In addition, a greater number of patients in the primary chemotherapy group avoided mastectomy ($p = 0.007$). The difference in breast conservation was particularly striking in patients with tumors measuring 5.1 cm or more (8% versus 22%). In addition, patients with clinically positive lymph nodes who received primary chemotherapy had a statistically significant decrease in pathologically positive lymph nodes compared with those who received postoperative chemotherapy (41% versus 57%) (27). Primary chemotherapy did not improve disease-free or overall survival through 6 years of follow-up compared with postoperative treatment (67 and 80% respectively, in both groups).

Mauriac et al. (28) recently published an updated analysis of a randomized trial of primary chemotherapy conducted at the Institute Bergonie. Women with tumors larger than 3 cm ($n = 272$) were randomized between 1985 and 1989 to mastectomy followed by adjuvant chemotherapy in patients with pathologically confirmed node-positive disease or ER/PR-

Table 1
Trial Designs of Randomized Clinical Trials of Primary Chemotherapy

Author	No. of patients	Stage or T size	Arm of trial	Treatment design
Fisher et al. (27)	1523	T1–3N0–1	Primary chemotherapy	AC × 4 → MRM or
			Standard therapy	SEG + RT
				MRM or SEG + XRT
				→ AC × 4
Mauriac et al. (28)	272	T > 3 cm	Primary chemotherapy (group B)	EVM + MTV (if T = CR → RT alone; T < 2cm → SEG + RT; T > 2 cm → MRM
			Standard therapy (group A)	MRM if N– and ER+ → no Rx
				If N+ or ER– → EVM ×3 + MTV ×3
Scholl et al.	414	T = 3–7 cm	Primary chemotherapy (group 1)	FAC × 4–6 → RT → surgery if patient operable
			Primary RT + adjuvant chemotherapy (group 2)	RT → surgery → FAC × 4
Semiglazov et al. (29)	271	Stage IIB–IIIA T3N1, 50%	Primary chemotherapy (group 1)	TMF × 3 + RT → MRM → TMF × 3
			Primary RT (group 2)	RT → MRM → TMF × 6
Powles et al. (5)	212	T1–2, 92–97%	Primary chemo-endocrine therapy	3M (2M × 4 + TAM → surgery ± RT → 3M (2M) × 4
			Standard adjuvant chemoendocrine therapy	Surgery ± RT → 3M (2M) × 8 + TAM

MRM, modified radical mastectomy; RT, radiotherapy; SEG, segmental mastectomy; T, tumor; AC, doxorubicin/cyclophosphamide; FAC, 5-fluorouracil/doxorubicin/cyclophosphamide; TMF, thiotepa/methotrexate/5-fluorouracil; EVM, epirubicin/vincristine/methotrexate; MTV, mitomycin/thiotepa/vinblastine; 3M, methotrexate/mitoxantrone/mitomycin C; 2M, methotrexate/mitoxantrone; TAM, tamoxifen; ER, estrogen receptor; CR, complete response

negative tumors (group A) versus primary chemotherapy followed by definitive local therapy (group B). Both groups received three cycles of epirubicin, vincristine, and methotrexate followed by three cycles of vincristine, thiotepa, and vindesine. Local-regional treatment options in the neoadjuvant chemotherapy group included 1) exclusive irradiation of breast and nodal areas in cases of clinical complete regression; 2) lumpectomy and breast irradiation in cases of residual tumor smaller than 2 cm; or 3) mastectomy without irradiation in cases of residual tumor larger than 2 cm. After 124 months of follow-up, there was no difference in relapse-free or overall survival between the two groups. However, 24% of patients in group A received no adjuvant therapy based on the initial treatment design. Local-regional recurrences were more common in the primary chemotherapy group (23%) than in the adju-

Table 2
Results of Randomized Clinical Trials of Primary Chemotherapy

Author	Arm of trial	Response rate	Breast conservation rate (%)	Local control rate (%)	Survival
Fisher et al. (27)	Primary chemotherapy	CR = 35 RR = 79	67*		DFS = 67 OS = 80
	Standard therapy	NA	60*		DFS = 67 OS = 80
Mauriac et al. (28)	Primary chemotherapy (group B)	CR = 33 RR = 63	45 at 124 mo	77	DFS = ND OS = 53
	Standard therapy (group A)	NA		91	DFS = ND OS = 53
Scholl et al.	Primary chemotherapy (group 1)	CR = 30 RR = 82	61	73	DFS = 59 OS = 86*
	Primary RT + adjuvant chemotherapy (group 2)	CR = 41 RR = 85	63	81	DFS = 55 OS = 78*
Semiglazov et al. (29)	Primary chemotherapy (group 1)	CR = 35	All MRM by trial design		DFS = 81 OS = 86
	Primary RT (group 2)	CR = 28	All MRM by trial design		DFS = 71 OS = 78
Powles et al. (5)	Primary chemoendocrine therapy	CR = 19 RR = 85	87		DFS = 89 OS = 87
	Standard adjuvant chemoendocrine therapy	NA	72		DFS = 87 OS = 90

CR, complete response; RR, response rate; RT, radiotherapy; MRM, modified radical mastectomy; DFS, disease-free survival; OS, overall survival; *, statistically significant, ND, no difference between the two groups; NA, data not provided.

vant group (8.8%). Thirty-three percent of patients in the primary chemotherapy group received radiation alone, 30% had lumpectomy and radiation, and 37% had a modified radical mastectomy. This type of local-regional therapy had an important impact on outcome. The failure rate was 34% in the radiation-alone group and 22 and 22% in the lumpectomy plus radiation and modified radical mastectomy groups, respectively. The overall breast conservation rate was 45% for the primary chemotherapy group (28).

Scholl et al. from the Institut Curie reported similar results. Primary end points in this randomized study of primary chemotherapy plus radiation (group 1) versus primary radiation followed by adjuvant chemotherapy (group 2) included overall survival and breast conservation rate. The targeted patient population was premenopausal women with breast tumors not amenable to breast conservation (3–7 cm). Surgery was performed in both groups after maximal tumor response, and patients on the radiotherapy arm received postoperative chemotherapy (group 2). The objective response rate to primary chemotherapy was 82%, with a 30% complete response rate. High response rates were also demonstrated in patients treated with primary breast irradiation, with 41% complete responses and an overall response rate of 85% (group 2). The combination of chemotherapy and radiation increased complete responses to 61% in the primary chemotherapy group (group 1). The 5-year breast preservation rates were 61 and 63% for groups 1 and 2, respectively. Five-year local control rates were not statistically different, at 73% in group 1 and 81% in group 2. However, this is the only randomized study to demonstrate a survival advantage for primary chemotherapy with a 5-year overall survival of 86% compared with 78% for adjuvant chemotherapy, suggesting a potential impact on the early treatment of micrometastatic disease *(6)*.

Semiglazov et al. *(29)* demonstrated added benefit from primary chemotherapy when given with concurrent radiation therapy in 271 patients with stage IIb–IIIA disease. Patients were randomized to receive radiation therapy with (group 1) or without (group 2) concurrent chemotherapy followed by modified radical mastectomy. Following surgery, both groups received a total of six cycles of thiotepa, methotrexate, and 5-fluorouracil. The clinical complete response rate was similar in both groups (35% verses 27.6%) whereas the pathologic complete response rate was significantly increased in the primary chemotherapy arm (29% versus 19%). Although relapse-free-survival was better in the primary chemotherapy arm (81% verses 71.6%), there was no difference in overall survival *(6,29)*.

The only randomized study to evaluate systemic chemotherapy plus endocrine therapy as primary treatment was initiated by Powles et al. *(5)* at the Royal Marsden Hospital in 1990. Patients ($n = 212$) younger than 70 years of age with a clinically palpable, operable breast cancer were randomized to neoadjuvant or adjuvant chemoendocrine treatment with methotrexate, mitoxantrone, and mitomycin C plus tamoxifen. Following a confirmed diagnosis of breast cancer by FNA or Trucut biopsy, women were randomized to 1) chemoendocrine therapy for 3 months before and 3 months after surgery plus radiotherapy if required; or 2) surgery followed by radiation and adjuvant chemoendocrine therapy for 6 months. The first 59 patients received mitomycin C, mitoxantrone, and methotrexate plus tamoxifen. The regimen was subsequently modified to exclude mitomycin with an increase in the dose of mitoxantrone because of an unanticipated serious interaction between mitomycin and tamoxifen manifested as anemia, thrombocytopenia, and renal dysfunction. Two hundred patients were evaluable for response. Primary chemoendocrine therapy produced an objective response in 86/101 patients (85%), with a complete clinical response in 19% and a pathologic complete response in 10%. Primary therapy also improved the rate of breast conservation compared with adjuvant therapy (87% verses 72%, respectively). At 28 months of follow-up, no difference in relapse-free or overall survival was seen. Longer term follow-up will be needed to assess the impact of primary therapy on mortality *(5)*.

4.2. Nonrandomized Clinical Trials of Primary Chemotherapy

Several nonrandomized clinical trials address the issue of primary chemotherapy (Table 3). Because of the diverse design and conduct of these studies, definitive conclusions regarding survival cannot be drawn.

The initial reports of primary chemotherapy in operable breast cancer were published by Bonnadonna et al. in 1990. Women with resectable tumors larger than 3 cm ($n = 161$) were given one of five different neoadjuvant regimens for three or four cycles. The overall response rate was 77%, with no difference between regimens. The magnitude of response was inversely proportional to the initial tumor size and was greater in ER-negative tumors. These authors concluded that primary chemotherapy produced significant downstaging, converting the definitive surgical treatment from mastectomy to breast conservation in 79% of cases *(30,31)*.

Similarly, other studies of primary chemotherapy demonstrated increased breast conservation (86–96%) and response rates ranging from 60 to 90% *(32–36)* (Table 4). Because of the design of these studies, it is difficult to comment on the impact of primary chemotherapy

Table 3
Trial Designs of Nonrandomized Clinical Trials of Primary Chemotherapy

Author	No. of patients	Tumor size	Treatment regimen
Bonadonna et al. (32) Trial 1, phase II	227	>3 cm	CMF or FAC × 3–4 cycles; or FEC or FNC or D × 3 cycles → QUAD + XRT or MRM → 2–3 adjuvant cycles using same preop regimen in N+ or ER–
Belembaogo et al. (35) phase II	126	≥3 cm or central location	AVcrCF ± M × 6 → if CR → RT → if not CR → SEG + RT → if tumor >3 cm → MRM
Calais et al. (33) phase II	158	>3 cm	MVCF or EVCF × 3 cycles → SEG + XRT or MRM or RT without surgery
Jacquillant et al. (34) phase II	250	T1–4	VTMFP ± A q 7–14 days × 3–6 cycles Plus external RT Plus iridium implant RT Plus 6–12 cycles of chemotherapy Plus tamoxifen Plus surgery if relapse
Smith et al. (36)	64	"MRM deemed necessary"	CMF × 6 or MMM × 8 + RT + surgery if necessary

MRM, modified radical mastectomy; RT, radiotherapy; SEG, segmental mastectomy; T, tumor; AVcrCF, doxorubicin/vincristine/cyclophosphamide/5-fluorouracil; D, doxorubicin; EVCF, epirubicin/vindesine/cyclophosphamide/5-fluorouracil, FAC, 5-fluoro-uracil/doxorubicin; FEC, 5-FU, etoposide/cyclophosphamide; FNC, 5-fluorouracil/mitoxantrone/cyclophosphamide; MMM, mitomycin C/mitoxantrone/methotrexate; VTMFP ± A, vinblastine/thiotepa/methotrexate/5-fluorouracil/prednisone ± doxorubicin; MVCF, mitoxantrone/vindesine/cyclophosphamide/5-fluorouracil; MTV, mitomycin/thiotepa/vinblastine; ER, estrogen receptor; QUAD, quadrantectomy; N, node.

Table 4
Results of Nonrandomized Clinical Trials of Primary Chemotherapy

Author	Median follow-up	Response rate (%)	Breast conservation rate (%)	Local control rate (%)	Survival (%)
Bonadonna et al. (32)	6 yr	CR = 21 RR = 78	91	94	DFS = 56 OS = 75
Belembaogo et al. (35)	30 mo	CR = 36 RR = 85	85	NA	NA
Calais et al. (33)	NA	CR = 20 RR = 61	49	NA	NA
Jacquillant et al. (34)	62 mo	CR = 100	96	NA	OS Stage I = 95 Stage IIA = 94 Stage IIB = 80 Stage IIIA = 60 Stage IIIB = 58
Smith et al. (36)	NA	Chemo alone = 67 Chemo + RT = 94	86	NA	NA

CR, complete response; RR, response rate; NA, not available; DFS, disease-free survival; OS, overall survival; RT, radiotherapy.

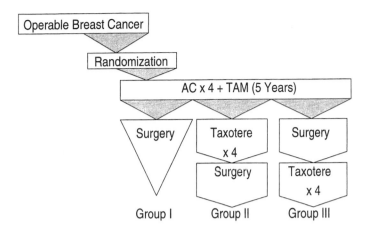

Fig. 1. NSABP trial, B-27, design.

on survival *(31)*. Various chemotherapy regimens, schedules, and treatments were used. Furthermore, the major limitation to interpreting these single-institution studies is the lack of well-defined criteria of patient selection for breast conserving therapy.

5. CURRENT AND FUTURE DIRECTIONS IN NEOADJUVANT THERAPY

The objectives of ongoing and anticipated trials of primary chemotherapy are to determine the effect of altering dose density or sequence of standard agents and the value of incorporating the class of taxanes, found to be highly effective in the metastatic setting, in the primary regimen.

The taxanes are active when used in first- and second-line treatment of metastatic breast cancer. The combination of anthracyclines and taxanes produced significantly greater response rates than either agent alone in previously untreated patients with metastatic breast cancer. Taxanes appear to add benefit in the adjuvant setting when given with AC in women with node-positive breast cancer *(20)*. The next logical step is to study the taxanes as primary therapy. The NSABP trial, B-27, exemplifies this principle and involves randomizing patients to four cycles of preoperative or postoperative docetaxel (100 mg/m^2) following four cycles of AC. AC followed by surgery will serve as the control arm (Fig. 1). The primary objectives are to determine the value and optimal sequencing of docetaxel in the adjuvant setting with the primary end points being disease-free and overall survival. Secondary end points will include rates of breast conservation, local-regional response, and pathologic response rates. The choice of surgical procedure will be left to the discretion of the surgeon, with the intended procedure noted before randomization; the control arm will not receive preoperative chemotherapy. Patients who undergo lumpectomy will receive standard postoperative radiation therapy. It is anticipated that 1606 patients will be accrued over the next 5 years *(21)*.

Two ancillary studies to B-27 will attempt to evaluate the role of serum and tumor biomarkers as they relate to outcome and response to preoperative AC and/or docetaxel chemotherapy. The objective of the first study is to determine the predictive value of serum HER-2/*neu* extracellular domains and HER-2/*neu* antibodies on response to chemotherapy and on long-term outcome. The second study will examine whether chemotherapy induces changes in select tumor biomarkers (i.e., nuclear grade, ER and PR, p53 and HER-2/*neu* expression, P-glycoprotein, and indices of proliferation) and whether these changes are correlated with tumor response and other outcome measures including survival. Therefore, B-27 and the companion studies should provide insight into the biologic and clinical effect of preoperative chemotherapy, especially as it relates to the evaluation of new agents in the adjuvant setting and the interaction of treatment with well-established and novel bio-markers *(21)*.

6. CONCLUSIONS

Primary chemotherapy offers several advantages over adjuvant chemotherapy, including the ability to assess response to individual drugs or combinations. The response to chemotherapy is an excellent indicator of survival *(3,34,37)*. Lack of response to chemother-apy identifies a patient population of potential candidates for investigational agents. Primary chemotherapy allows the investigators to follow histopathologic and molecular markers to determine whether they have any impact on drug sensitivity. For example, both mutant p53 and bcl-2 expression are correlated with resistance to chemotherapy, and HER-2/*neu* overex-pression may be responsible for resistance to CMF chemotherapy *(6)*. The lack of decreased expression of Ki67 following the administration of chemotherapy may also predict for drug resistance. These types of studies will ultimately help tailor therapies and strategically target new therapeutic interventions.

The theoretical advantage of increasing survival in women with breast cancer by giving chemotherapy before surgery has not been realized. Nonetheless, a major advantage to pri-mary chemotherapy is the ability to decrease the size of tumors so that more patients can receive breast-conserving surgery. Despite initial concerns, the rate of in-breast recurrence is not increased when primary chemotherapy is given followed by breast-conserving treatment and radiation therapy.

Disadvantages of primary chemotherapy include the risk of losing prognostic information including histologic markers and accurate evaluation of axillary lymph nodes. This will result in undertreating some patients and overtreating others. In addition, lack of this infor-mation will disqualify patients from many clinical trials.

With few exceptions, primary chemotherapy outside of a clinical trial should not be con-sidered standard treatment, rather, oncologists should enroll eligible patients in well-designed clinical trials testing new agents and sequences and assessing molecular markers so that the full potential of this approach can be explored.

REFERENCES

1. Swain S, Lippman M (1989) Systemic therapy of locally advanced breast cancer: review and guidelines. *Oncology* **3,** 21–28.
2. Gradishar W (1998) Primary chemotherapy regimens and schedules. *Semin. Oncol.* **25,** 25–30.
3. Schwartz GF, Birchansky CA, Komarnicky LT, et al. (1994) Induction chemotherapy followed by breast con-servation for locally advanced carcinoma of the breast. *Cancer* **73,** 362–369.
4. Chang J, Powles TJ, Allred DC, et al. (1999) Biologic markers as predictors of clinical outcome from sys-temic therapy for primary operable breast cancer. *J. Clin. Oncol.* **17,** 3058–3063.
5. Powles T, Hickish T, Makris A, et al. (1995) Randomized trial of chemoendocrine therapy started before or after surgery for treatment of primary breast cancer. *J. Clin. Oncol.* **13,** 547–552.
6. Harris L, Swain S (1996) The role of primary chemotherapy in early breast cancer. *Semin. Oncol.* **23,** 31–42.
7. Nissen-Meyer R, Kjellgren K, Mansson B (1982) Adjuvant chemotherapy in breast cancer. *Cancer Res.* **80,** 142–148.

8. Combination adjuvant chemotherapy for node-positive breast cancer: inadequacy of a single perioperative cycle (1988) Ludwig Breast Cancer Study Group. *N. Engl. J. Med.* **319,** 677–683.

9. Legler C, Shapiro C, Harris J, Hayes D (1995) Primary chemotherapy of resectable breast cancer. *Breast J.* **1,** 42–51.

10. Fisher B, Gunduz N, Saffer E (1983) Influence of the interval between primary tumor removal and chemotherapy on kinetics and growth of metastases. *Cancer Res.* **43,** 1488–1492.

11. Fisher B, Gundu N, Coyle J, Rudock C, Saffer E (1989) Presence of a growth-simulating factor in serum following primary tumor removal in mice. *Cancer Res.* **49,** 1996–2001.

12. Layfield L, Glasgow GJ, Cramer H (1989) Fine needle aspiration in the management of breast masses. *Pathol. Annu.* **24,** 23–62.

13. Donegan WL (1992) Evaluation of a palpable breast mass. *N. Engl. J. Med.* **327,** 937–942.

14. Minkowitz S, Moskowitz R, Khafif RA, Alderete MN (1986) Trucut needle biopsy of the breast. An analysis of its specificity and sensitivity. *Cancer* **57,** 320–323.

15. Hait WN, Toppmeyer DL, Dipaola RS (1999) Medical treatment of breast cancer. In: Hait WN (ed.) *Expert Consulations in Breast Cancer.* Marcel Dekker, New York, pp. 69–88.

16. Muss H, Thor A, Berrtm D, et al. (1994) c-erbB-2 expression and response to adjuvant therapy in women with node-positive early breast cancer. *N. Engl. J. Med.* **330,** 1260–1266.

17. Gusterson BA, Gelber RD, Goldhirsch A, et al. (1992) Prognostic importance of c-erB-2 expression in breast cancer. *J. Clin. Oncol.* **10,** 1049–1256.

18. Vera R, Albanell J, Lirola JL, et al. (1999) HER2 overexpression as a predictor of survival in a trial comparing adjuvant FAC and CMF in breast cancer. *Proc. Am. Soc. Clin. Oncol.* **18,** 71a (Abst 265).

19. Menard S, Valaguss P, Pilotti S, et al. (1999) Benefit of CMF treatment in lymph node-positive breast cancer overexpressing HER2. *Proc. Am. Soc. Clin. Oncol.* **18,** 69a (Abst 257).

20. Henderson IC, Berry D, Demetri G, et al. (1998) Improved disease-free and overall survival from the addition of sequential paclitaxel but not from the escalation of doxorubicin dose level in the adjuvant chemotherapy of patients with node-positive primary breast cancer. *Proc. Am. Soc. Clin. Oncol.* **17,** 101a (Abst 390A).

21. Mamounas E (1998) Overview of national surgical adjuvant breast project neoadjuvant chemotherapy studies. *Semin. Oncol.* **25,** 31–35.

22. Peters W, Rosner G, Vrenenburgh J, et al. (1999) A prospective randomized comparison of two doses of combination alkylating agents as consolidation after CAF in high-risk primary breast cancer involving ten or more axillary lymph nodes: preliminary results of CALGB 9082/SWOG9114/NCIC MA-13. *Proc. ASCO* **18,** 1a.

23. Results from a randomized adjuvant breast cancer study with high dose chemotherapy with CTCb supported by autologous bone marrow stem cells versus dose escalated and tailored FEC therapy (1999) The Scandinavian Breast Cancer Study Group 9401. *Proc. ASCO* **18,** 2a.

24. Bezwoda WR (1999) Randomized, controlled trial of high dose chemotherapy (HD-CNVp) versus standard dose (CAF) chemotherapy for high risk, surgically treated, primary breast cancer. *Proc. ASCO* **18,** 2a.

25. Kuerer HM, Newman LA, Smith TL, et al. (1999) Clinical course of breast cancer patients with complete pathologic primary tumor and axillary lymph node response to doxorubicin-based neoadjuvant chemotherapy. *J. Clin. Oncol.* **17,** 460–469.

26. Ferriere JP, Assier I, Cure H, Charrier S, Kwiatkowski F (1998) Primary chemotherapy in breast cancer correlation between tumor response and patient outcome. *Am. J. Clin. Oncol.* **21,** 117–120.

27. Fisher B, Brown A, Mamounas E, et al. (1997) Effect of preoperative chemotherapy on local-regional disease in women with operable breast cancer: findings from National Surgical Adjuvant Breast and Bowel Project B-18. *J. Clin. Oncol.* **15,** 2483–2493.

28. Mauriac L, MacGrogan G, Avril A, et al. (1999) Neoadjuvant chemotherapy or operable breast carcinoma larger than 3 cm: a unicentre randomized trial with a 124-month median follow-up. *Ann. Oncol.* **10,** 47–52.

29. Semiglazov V, Topuzov E, Bavli J, et al. (1994) Primary (neoadjuvant) chemotherapy and radiotherapy compared with primary radiotherapy alone in stage IIb-IIIb breast cancer. *Ann. Oncol.* **5,** 591–595.

30. Bonnadonna G, Valagussa P (1996) Primary chemotherapy in operable breast cancer. *Semin. Oncol.* **23,** 464–474.

31. Brenin D, Morrow M (1998) Breast-conserving surgery in the neoadjuvant setting. *Semin. Oncol.* **25,** 13–18.

32. Bonnadonna G, Veronesi U, Brambilla C, et al. (1990) Primary chemotherapy to avoid mastectomy in tumors with diameters of three centimeters or more. *J. Natl. Cancer Inst.* **82,** 1539–1545.

33. Calais G, Berger C, Descamps P, et al. (1994) Conservative treatment feasibility with induction chemotherapy, surgery, and radiotherapy for patients with breast carcinoma larger than 3 cm. *Cancer* **74,** 1283–1288.

34. Jacquillat C, Weil M, Baillet R, et al. (1990) Results of neoadjuvant chemotherapy and radiation therapy in the breast conserving treatment of 250 patients with all stages of infiltrative breast cancer. *Cancer* **66,** 119–129.

35. Belembaogo E, Feillel V, Chollet P, et al. (1992) Neoadjuvant chemotherapy in 126 operable breast cancers. *Eur. J. Cancer Clin. Oncol.* **28A,** 896–900.

36. Smith I, Jones A, O'Brien M, McKinna J, Sacks N, Baum M (1993) Primary medical (neoadjuvant) chemotherapy for operable breast cancer. *Eur. J. Cancer Clin. Oncol.* **29A,** 1796–1799.

37. Bonadonna G, Valagussa P, Zucali R, et al. (1995) Primary chemotherapy in surgically resectable breast cancer. *CA Cancer J. Clin.* **45,** 227–243.

15

Axillary Adenopathy as the Initial Presentation of Breast Cancer

Shirley Scott, MD, and Monica Morrow, MD

CONTENTS

INTRODUCTION
DIAGNOSTIC INTERVENTION
MANAGEMENT
PROGNOSIS
CONCLUSIONS
REFERENCES

1. INTRODUCTION

Breast cancer presenting as axillary adenopathy without clinical or radiologic breast findings is a rare clinical entity first described by Halsted in 1907 *(1)*. These occult primary cancers are staged as TON1, stage II breast cancer when thorough clinical and radiologic investigations do not reveal the presence of a primary breast tumor. The reported incidence of this phenomenon ranges from 0.3 to 0.8% *(2–5)*. The mean age at presentation is approximately 50 years in most series, which is similar to that of the general breast cancer population *(3,5–10)*. This rare, but well-recognized phenomenon can present both a diagnostic and therapeutic dilemma because other occult malignancies may present as axillary adenopathy, including melanoma and carcinomas of the thyroid, lung, gastrointestinal tract, ovary, and genitourinary tract. However, the most common source of adenocarcinoma in axillary lymph nodes in women is the breast *(6,11–14)*.

2. DIAGNOSTIC INTERVENTION

The initial workup of a patient presenting with axillary lymphadenopathy begins with a careful history and physical examination. The patient should be evaluated for adenopathy in other nodal regions, as generalized lymphadenopathy may suggest other etiologies such as lymphoma or a viral source. The skin of the patient should also be carefully evaluated to search for pigmented skin lesions, and a history of skin lesions removed by cautery or freezing without pathologic examination should be sought. A complete physical exam with special attention directed toward examination of the thyroid gland, lungs, abdomen, and pelvis should be performed since adenocarcinomas in areas other than the breast may also present in this manner *(8,15)*.

From: *Current Clinical Oncology:*
Breast Cancer: A Guide to Detection and Multidisciplinary Therapy
Edited by: M. H. Torosian © Humana Press Inc., Totowa, NJ

Frequently, adenocarcinomas originating in areas other than the breast will be symptomatic, and a thorough history and physical exam will direct the examiner to the primary site *(15,16)*. In the absence of suggestive history and physical findings, an extensive search for extramammary primary adenocarcinomas is not indicated *(3,5,16–18)*. In fact, Patel et al. *(18)* demonstrated that the yield for multiple investigations in search of other primary sites is invariably low. Investigative procedures in 29 patients were normal except for one suspicious liver scan that was later found to be falsely positive after surgical exploration *(18)*. Kemeny et al. *(17)* also found that extensive investigations have a high incidence of false-positive results and rarely result in the identification of a primary tumor site. Their study revealed that of 74 radiographic or nuclear imaging tests performed, 16 tests were read as positive. Five of the 16 positive tests were true positive, and 11 were false positive. An extensive radiologic workup had a true-positive rate of less than 7%. This general rule, however, does not hold true for men because male patients with axillary nodal metastases have a higher likelihood of an extramammary primary. To date, only one male patient has been reported in the literature as presenting with isolated axillary lymphadenopathy from an occult breast primary *(5)*.

2.1. Biopsy

The initial diagnostic maneuver in patients presenting with isolated axillary lymphadenopathy should be a biopsy of the palpable lymph node. This may consist of fine needle aspiration biopsy (FNAB), core needle biopsy, or excisional biopsy. In general, FNA is not adequate to determine the primary site, and excision of the node should be undertaken. The pathologist should be informed that the primary site is unknown, and the specimen should be sent fresh to the pathologist so that special stains can be performed and estrogen and progesterone receptor (ER/PR) status can be evaluated *(7,14,19)*. Haupt et al. *(19)* studied the histologic appearance associated with occult breast cancer metastatic to the axilla and found that the most common pattern observed in their series of 37 patients was characterized by "sheets of large, apocrine-like pleomorphic cells with pale to granular pink cytoplasm, large nuclei and prominent nucleoli." Two less common histologic patterns were architecturally more suggestive of breast cancer, with glandular, cribriform, or papillary elements. Pathologically, 73% of cases of occult carcinoma are classified as infiltrating ductal carcinoma *(20)*. Special stains such as immunoperoxidase staining for lactalbumin may be valuable to help make the diagnosis of metastatic breast cancer *(21)*. ER/PR analysis should be performed routinely in this clinical circumstance *(8,19,21–23)*. Positive findings are suggestive of breast cancer and occur in approximately 50% of female patients *(8,24)*. Negative ER/PR status does not exclude the diagnosis of breast cancer, and it is important to realize that carcinomas of the kidney, colon, ovary, endometrium, and melanoma may demonstrate ER/PR activity *(19,22)*. Another important reason for obtaining ER/PR studies on the initial biopsy is that the primary tumor may be too small to perform ER/PR assays or may not be found at all *(18,21)*.

2.2. Mammography

All patients presenting with isolated axillary lymphadenopathy should undergo bilateral mammography with two or more views of each breast using state of the art equipment, prior to biopsy of the axillary node. If a mammographic abnormality is found, it, rather than the node should be the initial biopsy target. However, even the highest quality mammogram will not always demonstrate a lesion, and mammography has been reported to be positive in only 12–25% of cases *(15,25)*. Patel et al. *(18)* reported on 17 patients with breast exams that were clinically normal who had metastatic adenocarcinoma to the axilla. All patients underwent mammography and mastectomy, and six of eight patients with positive or suspicious mammograms had cancer found on specimen examination, whereas only four of nine patients with negative mammograms had a primary tumor identified. With the widespread availability of image-guided core biopsy, any suspicious mammographic lesion should be sampled since identification of the primary site in the breast will facilitate breast-conserving therapy. Despite a negative mammogram, an occult primary breast cancer should be considered the source of the adenocarcinoma found in the axilla.

2.3. Magnetic Resonance Imaging

Recent studies have evaluated the use of magnetic resonance imaging (MRI) to identify breast cancers not seen on mammogram (26). MRI of the breast with paramagnetic contrast has been shown to have a sensitivity for breast cancer of 86–100% (27–32). However, the specificity for cancer is lower and more variable, ranging from 37 to 97% (26,28,29,33–36). Owing to the current expense of MRI, as well as the low specificity, it is not appropriate for evaluation of all patients. However, the high sensitivity of MRI makes it an attractive diagnostic modality for use in the patient thought to have occult primary breast carcinoma (37). Harms and Flamig (38) and Davis et al. (39) have reported individual cases in which MRI has been valuable in identifying the primary tumor site in the breast. Porter et al. (40) reported the efficacy of varying breast MRI parameters at a single institution in six patients with occult primary breast cancer. Histologically confirmed primary carcinomas were detected in four of the six patients. A study performed by Morris et al. (37) reported contrast-enhanced foci on MRI of the breast in 9 of 12 patients with occult primary tumors. Eight of the nine were subsequently confirmed to have breast cancer. Two patients had a negative MR study, and no identifiable tumor was found in either case after histologic examination of the mastectomy specimen. Since the actual false-negative rate of MRI is unknown, it remains unclear how patients with negative MR examinations should be treated.

Identification of an abnormal area on MRI also allows a focused mammographic and ultrasound examination. Brenner and Rothman (41) reported on four patients with occult carcinoma metastatic to axillary nodes. After detecting foci of enhancement on MRI, ultrasound-guided biopsy was successful in all cases. A similar finding was reported by Tilanus-Linthorst et al. (42) in four cases. The available data on the use of MRI for the detection of occult primary breast cancer are summarized in Table 1.

Breast MRI is a promising tool, but owing to problems with specificity and the difficulty in sampling small lesions not seen with other imaging modalities, it remains investigational.

2.4. Positron Emission Tomography

Since standard imaging techniques do not always demonstrate a lesion in the breast in patients with adenocarcinoma involving axillary lymph nodes, other diagnostic modalities are being investigated. Positron emission tomography (PET) is an imaging technique that evaluates the metabolic activity of tumors using radiopharmaceuticals labeled with isotopes that undergo radioactive decay by positron emission. The sensitivity and specificity of PET in the evaluation of suspicious breast masses is as high as 96–100% (43). Avril et al. (44) demonstrated that PET could be used to evaluate women with breast cancer and to assess axillary metastases. They reported a sensitivity of 95% and specificity of 65%. Block and Meyer (45) recently reported a case in which PET was useful in demonstrating an occult breast malignancy presenting with axillary metastases, allowing for treatment of the primary tumor. Scoggins et al. (46) reported on a case using PET and single-photon emission com-

Table 1
MRI Findings for Clinically and Mammographically Occult Breast Cancer

| Author | No. of cases | No. of cancers identified on MRI | | Cytologic/ pathologic confirmation | Size range of lesions (cm) |
		True +	False +		
Tilanus-Linthorst et al. *(42)*	4	4	0	4[a]	1–2
Morris et al. *(37)*	12	9[b]	1	9	0.4–1.5
Brenner and Rothman *(41)*	4	4	0	4	Microscopic–1.2
Porter et al. *(40)*	6	4	NA	4	0.8 or NA

NA, not available.

[a] Confirmation obtained by FNAC in all; pathologic confirmation obtained by lumpectomy in three; one patient did not have surgery.

[b] Two patients had negative MRIs and no tumor was found at mastectomy.

puter tomography that also localized an occult breast carcinoma. Although these findings suggest that PET may be a useful diagnostic tool in localizing occult breast carcinoma presenting with metastatic axillary lymph nodes, more data are needed to determine the actual value of this modality.

2.5. Other Evaluations

A chest X-ray should be performed on all patients to exclude the lung as a primary site. Blood tests including a complete blood count, chemistry profile, and liver function studies should be performed and are also useful screening modalities. Any abnormalities noted can determine the need for further investigation. A bone scan as a baseline study, as might be indicated for any node-positive breast cancer, can be considered, although the value of this is undocumented.

3. MANAGEMENT

The management of women presenting with adenocarcinoma in an axillary lymph node and no obvious primary tumor is controversial. Management options include mastectomy, breast irradiation, or observation. Other management considerations include the role of completion axillary dissection and adjuvant chemotherapy/hormonal therapy.

3.1. Mastectomy

The standard treatment for occult primary carcinoma has been mastectomy of the ipsilateral breast *(3,5,9,10,18,25,47)*. Although this approach was logical before the availability of high-quality breast imaging studies, it is more difficult to justify today. In addition, the acceptance of breast conservation for clinically evident tumors makes routine mastectomy for occult tumors somewhat irrational. A review of the pathology findings at mastectomy in 11 series is shown in Table 2. Breast cancer was found in the mastectomy specimens of 128 of 185 patients (69%) *(2–5,12,16–18,21,25,48,49)*. In general, the highest rates of tumor identification are in older series. More recently, Ellerbroek et al. *(48)* reported that no tumor was found in any of 10 mastectomy specimens, and Kemeny et al. *(17)* reported on 6 of 11 mastectomy specimens with no cancer detected. Most tumors are invasive, although in 8–20% of cases only ductal carcinoma *in situ* was noted. The size of the tumors identified

Table 2
Pathologic Findings after Mastectomy

Author	No. of Cases	% Tumor Identified	Size range (cm)
Ashikari et al. (25)	34	67	<1->2
Bhatia et al. (21)	10	100	$0.6–6 \times 5 \times 2^{a}$
Baron et al. (2)	28	71	<1->2
Ellerbroek et al. (48)	10	0	N/A
Feigenberg et al. (12)[b]	4	75	NA
Feurman et al. (16)	10	70	NA
Fitts et al. (3)	11	100	Microscopic–$5.5 \times 4 \times 2$
Haagensen (7)	13	92	5 mm–1.8
Kemeny et al. (17)	11	45	Microscopic–3×5
Owen et al. (5)	25	92	<5 mm–2
Patel et al. (18)	29	55	Microscopic–5
Weinberger and Stetten (49)	5	100	NA

N/A, not applicable; NA, not available.

[a] Mastectomy 6 months after axillary dissection.

[b] Eight patients were reviewed. Four of the eight had mastectomy (three sector mastectomies and one modified radical mastectomy). The remaining four patients had excisional biopsies.

ranged from less than 1 to 5 cm, emphasizing that even very large tumors may not be identified preoperatively.

3.2. Breast-Conserving Therapy

Recently, the role of breast-conserving therapy with or without breast radiation for TON1 cancers has been investigated. In a report from the M.D. Anderson (48), Cancer Center 25 of 35 patients were treated with breast preservation. The breast was irradiated in 16 patients, and no breast treatment was given to 9 patients. Breast recurrences occurred in 12% of patients receiving radiation and in 56% of patients not receiving radiation. There was no difference in survival between those who underwent mastectomy and those who did not. Baron et al. (2) found no difference in survival between 7 patients treated with breast conservation (6 with irradiation) and 28 treated by mastectomy. The Institut Curie Series (50) consisted of 59 patients treated between 1960 and 1997. Three patients underwent mastectomy, 54 patients received whole breast irradiation to a median dose of 59 Gy, and 2 patients had no treatment. Both of the untreated patients developed detectable breast cancer at 9 and 67 months, respectively. Of the 54 patients receiving whole breast irradiation, 9 patients had breast recurrence and were treated by mastectomy. The 8-year risk for ipsilateral breast recurrence was 12%, and the 8-year breast preservation rate was 93%.

The results of these studies support the use of breast conservation with irradiation as an alternative to mastectomy. Observation alone as a treatment modality carries a high risk of the clinical development of a breast primary tumor. Twenty of 53 patients described in the literature (1,4,12,16,17,48,51–54) developed detectable breast cancer in the untreated breast with recurrence intervals ranging from 5 to 64 months. Although this approach may avoid the removal of a clinically and mammographically "normal" breast, the opportunity for cure may be lost as the untreated primary acts as a source of additional metastatic disease.

3.3. Management of the Axilla

Completion axillary node dissection has been considered standard management of these cases. The benefits of completion axillary dissection include provision of prognostic information based on the total number of positive lymph nodes and the maintenance of local control. In patients with one clinically evident node, there is a significant risk for nodal involvement of the upper axilla, and half of these patients will have three or four involved nodes *(55)*. Overall, approximately 70% of patients are found to have additional positive nodes at completion of axillary dissection *(2,10,17,24,25,56)*.

3.4. Adjuvant Therapy

Specific data on the efficacy of systemic therapy in patients with TON1 breast cancer are difficult to obtain owing to the rarity of this disease process. The general tendency is to use the same criteria as are used for nonoccult stage II, node-positive patients to recommend systemic chemotherapy or hormonal therapy. Jackson et al. *(24)* suggest that treatment with chemotherapy is not an acceptable substitute for definitive control of primary lesions and believe that in order to obtain long-term survival, aggressive treatment of the primary lesion is of critical importance. Although larger series are necessary to confirm the benefits of adjuvant therapy in this patient population, the common policy in most institutions is to give adjuvant therapy to patients with involved axillary nodes despite the slightly better outcome reported in these patients when compared with other stage II, node-positive patients.

4. PROGNOSIS

The prognosis of clinical stage II breast cancers is determined by the number of involved lymph nodes and the biologic behavior of the tumor. Prognosis in patients with occult breast cancer with axillary metastases has been slightly better than that of patients with stage II breast cancers in most series *(5,12,17,22)*, possibly because of the small size of many of the primary tumors, since even in node-positive patients, tumor size influences prognosis *(57)*.

The reported 5-year actuarial survival rates after treatment of occult breast cancer with axillary metastases range between 36 and 79% *(2,16,17,25,48)*. The 5-year survival rate estimate in the 59 patients treated at the Institut Curie was 84%; at 8 years, it was 76% *(50)*. Rosen and Kimmel *(56)* evaluated patients more precisely by matching a series of 48 patients who had occult breast cancer and axillary metastases with patients diagnosed with stage II breast cancer presenting with palpable breast tumors. They found a higher overall survival in the group of patients with occult primary tumors. After adjusting for tumor size and nodal status, this difference persisted, although it was not statistically significant. Standard prognostic factors such as number of involved axillary nodes *(56)* and hormone receptor status *(2)* have been shown to be predictive of outcome in occult primary breast cancer in many series, although Forquet et al. *(55)* were unable to identify any predictors of overall survival.

5. CONCLUSIONS

Occult primary breast carcinoma with axillary metastases is rare. Diagnostic intervention with attempts to localize the lesion in the breast is indicated. A bilateral mammogram should be obtained, and MRI may be considered in institutions with experience with this technique. Extensive studies to locate an extramammary primary are not indicated. Ipsilateral mastectomy has been the standard treatment, but recent studies have shown no survival benefit of mastectomy over breast-conserving therapy using breast irradiation. Completion axillary dissection should be done for local control and prognostic information. Although most studies report that the overall survival for TON1 cancers is slightly better than that for other stage II cancers, these two disease processes are generally managed similarly.

REFERENCES

1. Halsted W (1907) The results of radical operations for the cure of carcinoma of the breast. *Ann. Surg.* **46,** 1–18.
2. Baron PL, Moore MP, Kinne DW, et al. (1990) Occult breast cancer presenting with axillary metastases: updated management. *Arch. Surg.* **125,** 210.
3. Fitts WT, Steiner GC, Enterline HT (1963) Prognosis of occult carcinoma of the breast. *Am. J. Surg.* **106,** 460–463.
4. Haagensen CD (1971) The diagnosis of breast carcinoma. In: Haagensen CD (ed.) *Diseases of the Breast.* WB Saunders, Philadelphia, p. 486–488.
5. Owen HW, Dockerty MB, Gray HK (1954) Occult carcinoma of the breast. *Surg. Gynecol. Obstet.* **98,** 302.
6. Copeland EM, McBride CM (1973) Axillary metastases from unknown primary sites. *Ann. Surg.* **178,** 25–28.
7. Haagensen CD (1986) *Diseases of the Breast,* 3rd ed. WB Saunders, Philadelphia, pp. 548–555.
8. Knapper WH (1991) Management of occult breast cancer presenting as an axillary metastasis. *Semin. Surg. Oncol.* **7,** 311–313.
9. Patterson WB (1987) Occult primary tumor with axillary metastases. In: Harris JR, Hellman S, Henderson IC, et al. (eds.) *Breast Diseases.* JB Lippincott, Philadelphia, pp. 608–613.
10. Westbrook KC, Gallagher HS (1971) Breast cancer presenting as an axillary mass. *Am. J. Surg.* **122,** 607–611.
11. Albers CA, Johnson RH, Mansburger AE (1981) The management of patients with metastatic cancer from an unknown primary site. *Am. Surg.* **47,** 162–166.
12. Feigenberg Z, Zer M, Dintsman M (1976) Axillary metastases from an unknown primary source. *Israel J. Med. Sci.* **12,** 1153–1158.
13. Kern WH, Abbott M (1980) The determination of unknown primary sites based upon the histologic appearance of metastases. *Surg. Gynecol. Obstet.* **151,** 73–76.
14. Rosen PP (1980) Axillary lymph node metastases in patients with occult noninvasive breast carcinoma. *Cancer* **46,** 1298–1306.
15. Tench DW, Page DL (1991) The unknown primary presenting with axillary lymphadenopathy. In: Bland KI, Copeland EM III (eds.) *The Breast:Comprehensive Management of Benign and Malignant Diseases.* WB Saunders, Philadelphia, pp. 1041–1045.
16. Feurman L, Attie JN, Rosenberg B (1962) Carcinoma in axillary lymph nodes as an indicator of breast cancer. *Surg. Gynecol. Obstet.* **114,** 5–8.
17. Kemeny MM, Rivera DE, Teri JJ, et al. (1986) Occult primary adenocarcinoma with axillary metastases. *Am. J. Surg.* **152,** 43–47.
18. Patel J, Nemoto T, Rosner D, et al. (1981) Axillary lymph node metastasis from an occult breast cancer. *Cancer* **47,** 2923–2927.
19. Haupt HM, Rosen PP, Kinne DW (1985) Breast carcinoma presenting with axillary lymph node metastases. *Am. J. Surg. Pathol.* **9,** 165–175.
20. Merson M, Andreola S, Galimberti V, et al. (1992) Breast carcinoma presenting as axillary metastases without evidence of a primary tumor. *Cancer* **70,** 504–508.
21. Bhatia SK, Saclarides TJ, Witt TJ, et al. (1987) Hormone receptor studies in axillary metastasis from occult breast cancers. *Cancer* **59,** 1170–1172.
22. High RM, Watne AL (1984) The axillary mass in occult breast carcinoma: case reports and overview. *Am. Surg.* **50,** 630–636.
23. Iglehart JD, Ferguson BJ, Shingleton WW, et al. (1982) An ultrastructural analysis of breast carcinoma presenting as isolated axillary adenopathy. *Ann. Surg.* **196,** 8–13.
24. Jackson B, Scott-Conner C, Moulder J (1995) Axillary metastasis from occult breast carcinoma: diagnosis and management. *Am. Surg.* **61,** 431–434.
25. Ashikari R, Rosen PP, Urban JA, et al. (1907) Breast cancer presenting as an axillary mass. *Ann. Surg.* **46,** 1–19.
26. Orel SG, Hochman MG, Schnall MD, et al. (1996) High-resolution MR imaging of the breast: clinical context. *Radiographics* **16,** 1385–1401.
27. Harms SC, Flamig DP, Hesley KL, et al. (1993) Fat suppressed three-dimensional MR imaging of the breast. *Radiographics* **13,** 247–267.
28. Harms SE, Flamig DP, Hesley KL, et al. (1993) MR imaging of the breast with rotating delivery of excitation of resonance: clinical experience with pathologic correlation. *Radiology* **187,** 493–501.
29. Heywang SH, Wolf A, Pruss E, et al. (1989) MR imaging of the breast with Gd-DTPA: use and limitations. *Radiology* **171,** 95–103.

30. Kaiser WA (1992) MRI promises earlier breast cancer diagnosis. *Diagn. Imaging Int.* **Nov/Dec,** 44–50.
31. Obdeijn AIM, Kuijpers TJA, van Dijk P, et al. (1996) Limited indications for MR mammography. In: *Advances in Magnetic Resonance Imaging.* Blackwell Science, London.
32. Pierce WP, Harris SE, Fleming DP, et al. (1991) Three dimensional gadolinium-enhanced MR imaging of the breast: pulse sequence with fat suppression and magnetization transfer contrast. *Radiology* **181,** 757–763.
33. Gilles R, Guinebretiere JM, Lucidarme O, et al. (1994) Nonpalpable breast tumors: diagnosis with contrast-enhanced subtraction dynamic MR imaging. *Radiology* **191,** 625–631.
34. Hulka CA, Smith BL, Sgroi DC, et al. (1995) Benign and malignant breast lesions: differentiation with echo-planar MR imaging. *Radiology* **197,** 33–38.
35. Kaiser WA, Zeitler E (1989) MR imaging of the breast: fast imaging sequences with and without Gd-DTPA-preliminary observations. *Radiology* **170,** 681–686.
36. Stomper PC, Herman S, Klippenstein DL, et al. (1995) Suspect breast lesions: findings at dynamic gandolinium-enhanced MR imaging correlated with mammographic and pathologic features. *Radiology* **197,** 387–395.
37. Morris EA, Schwartz LH, Dershaw DD, et al. (1997) MR imaging of the breast in patients with occult primary breast carcinoma. *Radiology* **205,** 437–440.
38. Harms SC, Flamig DP (1994) Staging of breast cancer with MR imaging. *Magn. Reson. Imaging Clin. N. Am.* **2,** 573–584.
39. Davis PL, Julian TB, Staiger M, et al. (1994) Magnetic resonance imaging detection and wire localization of an "occult" breast cancer. *Br. Cancer Res. Treat.* **32,** 327–330.
40. Porter BA, Smith JP, Borrow JW (1995) MR depiction of occult breast cancer in patients with malignant axillary adenopathy (abstr). *Radiology* **197,** 130.
41. Brenner RJ, Rothman BJ (1997) Detection of primary breast cancer in women with known adenocarcinoma metastatic to the axilla: use of MRI after negative clinical and mammographic examination. *J. Magn. Reson. Imaging* **7,** 1153–1158.
42. Tilanus-Linthorst MMA, Obdeijn AIM, Bontenbal M, et al. (1997) MRI in patients with axillary metastases of occult breast carcinoma. *Breast Cancer Res. Treat.* **44,** 179–182.
43. Adler LP, Crowe JP, al-Kaisi NK, et al. (1993) Evaluation of breast masses and axillary lymph nodes with [F-18] 2-deoxy-2-fluoro-D glucose PET. *Radiology* **187,** 743–750.
44. Avril N, Dose J, Janicke F, et al. (1996) Assessment of axillary lymph node involvement in breast cancer patients with positron emission tomography using radiolabeled 2- (fluorine-18)-fluoro-2-deoxy-D-glucose. *J. Natl. Cancer Inst.* **88,** 1204–1209.
45. Block EFJ, Meyer MA (1998) Positron emission tomography in diagnosis of occult adenocarcinoma of the breast. *Am. Surg.* **64,** 906–908.
46. Scoggins CR, Vitola JV, Sandler MP, et al. (1999) Occult breast carcinoma presenting as an axillary mass. *Am. Surg.* **65,** 1–5.
47. McLeod MK (1988) Dilemmas in breast cancer: occult carcinoma and Paget's disease of the breast. In: Harness JK, Oberman HA, Lichter AS, et al. (eds.) *Breast Cancer: Collaborative Management.* Lewis, Chelsea MI, pp. 211–232.
48. Ellerbroek N, Holmes F, Singletary E, et al. (1990) Treatment of patients with isolated axillary nodal metastases from an occult primary consistent with breast. *Origin. Cancer* **125,** 43–47.
49. Weinberger HA, Stetten D (1951) Extensive secondary axillary lymph node carcinoma without clinical evidence of primary breast lesion. *Surgery* **29,** 217–223.
50. Forquet A, de la Rochefordiere A, Campana F (in press) Occult primary cancer with axillary metastases. In: Harris JR, Lippman ME, Morrow M, et al. (eds.) *Diseases of the Breast.* Lippincott-Raven, Williams & Wilkins, Philadelphia, pp. 703–707.
51. Atkins H, Wolff B (1960) The malignant gland in the hospital. *Guys Hosp. Rep.* **1,** 109–113.
52. Campana F, Forquet A, Ashby MA, et al. (1989) Presentation of axillary lymphadenopathy without detectable breast primary (TON1b breast cancer): experience at Institut Curie. *Radiother. Oncol.* **15,** 321–325.
53. Klopp CT (1950) Metastatic cancer of axillary lymph node without a demonstrable primary lesion. *Ann. Surg.* **131,** 437.
54. Van Ooijen B, Bontenbal M, Henzen-Logmans SC, et al. (1993) Axillary nodal metastases from an occult primary consistent with breast carcinoma. *Br. J. Surg.* **80,** 1299–1300.
55. Forquet A, de la Rochefordiere A, Campana F (1996) Occult primary cancer with axillary metastases. In: Harris JR, Lippman ME, Morrow M, et al. (eds.) *Diseases of the Breast.* Lippincott-Raven, Philadelphia, pp. 892–896.
56. Rosen PP, Kimmell M (1990) Occult breast carcinoma presenting with axillary lymph node metastases: a follow up study of 48 patients. *Hum. Pathol.* **21,** 518–523.
57. Quiet CA, Ferguson DJ, Weichselbaum RR, et al. (1996) Natural history of node-positive breast cancer: the curability of small cancers with a limited number of positive nodes. *J. Clin. Oncol.* **14,** 3105–3111.

16 Breast Cancer During Pregnancy

Mary L. Gemignani, MD,
and Jeanne A. Petrek, MD

CONTENTS

INTRODUCTION
DIAGNOSIS OF BREAST CANCER DURING PREGNANCY
TREATMENT
PROGNOSIS
THERAPEUTIC ABORTION
CONCLUSIONS
REFERENCES

1. INTRODUCTION

Ten to 20% of the 178,700 new cases of breast cancer occurring yearly (1998 estimates) are found in women of childbearing age *(1)*. The issue of pregnancy-associated breast cancer is very important, particularly as more women delay childbearing for personal or professional reasons. The delay in childbearing to the 30s or 40s occurs concordantly with an increasing incidence of breast cancer in those ages. Pregnancy-associated breast cancer has been traditionally defined as the diagnosis of breast cancer made during pregnancy or within 1 year afterward. It is estimated to have an incidence of 0.2–3.8% *(2)* and is reported to occur in 1/10,000–1/3000 pregnancies *(3,4)*.

2. DIAGNOSIS OF BREAST CANCER DURING PREGNANCY

Pregnancy causes many changes in the breast. The intense hormonal milieu progressively causes greater breast volume and firmness. Physical examination of the breast becomes increasingly more difficult as pregnancy advances. Ideally a good prepregnancy baseline examination and a mammogram, as indicated by the patient's age and risk factors, would be most beneficial. However, the first obstetric visit does provide a good opportunity for screening as the breasts have undergone the least physiologic changes and an adequate exam can be performed. The finding of a thickness or a possible mass usually requires a short-interval follow-up as the mass may be hidden by the normal hypertrophic thickness as pregnancy advances.

From: *Current Clinical Oncology:*
Breast Cancer: A Guide to Detection and Multidisciplinary Therapy
Edited by: M. H. Torosian © Humana Press Inc., Totowa, NJ

2.1. Breast Imaging

Besides the drawback of possible exposure to ionizing radiation to a fetus from mammography, it has been intuitive to believe that little information can be gained from this study during pregnancy. Increased parenchymal density may result from all the breast changes that accompany pregnancy, i.e., increased vascularity, cellularity, water content, and possibly the presence of milk in the lactating breast. However, a recent study on a small series of 18 patients compared mammograms obtained during pregnancy, lactating, or recently lactating with mammograms obtained before pregnancy. Against conventional wisdom, using the four categories of breast density from the Breast Imaging Reporting and Data System (BIRADS) few women were noted to have an increased density category compared with their baseline (5). More studies are needed to address this issue.

There are several small series of breast imaging in pregnancy-associated breast cancer. At Sloan-Kettering Memorial Hospital 78% of mammograms in 23 women with clinically evident pregnancy-associated breast cancer demonstrated radiologic signs of the cancer (6). All of six ultrasonographic examinations performed in these patients with a palpable abnormality revealed a solid mass. If mammography is necessary in the lactating woman, it should be performed immediately after emptying the breast by nursing or pumping.

Breast ultrasonography in pregnancy is safe and helpful in differentiating between a cystic or solid mass. It is not possible to distinguish benign solid masses from malignant masses. Little is known about the ultrasonographic appearance of normal breasts during pregnancy.

Although there are no published data on the normal magnetic resonance image of the pregnant or lactating breast, such imaging has been used in pregnancy and seems safe for the fetus. Recent studies on its use for fetal imaging in prenatal diagnosis, with limited follow-up of the infants, report no untoward effects. It does not expose the fetus to ionizing radiation and has been used in pregnancy (7,8). However, little has been reported on the use of gadolinium in pregnancy.

2.2. Biopsy

Fine needle aspiration (FNA) cytology is commonly used for evaluating routine breast masses. There are several small reports concerning pregnancy/lactation and problems associated with FNA diagnosis (9–11). The largest series, from New Zealand, reports the successful use of FNA in 331 women, ranging from 8 weeks of gestation to lactation 30 weeks postpartum. None of the cases with benign FNA diagnosis developed cancer in the follow-up of 1.5–2 years. Ten women with a cytodiagnosis of cancer were confirmed with surgical excision (12). False-positive diagnoses can occur particularly because of the increased cellularity and frequent mitoses that can be seen during gestation; an experienced cytopathologist is very important for establishing an accurate diagnosis. Core biopsies are more accurate, but a milk fistula, a complication seen with a surgical biopsy, has recently been reported (13).

Many authors have attributed the advanced disease and poor prognosis often characteristic of gestational breast cancer to delay in diagnosis (14–16). After a thickness or possible mass is found, surgical biopsy may be postponed owing to the greater complication rate expected in the pregnant/lactating woman. A study of 63 patients diagnosed while pregnant or within 1 year postpartum at Memorial Hospital suggests a reluctance to biopsy during pregnancy (16). Less than 20% of such patients were diagnosed during pregnancy. Almost half were diagnosed within 12 weeks after delivery for a mass noted during pregnancy. The large size of the cancers at the time of postpartum diagnosis (median of 3.5 cm) makes it likely that a smaller mass was palpable during pregnancy.

3. TREATMENT

Modified radical mastectomy is the preferred local management of a breast cancer patient during pregnancy. There is much experience regarding pregnancy and general anesthesia because many different surgical procedures are performed on pregnant women. A population–based study from Sweden studied 5405 nonobstetric operations during pregnancy and compared the results with 720,000 pregnancies in women who had not had general anesthesia. Adverse effects reported included low birth weight, prematurity, intrauterine growth retardation, and early neonatal death; such effects are thought to correlate with the underlying condition that necessitated the surgical procedure. The incidence of congenital anomalies was not increased in women who had general anesthesia during the first trimester *(17)*.

3.1. Adjuvant Treatment

In cancer diagnosis and treatment, radiation and chemotherapy may affect the risk of teratogenicity and subsequent fetal development. Although the risk of congenital abnormalities is the most common concern, intrauterine growth retardation, premature birth, and subsequent neoplasia in the newborn pose a significant risk.

3.1.1. RADIATION

The risk to the fetus from radiation depends on the period of gestation during the exposure. The principal effect during the preimplantation period (from conception to days 10–14) is embryo death. The period of organogenesis (second through eighth week) is the most sensitive, and the greatest risk for congenital malformation is found at this time *(18)*. Radiation exposure beyond 8 weeks is less likely to produce abnormalities; however, concerns about neurologic development have been reported *(18,19)*. Subsequent increased risks of childhood cancers in these newborns were reported in a recent review of published data *(20)*.

The atomic bomb experience at Hiroshima and Nagasaki led to the conclusion that 5 cGy is the dose level for early pregnancy at which radiation-induced anomalies become significant *(2)*. The standard breast radiotherapy course of about 5000 cGy will expose the fetus to 10 cGy early in pregnancy and 200 cGy or more late in pregnancy and therefore should be rejected as a treatment option. The developing fetus receives a small percentage of the total dose of radiation given to the breast. The radiation leakage from the radiotherapy unit should not exceed 0.1% of the direct beam exposure rate, as measured at a distance of 1 m from the radiation source *(21)*. A larger amount of radiation, however, reaches the fetus from internal scatter by the mother's tissues. External shielding cannot reduce this. Chest wall irradiation after mastectomy poses the same hazard to the fetus as breast irradiation would and should be delayed until after childbirth.

To accomplish breast preservation in the pregnant woman, a plan for lumpectomy during pregnancy followed by radiation therapy after delivery has been suggested. To advocate this approach, one must extrapolate from the data obtained in the nonpregnant woman. However, the pregnant woman's breast is very different. The increase in size of the ducts, as well as increased blood supply, may predispose to lengthy intraductal spread. It is thus not certain that local control and survival results using this approach would be the same in the pregnant woman as would be obtained after standard lumpectomy and irradiation. Limited experience, with a median follow-up of 24 months, has been reported in nine women with pregnancy-associated breast cancer who were treated conservatively. Two of the nine were in the first trimester and underwent abortion; perhaps they should not be included, as the breast would have undergone minimal physiologic change. Median tumor size was 1.5 cm. There were no local recurrences and three distant recurrences in this short follow-up *(22)*.

3.1.2. CHEMOTHERAPY

The decision to recommend chemotherapy to a pregnant woman is one of the most difficult in the management of women with breast cancer. The treatment involves not only the patient and the medical oncologist but also the family, the obstetrician, the neonatolgist, and of course the unborn fetus.

Chemotherapeutic drugs exert their effect by inhibiting cell division. With pregnancy there are physiologic changes in blood volume, glomerular filtration rate, and other parameters that may affect maternal chemotherapy drug metabolism. There are a few pharmacokinetic studies of chemotherapy in pregnant patients. Although most drugs cross the placenta, detailed studies of transplacental passage of chemotherapeutic agents to human fetuses are not available. The potential adverse effects of antineoplastic agents on the fetus and neonate are either immediate (such as spontaneous abortion, teratogenesis, or organ damage) or delayed (such as growth retardation or gonadal dysfunction). Administration of chemotherapy in the first trimester is associated with an increased incidence of stillbirths and congenital malformations because it is the period of organogenesis and limb formation *(23)*. In one series of 13 women exposed to chemotherapy during the first trimester, there were four spontaneous abortions, four therapeutic abortions, and two major fetal malformations among the five term infants *(24)*. Delayed cognitive disability is a theoretical concern with administration of chemotherapy in the second trimester because of ongoing central nervous system development. The long-term follow-up of children exposed to *in utero* chemotherapy during maternal treatment for breast cancer is important.

The chemotherapy agents most commonly used in the initial management of a woman with breast cancer are relatively safe to administer during the second and third trimesters. Drugs that have been given after the first trimester without a reported increased risk of birth defects include cyclophosphamide, doxorubicin, and 5-fluorouracil (5-FU) *(25–27)*. Methotrexate, a folic acid antagonist, has also been given without serious sequelae in the second and third trimesters. Because of the association with fetal abnormalities in the first trimester and concern over its metabolism in the presence of third-space (amniotic) fluid, most oncologists prefer to avoid methotrexate during pregnancy. Taxanes have not been studied and for that reason should be avoided during pregnancy. Since laboratory studies have suggested that tamoxifen is teratogenic, it is contraindicated during pregnancy.

A recent prospective study of 24 women with breast cancer treated with chemotherapy during the second and third trimesters showed no evidence of fetal compromise or adverse effects on early development. Twenty-two women were treated for primary breast cancer, primarily stage II or III, including two women with inflammatory breast cancer. Cyclophosphamide, doxorubicin, and 5-FU were given every 21–28 days for a maximum of four treatments. The disease-free survival of the mothers was similar to that of nonpregnant patients and was dependent on the stage of the breast cancer at diagnosis *(27)*.

In planning chemotherapy for pregnant women, it is preferable to allow at least 2 weeks between the last dose and delivery. This minimizes the risk of delivering a neutropenic infant from a neutropenic mother. In addition, fetal drug metabolism switches from the placenta to the kidney and liver at delivery. If the fetus is delivered soon after chemotherapy, the drugs may persist for a prolonged period in the newborn *(28)*. Women who have recently received chemotherapy should be advised against breast-feeding.

The management of the pregnant woman with breast cancer involves close communication with the patient, her family, and the medical team involved in her care. A discussion of risks to the fetus versus possible maternal benefits is crucial.

4. PROGNOSIS

The earliest reports more than a century ago noted a dismal prognosis. Kilgore and Bloodgood *(29)* reported no survivors, and White's collective series *(30)* in 1929 reported a 17% 5-year survival rate. Haagensen and Stout *(31)* reported an only 8.6% overall 5-year survival rate.

Harrington *(32)*, at the Mayo Clinic in 1937, is credited with reviving optimism by finding a 61% 5-year survival rate among those with negative lymph nodes. Unfortunately, presentation with lymph node metastases was then, and remains, common in the pregnant woman. Eight papers published during the 1960s *(33–40)*, reporting numbers of patients ranging from 29 to 117, found positive lymph node rates of 53–74% (median of 65%). Four similar papers *(4,41–43)* published during the 1970s found positive lymph node rates of 56–81%. Few studies have attempted to put these percentages into the context of age, decade of diagnosis, and similar demographics by designating a nonpregnant comparison group.

At Memorial Hospital the author compared 56 pregnancy-associated breast cancer patients (American Joint Committee stages I/II/III) diagnosed between 1960 and 1980 with nonpregnant control patients from a consecutive mastectomy series of the same age, diagnosed and treated at the same hospital during the same period by the same physicians *(16)*. Sixty-two percent of the pregnancy-associated cancer patients had positive lymph nodes versus 39% of their nonpregnant counterparts. Only 31% of the pregnant patients had pathologic tumors less than 2 cm versus 50% of their counterparts. A more recent report *(44)* of a smaller series of women from Memorial Hospital had the same findings, which are similar to those of other studies *(37,45–48)* that also include a comparison group.

The pregnancy-associated breast cancer patients with negative lymph nodes had a 82% 5-year survival rate compared with 82% in their nonpregnant counterparts. The pregnancy-associated patients with positive lymph nodes had a 47% 5-year survival rate compared with 59% in their counterparts. Among pregnancy-associated patients who were eligible, there was a 77% 10-year survival rate for those with negative lymph nodes and a 25% rate for those with positive lymph nodes. In comparison, the 10-year survival rate was 75% for the nonpregnant patients with negative nodes and 41% for the nonpregnant patients with positive nodes. The differences in 5- and 10-year survival times in patients grouped by stage are not statistically significant.

There are only two modern case-control series indicating that pregnancy is a risk factor independent of stage at diagnosis. A small series from Norway contained 20 patients *(49)*. More important is the 1997 French study of 154 women, each matched with two controls *(50)*. In this countrywide group of patients, multivariate analysis demonstrated that pregnancy was an independent and significant prognostic factor.

Other recent reports indicate that pregnancy was associated with a more advanced stage at diagnosis, but not a worse survival within that stage. In Toronto, 118 women diagnosed with pregnancy-associated breast cancer from 1958 to 1987 were studied. No statistically significant difference in survival between pregnant and nonpregnant patients was found when patients matched by age, stage, and year of diagnosis *(15)*. Showing the tendency to present with advanced disease, the pregnant women had a 2.5-fold higher risk of diagnosis with metastatic breast cancer and a significantly decreased chance of a stage I diagnosis. A 1992 study published in a Japanese cancer journal, also with a large number of patients, shows similar findings *(51)*. A New Zealand report *(52)* of 20 women and a Saudi Arabian report *(53)* of 28 women showed the same findings. Table 1 lists six series giving data on long-term survival based on nodal status. Four of these are case-control studies.

In summary, almost all reports note a worse survival rate for pregnancy-associated breast cancer overall. However, when the pregnancy-associated breast cancer patients are evaluated with nonpregnant controls, the pregnancy-associated group has an equivalent survival rate, at least in the early stages. Overall, pregnancy-associated breast cancer bears a worse prognosis, since it is regularly associated with more advanced disease at presentation. It is unknown whether this is owing to 1) a more aggressive growth pattern secondary to the biologic effects of pregnancy; 2) delayed diagnosis secondary to the breast changes of pregnancy; or 3) a combination of the two.

5. THERAPEUTIC ABORTION

One of the most controversial issues in treating breast cancer during pregnancy is the question of therapeutic abortion. In the past century, therapeutic abortion was not uncommon and was often used in combination with oophorectomy. Haagansen and Stout *(54)* initially believed that any breast cancer diagnosed during pregnancy or lactation was incurable and could be used as a criterion for refusing mastectomy. They later changed their opinion. In 1953, Adair *(55)* at Memorial Hospital reported on a small series of patients who had longer crude survival rates after therapeutic abortion, especially those with positive axillary lymph nodes. These differences were not statistically different.

Gradually the opinion on the lethality of pregnancy-associated breast cancer as well as the value of therapeutic abortion began to change. In 1962 Holleb and Farrow *(56)* reported on 24 patients treated with radical mastectomy and abortion and did not find a survival advantage. Other recent reports found similar results *(45,46)*. Some authors have found that therapeutic abortion was associated with decreased survival *(48,57)*. In these studies, however, patients who underwent abortion appear to have had more advanced disease than those who delivered. Thus, any beneficial effect of abortion might be disguised by that selection factor.

In a series of 63 pregnant patients at the Mayo Clinic, a 5-year survival rate of 43% was reported in the interrupted group versus 59% in the full-term delivery group *(46)*. Of the 20 patients with stage I disease, only 3 were interrupted. Of those three patients, only one survived. Thus it is likely that patient selection influenced the survival statistics.

In summary, when combined with standard therapy, any additional benefit of routine therapeutic abortion cannot be demonstrated in the published reports. Because survival rates are generally equivalent among those continuing pregnancy and those aborted, and because patients with more advanced disease are generally aborted, patient selection affects the ability to determine the true value of therapeutic abortion. However, therapeutic abortion is strongly recommended if the issue is fetal damage from the necessary proposed chemotherapy or radiation treatment.

6. CONCLUSIONS

The various modalities used for screening, diagnosis, and staging of breast cancer are not always applicable during pregnancy. Often a delay in diagnosis may contribute to a more advanced stage at presentation. The management of breast cancer during pregnancy requires assessment of the risks to the fetus versus the maternal benefits gained. Pregnancy-associated breast cancer has a worse prognosis overall than nonpregnancy associ-

Table 1
Selected Retrospective Series with Survival Follow-Up Data

Author	Period/country	No.	Node-positive PA/ non-PA (%)	Node-positive		Node-negative	
				PA (%)	Non-PA (%)	PA (%)	Non-PA (%)
King et al., 1985 (46)	1950–1980 U.S.	63	62/—	82/71	—	36/36	—
Nugent and O'Connell, 1985 (45)	1970–1980 U.S.	19	74/37	100/—	70/—	50/—	48/—
Ribeiro et al., 1986 (47)	1941–1983 U.K.	121	72/—	79/—	—	—	—
Petrek et al., 1989 (16)	1960–1980 U.S.	63	62/39	82/77	82/75	47/25	59/41
Ishida et al., 1992 (51)	1970–1988 Japan	192[a]	58/46	—/85	—/93	—/37	—/62
Bonnier et al., 1997 (50)	1960–1993 France	154[b]	56/54	63/—	77/—	31/—	63/—

PA, pregnancy-associated breast cancer; Non-PA, non-pregnancy–associated cohort; —, data not available.

[a] Data from 18 institutions including lactating patients within 2 years of delivery in PA group.

[b] Survival data are for disease-free survival

ated breast cancer because a large proportion of patients present with more advanced disease. However, stage for stage, the prognosis is similar between pregnant and nonpregnant women with breast cancer.

REFERENCES

1. Landis SH, Murray T, Bolden S, Wingo PA (1990) Cancer statistics, 1999. *CA Cancer J. Clin.* **49,** 8–31.
2. Wallack MK, Wolf JA Jr, Bedwinek J, et al. (1983) Gestational carcinoma of the female breast. *Curr. Probl. Cancer* **7,** 1–58.
3. Saunders CM, Baum M (1993) Breast cancer and pregnancy: a review. *J. R. Soc. Med.* **86,** 162–165.
4. Anderson JM (1979) Mammary cancers and pregnancy. *BMJ* **1,** 1124–1127.
5. Swinford AE, Adler DD, Garver KA (1998) Mammographic appearance of the breasts during pregnancy and lactation: false assumptions. *Acad. Radiol.* **5,** 467–472.
6. Liberman L, Giess CS, Dershaw DD, Deutch BM, Petrek JA (1994) Imaging of pregnancy-associated breast cancer. *Radiology* **191,** 245–248.
7. Adzick NS, Harrison MR (1994) The unborn surgical patient. *Curr. Probl. Surg.* **31,** 1–68.
8. Mattison DR, Angtuaco T (1988) Magnetic resonance imaging in prenatal diagnosis. *Clin. Obstet. Gynecol.* **31,** 353–389.
9. Bottles K, Taylor RN (1985) Diagnosis of breast masses in pregnant and lactating women by aspiration cytology. *Obstet. Gynecol.* **66,** 76S–78S.
10. Gupta RK, McHutchinson AGR, Dowle CS, Simpson JS (1993) Fine-needle aspiration cytodiagnosis of breast masses in pregnant and lactating women and its impact on management. *Diagn. Cytopathol.* **9,** 156–159.
11. Novotny DB, Maygarden SJ, Shermer RW, Frable WJ (1991) Fine needle aspiration of benign and malignant breast masses associated with pregnancy. *Acta Cytol.* **35,** 676–686.
12. Gupta RK (1997) The diagnostic impact of aspiration cytodiagnosis of breast masses in association with pregnancy and lactation with an emphasis on clinical decision making. *Breast J.* **3,** 131–134.
13. Schackmuth EM, Harlow CL, Norton LW (1993) Milk fistula: a complication after core biopsy. *AJR* **161,** 961–962.
14. Haagenson CD (1971) Carcinoma of the breast in pregnancy. In: Haagensen CD (ed.) *Diseases of the Breast,* 2nd ed. WB Saunders, Philadelphia, p. 74–86.
15. Zemlickis D, Lishner M, Degendorfer P, et al. (1992) Maternal and fetal outcome after breast cancer in pregnancy. *Am. J. Obstet. Gynecol.* **166,** 781–787.
16. Petrek JA, Dukoff R, Rogatko A (1991) Pregnancy-associated breast cancer. *Cancer* **67,** 869–872.
17. Mazze RI, Kallen B (1989) Reproductive outcome after anesthesia and operation during pregnancy: a registry study of 5405 cases. *Am. J. Obstet. Gynecol.* **161,** 1178–1185.
18. Miller R, Mulvihill S (1976) Small head size after atomic radiation. *Teratology* **14,** 355–357.
19. Kimler BF (1998) Prenatal irradiation: a major concern for the developing brain. *Int. J. Radiat. Biol.* **73,** 423–434.
20. Doll R, Wakeford R (1997) Risk of childhood cancer from fetal irradiation. *Br. J. Radiol.* **70,** 130–139.
21. National Council on Radiation Protection and Measurements (1971) *Report #39: Basic Radiation Protection Criteria.* NCRP, Washington, DC.
22. Kuerer HM, Cunningham JD, Bleiweiss IJ, et al. (1998) Conservative surgery for breast carcinoma associated with pregnancy. *Breast J.* **4,** 171–176.
23. Doll DC, Ringenberg S, Yarbro JW (1989) Antineoplastic agents and pregnancy. *Semin. Oncol.* **16,** 337–346.
24. Zemlickis D, Lishner M, Degendorfer P, et al. (1992) Fetal outcome after in utero exposure to cancer chemotherapy. *Arch. Intern. Med.* **152,** 573–576.
25. Glantz JC (1994) Reproductive toxicology of alkylating agents. *Obstet. Gynecol. Surv.* **49,** 709–715.
26. Turchi JJ, Villasis C (1988) Anthracyclines in the treatment of malignancy in pregnancy. *Cancer* **61,** 435–440.
27. Berry DL, Theriault RL, Holmes FA, et al. (1999) Management of breast cancer during pregnancy using a standard protocol. *J. Clin. Oncol.* **17,** 855–861.
28. Buekers TE, Lallas TA (1998) Chemotherapy in pregnancy. *Obstet. Gynecol. Clin. North. Am.* **25,** 323–329.
29. Kilgore AR, Bloodgood JC Tumors and tumor-like lesions of the breast in association with pregnancy. *Arch. Surg.* **18,** 2079–2098.
30. White TT (1954) Carcinoma of the breast and pregnancy. *Ann. Surg.* **139,** 9–18.
31. Haagensen CD, Stout AP (1943) Carcinoma of the breast: criteria of operability. *Ann. Surg.* **118,** 859–870, 1032–1051.
32. Harrington SW (1937) Carcinoma of the breast: results of surgical treatment when the carcinoma occurred in course of pregnancy or lacation and when pregnancy occurred subsequent to operation, 1910–1933. *Ann. Surg.* **106,** 690–700.

33. Byrd BF, Bayer DS, Robertson JC, et al. (1962) Treatment of breast tumors associated with pregnancy and lactation. *Ann. Surg.* **155,** 940–947.
34. Bunker ML, Peters MV (1963) Breast cancer associated with pregnancy or lactation. *Am. J. Obstet. Gynecol.* **85,** 312–321.
35. Montgomery TL (1961) Detection and disposal of breast cancer in pregnancy. *Am. J. Obstet. Gynecol.* **81,** 926–933.
36. Miller HK (1962) Cancer of the breast during pregnancy and lactation. *Am. J. Obstet. Gynecol.* **83,** 607–611.
37. Peters VM, Meakin JW (1965) The influence of pregnancy in carcinoma of the breast. *Prog. Clin. Cancer* **1,** 471–506.
38. Mickal A, Torres JE, Mule JG (1963) Carcinoma of breast in pregnancy and lactation. *Am. Surg.* **29,** 509–514.
39. Rosemond GP (1963) Carcinoma of the breast during pregnancy. *Clin. Obstet. Gynecol.* **6,** 994–1001.
40. DeVitt JE, Beattie WG, Stoddart TG (1964) Carcinoma of the breast and pregnancy. *Can. J. Surg.* **7,** 124–128.
41. Clark RM, Reid J (1978) Carcinoma of the breast in pregnancy and lactation. *Int. J. Radiat. Oncol. Biol. Phys.* **4,** 693–698.
42. Applewhite RR, Smith LR, DeVicenti F (1973) Carcinoma of the breast associated with pregnancy and lactation. *Am. Surg.* **39,** 101–104.
43. Crosby CH, Barclay THC (1971) Carcinoma of the breast: surgical management of patients with special conditions. *Cancer* **28,** 1628–1636.
44. Anderson BO, Petrek JA, Byrd DR, Senie RT, Borgen PI (1996) Pregnancy influences breast cancer stage at diagnosis in women 30 years of age and younger. *Ann. Surg. Oncol.* **3,** 204–211.
45. Nugent P, O'Connell TX (1985) Breast cancer and pregnancy. *Arch. Surg.* **120,** 1221–1224.
46. King RM, Welch JS, Martin JL, et al. (1985) Carcinoma of the breast associated with pregnancy. *Surg. Gynecol. Obstet.* **160,** 228–232.
47. Ribeiro GG, Jones DA, Jones M (1986) Carcinoma of the breast associated with pregnancy. *Br. J. Surg.* **73,** 607–609.
48. Deemarsky LJ, Neishtadt EL (1980) Breast cancer and pregnancy. *Breast* **7,** 17–21.
49. Tretli S, Kvalheim G, Thoresen S, Host H (1988) Survival of breast cancer patients diagnosed during pregnancy or lactation. *Br. J. Cancer.* **58,** 382–384.
50. Bonnier P, Romain S, Dilhuydy JM, et al. (1997) Influence of pregnancy on the outcome of breast cancer: a case-control study. Societé Française de Sénologie et de Pathologie Mammaire Study Group. *Int. J. Cancer* **72,** 720–727.
51. Ishida T, Yokoe T, Kasumi F, et al. (1992) Clinicopathologic characteristics and prognosis of breast cancer patients associated with pregnancy and lactation: analysis of case-control study in Japan. *Jpn. J. Cancer Res.* **83,** 1143–1149.
52. Lethaby AE, O'Neill MA, Mason BH, Holdaway IM, Harvey VJ (1996) Overall survival from breast cancer in women pregnant or lactating at or after diagnosis. Auckland Breast Cancer Study Group. *Int. J. Cancer* **67,** 751–755.
53. Ezzat A, Raja MA, Berry J, et al. (1996) Impact of pregnancy on non-metastatic breast cancer: a case control study. *Clin. Oncol.* **8,** 367–370.
54. Haagensen CD, Stout AP (1943) Carcinoma of the breast: criteria of operability. *Ann. Surg.* **118,** 859–870.
55. Adair FE (1953) Cancer of the breast. *Surg. Clin. North Am.* **33,** 313–319.
56. Holleb AI, Farrow JH (1962) The relation of carcinoma of the breast and pregnancy in 283 patients. *Surg. Gynecol. Obstet.* **115,** 65–71.
57. Clark RM, Chua T (1989) Breast cancer and pregnancy: the ultimate challenge. *Clin. Oncol.* **1,** 11–18.

17 Local-Regional Recurrence in Breast Cancer

Thomas J. Kearney, MD, FACS, and David A. August, MD, FACS

CONTENTS

INTRODUCTION
IN-BREAST RECURRENCE FOLLOWING BREAST CONSERVATION
CHEST WALL RECURRENCE FOLLOWING MASTECTOMY
AXILLARY RECURRENCE
CONCLUSIONS
BIBLIOGRAPHY

1. INTRODUCTION

The problem of local-regional recurrence of breast cancer confronts a substantial number of patients who are initially treated with apparent success. The percentage of patients who experience such recurrence varies depending on the initial stage of the disease and the form of initial breast treatment. Patients with stage I breast cancer treated with a clean margin lumpectomy and postoperative radiation therapy will have recurrence rates in the conserved breast of about 5%. In contrast, patients with Stage IIIB, initially inoperable, disease will have recurrence rates of greater than 25% on the chest wall even in the setting of successful neoadjuvant chemotherapy, mastectomy, and postoperative radiation. In patients who suffer a local-regional recurrence, one-third will have synchronous distant failure. Others subsequently develop distant disease following local-regional recurrence.

Local-regional recurrence should be considered within one of three contexts (Table 1). The first is in the setting of breast-conserving surgery. Since breast conservation is the preferred approach for early-stage breast cancer and now represents the approach taken in most patients, recurrences occur in this setting with some regularity. Second is the setting of postmastectomy chest wall recurrence after mastectomy. The increasing use of immediate reconstruction following mastectomy must also be considered in this scenario. The third scenario involves axillary recurrence. This is relatively unusual but may occur more frequently in the future if fewer patients undergo formal axillary dissection. Other forms of regional recurrence such as supraclavicular nodal disease are considered to be signs of distant disease. Their evaluation and treatment are discussed elsewhere.

From: *Current Clinical Oncology:*
Breast Cancer: A Guide to Detection and Multidisciplinary Therapy
Edited by: M. H. Torosian © Humana Press Inc., Totowa, NJ

Table 1
Patterns of Local-Regional Recurrence According to Initial Surgical Treatment

Initial surgery	Location of recurrence	Frequency (%)
Breast conservation	In-breast	5–15
Mastectomy	Chest wall	5–25
Axillary dissection	Axilla	2–3

As will become apparent, the treatment of local-regional recurrences is difficult and often fails. Therefore, the most effective approach is to prevent the situation from occurring through the use of appropriately aggressive initial local-regional surgery and irradiation.

2. IN-BREAST RECURRENCE FOLLOWING BREAST CONSERVATION

The pioneering work of Fisher and others has led to the acceptance of lumpectomy as the preferred surgical treatment for early-stage invasive breast cancer. There is broad agreement that lumpectomy should involve a negative margin excision with a rim of normal tissue surrounding the cancer. The minimum acceptable size of the margin is still debated. Some authors consider a margin to be free if there are no cancer cells right at the margin, whereas others require a specific distance in millimeters. Nevertheless, it is clear that a negative margin lumpectomy, however defined, often does not clear the entire breast of all malignant cells. An elegant pathologic and radiologic study by Holland and colleagues demonstrated that over 40% of mastectomy specimens contain residual invasive and/or noninvasive cancer cells 2 cm or more beyond what might have been the lumpectomy margin. This percentage is very similar to the in-breast recurrence rate observed when lumpectomy alone is used to treat invasive cancer. When an adequate dose of radiation is added to the treatment, the local recurrence rate in the breast falls to less than 10%. A negative margin lumpectomy does not mean that all cancer cells are gone from the breast. It should be viewed as a marker indicating that a minimal amount of cancer (and perhaps none) remains in the breast. The few remaining cells, if present, can be eliminated by adequate radiation in the vast majority of cases.

Therefore, adequate initial surgery for invasive breast cancer along with appropriate radiation will prevent most cases of local recurrence in the conserved breast. Some groups of patients will have higher rates of in-breast recurrence (Table 2). Diffuse disease, particularly with positive margins, is associated with higher failure rates. Diffuse disease and positive margins are contraindications to breast conservation. An extensive intraductal component (EIC) was considered by some to indicate a higher risk of local recurrence. EIC is defined as intraductal carcinoma prominently present within the tumor and intraductal carcinoma present in sections of grossly normal adjacent breast tissue. In addition, tumors that are predominantly intraductal but have foci of invasion are considered to have an EIC. However, the higher rate of local recurrence is probably related to the difficulty in achieving negative margins in this situation. Some studies have indicated a higher in-breast recurrence rate for younger women, under age 35, but this finding is not consistent. It may be that younger patients have smaller volume excisions owing to cosmetic concerns. In contrast, larger excisions provide better local control than smaller excisions, even with radiation.

Patients who are not irradiated have higher rates of local recurrence. There are some contraindications to breast radiation such as previous irradiation and pregnancy. Irradiating a

Table 2
Risk Factors for Local Recurrence Following
Breast-Conserving Surgery

Proven risk factors
    Positive margins
    No radiation
    Multicentric tumor
Possible risk factors
    Close margins
    Extensive intraductal component
    Young age

previously radiated breast causes unacceptable tissue damage, and radiation of pregnant women subjects the fetus to unacceptable levels of radiation scatter. Mastectomy is the treatment of choice in these settings. There may also be some groups who have lower rates of in-breast recurrence. Elderly women receiving tamoxifen with small, estrogen receptor-positive tumors excised with wide margins may be able to avoid radiation altogether. This concept is currently being tested in an Intergroup trial (C9343) that recently closed. Currently, to prevent local recurrence, radiation should be considered standard postoperative therapy following a negative margin lumpectomy in almost all women outside of clinical trials.

In the setting of noninvasive breast cancer (ductal carcinoma *in situ* [DCIS]), the situation is analogous. The largest prospective randomized trial performed in this disease, the National Surgical Adjuvant Breast and Bowel Project (NSABP) B-17, showed a clear reduction in local recurrence when radiation therapy followed lumpectomy. At 8 years of follow-up, the patients treated with postlumpectomy radiation had a 12% total in-breast recurrence rate (DCIS and invasive) compared with a 27% recurrence rate without radiation. In addition, a significantly higher proportion of the recurrences was invasive in the nonirradiated group. No subgroup, based on clinical or mammographic findings, had a low enough recurrence rate to justify avoiding radiation therapy in this study. Nonetheless, other investigators have retrospectively identified patients with a low risk of local recurrence. Patients with small (<2 cm) low-grade tumors excised with generous margins have very low rates of local recurrence in these highly selected series. Currently, about half of patients in the United States undergoing lumpectomy for DCIS receive postoperative radiation. Further studies are required to identify clearly those patients with DCIS who can be adequately treated with lumpectomy alone. With currently available information, breast irradiation should be considered for most women with DCIS to prevent recurrence in the breast.

Once a patient has undergone adequate lumpectomy and received adjuvant systemic therapy (if indicated) as well as adequate irradiation, she enters a period of surveillance. The detection and treatment of local recurrence is one of the goals of regular follow-up. Long-term studies suggest a local failure rate between 1 and 2% per year initially, with an ultimate rate of 15–20% if patients are followed for a lifetime. At follow-up, detailed breast examination is important. Because of postradiation changes, the physical exam can be difficult. Annual mammography is necessary. In the event of a suspicious finding, either mammographic or clinical, biopsy should be undertaken. The choice of biopsy (excisional, core, image-guided) should be based on the presentation of the abnormality and the skills of the clinician and institution. A high percentage of biopsies (perhaps 50%) for suspected local recurrence following breast conservation are positive. This rate is

Table 3
Ten-year In-Breast and Distant Recurrence Rate Following Breast Conservation

	No.	In-breast recurrence	Distant recurrence
All patients	973	73 (5.1%)	134 (14%)
Time to local recurrence			
<4 years	32		16 (50% of patients with IBTR)
>4 years	41		7 (17% of patients with IBTR)

IBTR, in-breast tumor recurrence.

higher then the positive rate for initial biopsy (about 20%). Once a positive biopsy has been obtained, a full staging workup should be undertaken because of the association of local recurrence with synchronous distant recurrence. This is particularly true for patients with a short disease-free interval (Table 3). It is also instructive to review the initial pathology reports to determine retrospectively whether there were factors suggesting a higher chance of local recurrence.

If the recurrence is local, with no sign of distant disease, a simple mastectomy is usually performed. There have been reports of selected patients treated with wide local reexcision, sometimes in combination with additional radiation. However, no prospective trials have examined this approach, and it should only be considered in unusual circumstances. At the time of salvage mastectomy, immediate reconstruction can be performed with autologous tissue. Saline implants can also be used, but the cosmetic outcome is not as good owing to the effects of the radiation delivered at the time of the initial breast conservation. The patient can also choose delayed reconstruction if desired.

The role of additional adjuvant therapy is controversial. Since the axilla was usually dissected at the original operation, nodal information is not available unless the patient has new signs of a clinically positive axilla. It is often not possible to determine whether the in-breast recurrence is a recurrence of the original cancer or the development of a new one. A different histology would confirm that the patient has two distinct primaries. A "recurrence" widely separated from the initial location would imply a new primary, as would a long disease-free interval. For a new cancer (different histology and location), adjuvant systemic therapy should be considered if the tumor is large or the histology aggressive. It is unclear whether a presumed local recurrence of the old cancer should be treated systemically. There are no prospective studies to guide decision making. It is reasonable to consider adjuvant therapy in patients, given the association with distant failure. It is also reasonable to consider tamoxifen in estrogen receptor-positive recurrences if the patient did not initially receive hormonal therapy. However, decisions to treat systemically should be made on an individual basis.

In general, recurrences after breast conservation for DCIS are treated the same as recurrences after breast conservation for invasive disease. In the face of prior lumpectomy with radiation, a salvage mastectomy is indicated. If the previous lumpectomy was not accompanied by radiation, reexcision to a clean margin with radiation is a reasonable alternative if the patient is highly motivated for breast conservation, realizing that there is still a significant chance for further local recurrence. This may represent a fair proportion of patients, given the increasing interest in avoiding radiation for low-risk patients with DCIS (low histologic grade, wide margin, and small size). Noninvasive recurrences would not require an

Table 4
Local-Regional Recurrence after
Mastectomy Without Radiation

Nodal status	Any local recurrence (%)
1–3 nodes +	13
4–7 nodes +	29

axillary dissection. Invasive recurrences should be staged with axillary dissection as for a patient presenting initially with an invasive cancer.

In summary, local recurrence following breast-conserving surgery with radiation for invasive and noninvasive cancer will occur in up to 20% of patients. The standard treatment includes restaging, a mastectomy, and possible systemic treatment. Continued breast conservation may be considered in special circumstances. The ultimate outcome for a patient initially making a choice between lumpectomy with radiation versus mastectomy is the same with regard to survival. However, in those patients who experience local failure following breast-conserving treatment, poorer survival at 10 years is seen.

3. CHEST WALL RECURRENCE FOLLOWING MASTECTOMY

Many patients and some physicians are surprised to learn that mastectomy is not a guarantee against local recurrence of invasive breast cancer. Depending on the initial stage at presentation, local recurrence after mastectomy can be seen in anywhere from 5 to 25% of patients. Several theories have been described to explain local failure after mastectomy. Residual bits of breast tissue always remain on mastectomy skin flaps, thus providing a potential source of residual tumor cells. More likely, systemically circulating cancer cells may implant at the site of the fresh wound, which is rich in growth factors. Thus, local recurrence after mastectomy is a marker for systemic disease.

Larger tumor size and an increasing number of involved nodes correlate with an increased local failure rate, even in the setting of adjuvant chemotherapy (Table 4). The coexistence of local and distant recurrence holds true for mastectomy patients as it does for breast conservation patients. Local recurrence after mastectomy is more ominous than local recurrence after breast conservation, particularly with a short disease-free interval. About 80% of local-regional recurrences after mastectomy will occur within the initial 5 years. For those patients who have chest wall recurrence within 2 years of their mastectomy, the median survival is poor at just over 1 year. Overall, about 90% of patients with local-regional recurrence after mastectomy have or will develop systemic disease, a rate much higher than that seen following in-breast recurrence after breast conservation.

Patients with local recurrence following mastectomy usually present with a skin nodule at or near the original mastectomy site. Some patients present with multiple nodules. A small number have diffuse chest wall involvement, known as *carcinoma en cuirasse*. The initial evaluation of suspected local recurrence must include biopsy. If possible, the surgeon should attempt a complete removal of the nodule with a clean margin, without resorting to a skin graft or vascularized flap. This helps establish the diagnosis and also provides fresh tumor for determination of hormone receptor status, her-2/neu status, and other molecular markers. Following a positive biopsy, complete restaging with computed tomography and bone scans should be undertaken to evaluate potential distant recurrence.

The mainstay of therapy for local recurrence after mastectomy is radiation therapy following excisional biopsy, when the latter can be accomplished without resorting to aggressive surgery. The doses are similar to those used during breast conservation. The chest wall and the supraclavicular fossa are treated. The axilla is not irradiated if an axillary dissection has been performed due to the risk of lymphedema. Most patients will have an initial complete response, but many tumors reoccur, often at the margins of the radiation field. There is an inverse relationship between the radiation dose and the subsequent local failure rate. Some reports suggest that patients who have and maintain a complete response to treatment have a longer survival time, but eventually up to 90% will have distant metastases by 10 years. There are reports of small series of patients being treated with repeat radiation following an initial radiation course. For selected patients with small areas of re-treatment, significant palliation can be achieved.

There is only a limited role for extensive surgery in the treatment of local recurrence following mastectomy. Most patients treated with local excision alone will relapse. Wide excision including chest wall resection has been reported, and some highly selected patients have good results. Morbidity from such a procedure can be high, and many of the patients will eventually have further local recurrence or the emergence of systemic disease. Some unfortunate patients present with chest wall recurrence that is beyond the scope of simple excision with primary closure. In this setting, a more extensive procedure with flap reconstruction is a reasonable alternative. The main goal of such an undertaking should be to maintain local control, even if systemic disease is present or anticipated.

On occasion, simple excision with chest wall irradiation is not possible, and an extensive resection with flap reconstruction is also not possible. This situation may occur with large, neglected fungating recurrences or with *carcinoma en cuirasse.* In such cases, treatment focuses primarily on managing local symptoms with adequate narcotic analgesia, dressing changes, control of local infection, and wound care. Photodynamic therapy using hematoporphyrin combined with laser or high-intensity light has been described. However, these reports describe heavily pretreated patients who have failed other modalities. Another modality, hyperthermia, has been used in conjunction with radiation therapy with similar mixed results.

The role of further systemic treatment is controversial. There are no large prospective randomized studies to guide the medical oncologist. A number of retrospective reviews are available. The results are in conflict. In theory, a patient with local recurrence after mastectomy without signs of systemic disease is similar to a high-risk patient following initial surgical therapy. If occult systemic disease is present, it should be most amenable to adjuvant therapy at that time. Therefore, it is reasonable to offer selected patients systemic chemotherapy, realizing that the data are quite limited. Observation is also a reasonable alternative. Patients with estrogen receptor-positive recurrences enjoy longer disease-free intervals with tamoxifen, although overall survival is similar. Given the acceptable toxicity, tamoxifen is a reasonable choice in this group of patients.

Given the devastating consequences of local recurrence after mastectomy, it is important to identify those patients at risk. Fowble and colleagues identified a group of patients at high risk of local recurrence following mastectomy despite the use of systemic adjuvant therapy (Table 5). A large tumor, 5 cm or greater, or the presence of four or more positive nodes conferred a high risk of local recurrence, almost equaling the risk of distant recurrence. These patients could expect a 25–30% local recurrence rate after mastectomy. The recommendation was to treat all such patients with radiation to the chest wall and supraclavicular area, lowering the local-regional recurrence rate to 10% or less. A number of studies have exam-

Table 5
Risk Factors for Local-Regional Recurrence
After Mastectomy

Tumor ≥5 cm
≥4 positive nodes
Pectoral fascia involvement

ined the role of radiation therapy following mastectomy for its effect on overall survival. Some hint at an effect but were hampered by small numbers or short follow-up. Two recent reports demonstrated a small but statistically significant improvement in survival in young, node-positive patients receiving postmastectomy radiation. This may lead to a greater use of postmastectomy radiation in the future.

4. AXILLARY RECURRENCE

The final clinical scenario involving local-regional recurrence is axillary recurrence. The usual presenting complaint is an asymptomatic mass in the axilla. About 30% of patients with axillary recurrence have or will develop symptoms. The most common complaints are arm edema and pain. The incidence of axillary recurrence in the past has been quite low (2–3%), given that most patients had formal axillary dissection. Patients who are truly node-negative (most patients today), presumably cannot have axillary nodal recurrence. Patients who are node-positive are at risk for axillary disease if not properly treated initially. Patients with clinically positive nodes almost invariably undergo formal axillary dissection. Patients who have microscopically positive nodes that are still clinically negative are at risk for axillary disease if not dissected initially. However, not all patients in this category (clinically negative but microscopically positive) will develop clinically palpable disease. The NSABP B-04 trial randomized patients with clinically negative axillary nodes to either radical mastectomy, total mastectomy with axillary radiation, or total mastectomy with no axillary treatment. Survival was the same in all three groups. About 40% of the patients in the radical mastectomy group had positive nodes at the time of surgery. Since the study was randomized prospectively, a similar percentage of pathologically node-positive patients should have been present in the mastectomy alone group. Only about 20% (half of the expected number of node-positive patients) of the patients who received no axillary treatment developed axillary disease requiring treatment in the future. This study is the basis for the current belief that axillary dissection is primarily a staging technique with no effect on survival.

As greater numbers of patients qualify for adjuvant therapy based on the pathologic and molecular characteristics of the primary tumor, some authors have questioned the role of axillary dissection. Currently, axillary dissection remains the standard of care for most patients because of its role in accurate staging and treatment choice. However, the evolving technique of lymphatic mapping and sentinel node biopsy in breast cancer surgery may impact on future rates of axillary recurrence. This technique promises to provide complete staging information while leaving most nodes in place (and at risk). Large prospective studies have been initiated, and it will be several years before the axillary recurrence rates in this setting are known.

As with local-regional recurrence elsewhere, diagnosis is the first step in evaluation. For patients with symptoms in the axilla but no mass, magnetic resonance imaging (MRI) may

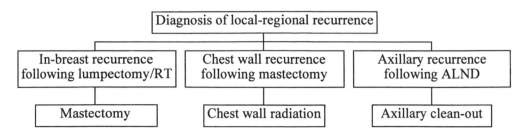

Fig. 1. Clinical pathways for treatment of local-regional recurrence. ALND, axillary lymph node dissection; RT, radiation therapy.

differentiate between posttreatment changes and tumor recurrence. In the setting of breast conservation, breast recurrence should be investigated. In the event of axillary lymphadenopathy following axillary dissection for breast cancer, a biopsy of the node should be performed (excisional or fine needle aspiration). This is indicated in both mastectomy and breast conservation patients. If the biopsy reveals recurrent cancer, a staging workup for systemic recurrence should be done. This situation is analogous to recurrence in the breast after breast conservation or on the chest wall after mastectomy.

If the recurrence is truly localized to the axilla, repeat axillary "clean-out" is the procedure of choice. This will provide the highest rate of long-term local control. Radiation to the axilla, without axillary dissection, will also provide control but not to the degree seen with complete excision. In general, if a complete dissection can be accomplished, the axillary nodes should not be radiated due to concerns about lymphedema. The supraclavicular area and the chest wall (if the patient had a mastectomy) should be radiated if not done initially. If the patient was initially treated with breast conservation and the axillary recurrence is confined to the axilla, the patient does not need a mastectomy. Mastectomy is only indicated for in-breast recurrence as outlined above. Overall, 60% of patients appropriately treated following local axillary failure will be alive at 5 years without disease.

The question of systemic therapy following complete excision is hampered by the lack of any prospective trials. Since patients with axillary recurrence are at increased risk for future systemic recurrence, it seems reasonable on theoretical grounds to offer systemic therapy. However, both the patient and physician should recognize that data are limited.

For patients with severe pain, parasthesias, weakness, and other signs of brachial plexus invasion, MRI is used initially for diagnosis. Brachial plexus invasion must be differentiated from radiation injury. Radiation therapy is the procedure of choice for the treatment of patients who have not been previously irradiated or who have rapidly progressing neurologic signs. Systemic therapy is the only other reasonable alternative in previously radiated patients or in patients with other sites of distant disease.

5. CONCLUSIONS

Local-regional recurrence, whether in the breast, the chest wall, or the axilla, is a clinical problem that will be encountered with some regularity. Surgery and radiation are the primary modalities used for treatment of local-regional recurrence (Fig. 1). However, the key to treatment is prevention. All the clinical scenarios described have risk factors that can be used to identify patients at increased risk of local-regional recurrence. Appropriate initial treatment with adequate surgery and postsurgical radiation when indicated are preferable to attempts at

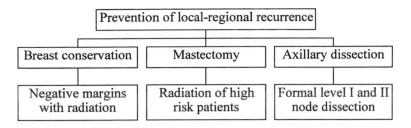

Fig. 2. Clinical pathways for prevention of local-regional recurrence

salvage after recurrence is present (Fig. 2). The association of distant disease with local-regional recurrence is high; in all three clinical scenarios, full reevaluation must be undertaken before beginning treatment for the local-regional problem.

BIBLIOGRAPHY

Albertini JJ, Lyman GH, Cox C, et al. (1996) Lymphatic mapping and sentinel node biopsy in the patient with breast cancer. *JAMA* **276**, 1818–1822.

Connolly JL, Harris JR, Schnitt SJ (1995) Understanding the distribution of cancer within the breast is important for optimizing breast-conserving treatment. *Cancer* **76**, 1–3.

Fisher B, Dignam J, Wolmark N, et al. (1998) Lumpectomy and radiation therapy for the treatment of intraductal breast cancer: findings from the National Surgical Adjuvant Breast and Bowel project B-17. *J. Clin. Oncol.* **16**, 441–452.

Fisher B, Redmond C, Fisher E (1985) Ten-year results of a randomized clinical trial comparing radical mastectomy and total mastectomy with or without radiation. *N. Engl. J. Med.* **312**, 674–681.

Fisher B, Redmond C, Poisson R (1989) Eight year results of a randomized clinical trial comparing total mastectomy and lumpectomy with or without irradiation in the treatment of breast cancer. *N. Engl. J. Med.* **320**, 822–828.

Fortin A, Larochelle M, Laverdiere J, Lavertu S, Tremblay D (1999) Local failure is responsible for the decrease in survival for patients with breast cancer treated with conservative surgery and postoperative radiotherapy. *J. Clin. Oncol.* **17**, 101–109.

Fowble B (1997) Postmastectomy radiation: then and now. *Oncology* **11**, 213–228.

Fowble B, Gray R, Gilchrist K, Goodman RL, Taylor S, Tormey DC (1988) Identification of a subgroup of patients with breast cancer and histologically positive axillary nodes receiving adjuvant chemotherapy who may benefit from postoperative radiotherapy. *J. Clin. Oncol.* **6**, 1107–1117.

Giuliano AE, Kirgan DM, Guenthler JM, Morton DL (1994) Lymphatic mapping and sentinel lymphadenectomy for breast cancer. *Ann. Surg.* **220**, 391–401.

Haffty BG, Reiss M, Beinfield M, Fischer D, Ward B, McKhann C (1996) Ipsilateral breast tumor recurrence as a predictor of distant disease: implications for systemic therapy at the time of local relapse. *J. Clin. Oncol.* **14**, 52–57.

Hait WN, August DA, Haffty BG (1999) *Expert Consultations in Breast Cancer — Critical Pathways and Clinical Decision Making*. Marcel Dekker, New York.

Holland R, Veling S, Mravunac M (1985) Histologic multifocality of Tis, T1–2 breast carcinomas: implication for clinical trials of breast conserving treatment. *Cancer* **56**, 979.

Kim SH, Simkovich-Heerdt A, Tran KN (1998) Women 35 years of age or younger have higher localregional relapse rates after undergoing breast conservation therapy. *J. Am. Coll. Surg.* **187**, 1–8.

Krag D, Weaver D, Ashikaga T, et al. (1998) The sentinel node in breast cancer—a multicenter validation trial. *N. Engl. J. Med.* **339**, 941–946.

Overgaard M, Hansen PS, Overgaard J, et al. (1997) Postoperative radiotherapy in high-risk premenopausal women with breast cancer who receive adjuvant chemotherapy. *N. Engl. J. Med.* **337**, 949–955.

Ragaz J, Jackson SM, Le N, et al. (1997) Adjuvant radiotherapy and chemotherapy in node-positive premenopausal women with breast cancer. *N. Engl. J. Med.* **337**, 956–962.

Recht A, Gray R, Davidson NE, et al. (1999) Local-regional failure 10 years after mastectomy and adjuvant chemotherapy with or without tamoxifen without irradiation: Experience of the Eastern Cooperative Oncology Group. *J. Clin. Oncol.* **17**, 1689–1700.

Schwartz GF, Finkel GC, Garcia JC, Patchefsky AS (1992) Subclinical ductal carcinoma in situ of the breast: treatment by local excision and surveillance alone. *Cancer* **15,** 2468–2474.

Silverstein MJ, Lagios MD, Craig PH, et al. (1996) A prognostic index for ductal carcinoma in situ of the breast. *Cancer* **77,** 2267–2192.

Veronesi U, Luini A, Galimberti V (1994) Conservative approaches for the management of stage I/II carcinoma of the breast: Milan Cancer Institute trials. *World J. Surg.* **18,** 70.

Winchester DJ, Menck HR, Winchester DP (1997) National treatment trends for ductal carcinoma in situ of the breast. *Arch. Surg.* **132,** 660–665.

18 Nipple Discharge

Marcia Boraas, MD

CONTENTS

INTRODUCTION
NORMAL PHYSIOLOGY
DISCHARGE OF EXTRINSIC/ENDOCRINE MEDIATED ORIGIN
DISCHARGE OF INTRINSIC/STRUCTURAL ORIGIN
EVALUATION STRATEGIES
FUTURE DIRECTIONS
BIBLIOGRAPHY

1. INTRODUCTION

Despite inclusion in the American Cancer Society's list of symptoms indicating possible malignancy, most women who present for evaluation of a nipple discharge will be found to have benign breast conditions or a cause extrinsic to the breast. Although approximately 5% of women presenting for breast evaluation will have a nipple discharge as their primary symptom, in most healthy women variable amounts of fluid can be obtained from the nipple with manual or mechanical stimulation. Of those presenting for evaluation of a nipple discharge, approximately 10–15% will be found to have an underlying breast malignancy. Patient age, characteristics of the discharge, and associated clinical and radiographic findings can be used to distinguish those who require specific evaluation to exclude carcinoma. To aid in this distinction, nipple discharge has been classified in the literature as *secretion,* which must be expressed, versus *discharge,* which is spontaneous (also termed *provoked* versus *spontaneous*). A classification of *galactorrhea* (milky) versus *physiologic* versus *pathologic* discharge has also been used. In the final analysis, the point of any classification is to identify patients whose symptoms indicate intrinsic breast pathology that requires a histologic diagnosis.

For purposes of clinical evaluation, which is the goal of this chapter, it is simplest to classify symptomatic nipple discharge by the underlying causative factors, which are either extrinsic to the breast and often endocrine mediated, or intrinsic to the breast and related to anatomic or structural abnormalities. Either type of discharge may be physiologic (an exaggeration of otherwise normal processes not requiring treatment) or pathologic (requiring a definitive diagnosis and therapeutic intervention). This chapter will not address conditions that may mimic a nipple discharge such as Paget's disease, eczema, periareolar infections, or obvious trauma. These can usually be identified with a careful history and physical examination, although findings suggestive of Paget's disease certainly require a biopsy for confirma-

From: *Current Clinical Oncology:*
Breast Cancer: A Guide to Detection and Multidisciplinary Therapy
Edited by: M. H. Torosian © Humana Press Inc., Totowa, NJ

tion. Similarly, a biopsy is mandatory for any nipple discharge in a male that is not readily explained by medication use or endocrine factors. In this setting, the likelihood of malignancy is high, a histologic diagnosis is necessary, and additional distinctions are of little value. Problems related to normal lactation are also excluded except for specific issues that may cause some diagnostic confusion. Finally, information regarding newer ductal imaging techniques that may prove clinically relevant in the future, and some information regarding current research directed at the use of ductal secretions in evaluating risk and screening for breast cancer is included at the conclusion of the chapter.

2. NORMAL PHYSIOLOGY

The normal nonlactating breast exhibits a balance of intraductal secretion and absorption, which may not be clinically apparent owing to the relatively small fluid volume and the presence of keratotic plugs within the distal nipple ducts. Using manual stimulation or mechanical aspiration, detectable fluid can be obtained in up to 90% of women depending on age, ethnic and hormonal factors, and the presence or absence of underlying breast disease. The appearance of nipple aspirate fluid varies with its composition from clear to yellow to dark green or blue-black and will contain variable amounts of exfoliated ductal cells as well as inflammatory cells and foam cells that share some characteristics with macrophages. In addition to endogenous substances such as cholesterol and proteins that reflect the character of colostrum and breast milk, exogenous substances can be secreted into ductal fluid including caffeine, nicotine, and pesticides. The presence of blood in nipple discharge fluid is not usually a normal finding and is one of the most critical factors in determining the need for further evaluation of a symptomatic discharge.

3. DISCHARGE OF EXTRINSIC/ENDOCRINE MEDIATED ORIGIN

This category of nipple discharge is essentially limited to *galactorrhea,* defined as a milky discharge in the absence of normal lactation. The stimulating factors are external to the breast and are often related to medications or to conditions that cause elevation of serum prolactin levels. Symptoms are typically bilateral, although the volume of discharge may be asymmetric, and usually the discharge is spontaneous and involves multiple ducts. Common medications associated with galactorrhea are listed in Table 1; the mechanism of action is typically mediated through an effect on pituitary dopamine receptors or direct hormonal activity, as is seen with oral contraceptives. Elevated prolactin levels causing galactorrhea may be caused by increased prolactin production, i.e., pituitary adenoma or bronchogenic carcinoma, or decreased renal clearance of prolactin, as in chronic renal failure. Treatment is directed at the underlying condition. Less commonly, galactorrhea has been reported with hypothyroidism, in which prolactin levels may be normal or increased, and rarely in other settings including chest trauma or following thoracotomy. Presumably this effect is caused by a transient elevation in serum prolactin levels, although the mechanism is not clear.

Occasionally women will experience persistent lactation following postpartum weaning and resumption of normal menstrual cycles, with a smaller number presenting an identical clinical picture in the absence of a history of recent breast-feeding. This form of idiopathic galactorrhea may be associated with normal prolactin levels, suggesting that the set point of breast response to prolactin has been altered. The symptoms may persist for years and are usually bilateral, although one breast may be more symptomatic. This condition is not related to intrinsic breast disease, although it may be aggravated by persistent mechanical stimulation if there is frequent checking to see whether a discharge is still present. Clinical

Table 1
Medications Associated with Galactorrhea

Hormones	Antidepressants
Estrogens	Amitriptyline (Elavil)
Progestins	Nortriptyline (Pamelor)
Combinations (oral contraceptives)	Doxepin (Sinequan)
Tamoxifen (Nolvadex)	Paroxetine (Paxil)
Phenothiazines and atypical antipsychotics	Fluoxetine (Prozac)
Prochlorperazine (Compazine)	Antihypertensives
Chlorpromazine (Thorazine)	Verapamil (Calan)
Trifluoperazine (Stclazine)	Methyldopa (Aldomet)
Thioridazine (Mellaril)	H_2 antagonists
Fluphenazine (Prolixin)	Cimetidine (Tagamet)
Risperidone (Risperdal)	Ranitidine (Zantac)
Clozapine (Clozaril)	Famotidine (Pepcid)
	Miscellaneous
	Metaclopramide (Reglan)
	Haloperidol (Haldol)
	Benzodiazepines
	Opiates
	Cannabis
	Amphetamines

monitoring is usually adequate, although if necessary the symptoms can be suppressed with bromocriptine despite normal prolactin levels. "Physiologic" galactorrhea may also be seen during times of rapid hormonal change such as puberty and menopause and is occasionally seen in neonates following withdrawal of maternal estrogen exposure. Persistent mechanical stimulation of the nipples may also produce some discharge in the absence of other hormonal changes.

4. DISCHARGE OF INTRINSIC/STRUCTURAL ORIGIN

A number of anatomic/structural changes within the breast ductal system may give rise to an increased volume of ductal secretions and subsequent nipple discharge, the most common of which are duct ectasia and cystic changes. In simple duct ectasia, there is dilation and thickening of multiple subareolar ducts with retained secretions that are opaque, often thick, and may range in color from creamy to blue-black. The findings are often bilateral, and the affected ducts may be intermixed with ducts of normal caliber. This finding occurs in at least 10% of the normal population and appears to increase with age. The discharge typically involves multiple ducts, may be bilateral, and is more often expressed than spontaneous. There may be associated periareolar cysts that serve as the source for the discharge, in which case the discharge itself will reflect the contents of the breast cyst. It has been suggested that this condition may lead to periductal inflammation and fibrosis, as bacteria can often be cultured from these ectatic ducts. In some patients, this may lead to chronic subareolar abscesses and fistula formation with progressive central nipple creasing and inversion. Treatment of any associated infection is certainly required, but the underlying duct ectasia and its associated discharge do not require intervention, although some of the darker fluids may require Hematest evaluation to exclude the presence of blood.

A bloody discharge that appears to be benign in character has been described by several authors as occurring during the second or third trimester of pregnancy. This discharge is characterized as spontaneous and "frankly bloody," unilateral, and involving multiple ducts. It usually is reported with a first pregnancy and follows a period of rapid physiologic breast enlargement. Breast examination is otherwise normal, and cytologic examination of the fluid will show only blood cells, foam cells, and benign epithelial cells. The discharge appears to be related to bleeding from fragile papillary tufts at the junction of the terminal ducts and newly formed lobules within the breast. It usually resolves within 2 months and has no effect on subsequent breast-feeding. Since carcinoma can occasionally present during pregnancy with a bloody discharge, care must be taken in making this diagnosis, and careful clinical monitoring is required if a benign etiology is suspected.

The most common cause of a spontaneous bloody or serous nipple discharge in the absence of pregnancy is an intraductal papilloma or papillomatosis. Forty to 50% of women who undergo surgery for a spontaneous nipple discharge will be found to have this condition, and ductal papillomas have been reported in 1.6% of the general population on autopsy. The nipple fluid is typically bloody, or serous but Hematest positive, originating from a single duct, and is not usually associated with a palpable mass. Several authors have made a distinction between single papillomas, which tend to be located in the large subareolar ducts, and peripheral papillomatosis, which may involve multiple smaller areas of intraductal proliferation. Peripheral papillomatosis has been reported to be associated with an increased risk of malignancy. In both cases, the histologic finding is of an epithelial lesion with a fibrovascular core. The central, solitary papillomas are typically located within 5 cm of the nipple and occasionally will produce a palpable mass if sufficiently large. Rarely, the papilloma may torse on its stalk and infarct, leading to spontaneous resolution of the discharge, but in most cases a surgical biopsy is required to exclude the small possibility of a papillary carcinoma.

An additional benign cause of a bloody nipple discharge is drainage of a posttraumatic or postoperative hematoma. There are anecdotal reports of spontaneous bloody nipple discharge occuring several weeks after documented surgery or trauma, although the exact frequency is unknown. It may be possible to demonstrate communication of the hematoma and ductal system by galactography. The antecedent history is usually quite helpful and there are often concordant clinical findings. After severe trauma with breast ecchymosis, such as a seat belt injury, mammography or physical examination may show a soft tissue density that should clear on follow-up several weeks later. This condition is self-limited, but if there is any question about the underlying diagnosis after short-term monitoring, more definitive evaluation including a biopsy may be necessary.

In the absence of a palpable mass, ductal carcinoma *in situ* or papillary carcinoma are the most common malignant diagnoses associated with nipple discharge. It is generally agreed that if the discharge is associated with a palpable mass, evaluation of the mass takes priority and should determine the appropriate workup. The likelihood of a malignant diagnosis nearly doubles under these circumstances. Similarly, a suspicious radiographic abnormality associated with a nipple discharge would dictate the course of evaluation. Nipple discharge associated with an underlying malignancy is typically unilateral, emanates from a single duct, and is bloody in up to 70% of cases. The discharge may also be serous, often Hematest-positive, and has rarely been reported to be watery or even "purulent," presumably related to underlying necrosis. The risk of any spontaneous discharge indicating malignancy increases with age over 40 years. Although the overall occurrence of nipple discharge decreases after menopause, the percentage of underlying malignancy may be as high as 30% after age 60.

Cytologic examination of the fluid may show suspicious cells, usually in the context of a bloody discharge, but a negative cytology cannot exclude an underlying carcinoma, and a biopsy is normally required.

There continues to be controversy regarding treatment of both *in situ* and invasive ductal carcinoma presenting with a nipple discharge. Typically a mastectomy is recommended, but there are some reports of treatment with lumpectomy with or without radiation. A higher rate of recurrence has been reported in these patients, which may be related to the completeness of the lumpectomy excision. More recently, a "duct-lobular segmentectomy" followed by radiation has been suggested as an effective breast-conserving approach if careful histologic mapping of the lumpectomy specimen is available. Excision of a portion or all of the nipple-areolar complex is normally required in any attempt at breast preservation, as well as meticulous attention to the surgical margins. Further investigation in this area is certainly required to determine whether breast preservation can equal the treatment results with mastectomy.

5. EVALUATION STRATEGIES

Whether a nipple discharge is the presenting symptom or is noted incidentally on a routine physical examination, further evaluation is directed by a careful medical history, including all current medications, and a thorough clinical breast examination. The character of the fluid should be noted (whether it is unilateral or bilateral, involves a single or multiple ducts, is milky or opaque versus serous or bloody) and whether there are any associated abnormalities on physical examination such as an underlying mass or nipple retraction. Mammography should be routinely performed, especially if there is a question of intrinsic breast disease, and a directed breast ultrasound may also prove helpful to clarify any questionable findings. As previously stated, a suspicious palpable or radiographic abnormality should take precedence over the nipple discharge and should determine further diagnostic testing. When the discharge appears to be of endocrine origin (milky, multiple ducts, usually bilateral) and not related to intrinsic breast disease, it should be addressed according to the potential underlying causes. In this case, a careful medication review as well as prolactin level and thyroid function tests are appropriate, and often a change in medication combined with education and reassurance is adequate. A confirmed endocrine abnormality should be referred to the appropriate specialist.

Nipple discharge that arises from intrinsic breast disease requires clarification of the underlying structural abnormality but may not require specific treatment. An opaque discharge secondary to underlying ectasia is often bilateral, involves multiple ducts, and may exhibit variable colors even within the same breast. The fluid should be Hematest-negative and often is expressed rather than spontaneous. If there is no associated clinical or radiographic finding other than ductal dilation or cysts confirmed on ultrasound, no further treatment is required. In the presence of an associated periareolar infection or abscess, treatment is directed at the underlying infection.

Serous or bloody fluid seen late in pregnancy involving multiple ducts, or following a documented history of trauma or surgery, can be managed conservatively if there are no inconsistent clinical findings. Further workup and consideration of a biopsy can usually be delayed for 6–8 weeks to allow spontaneous resolution. If symptoms persist or there is an associated breast abnormality, more immediate workup including a biopsy may be necessary. All other cases of serous or bloody discharge should be evaluated specifically to exclude an underlying malignant etiology, and surgery will often be required to provide a definitive diagnosis. This discharge typically is unilateral from a single duct, and it is frequently possible on physical examination to isolate the radiant of origin by serial compression around the circumference of the areola border. If the discharge is nonfocal, galactography may be helpful in clarifying the underlying ductal anatomy and in planning the surgical approach. As a diagnostic study, galactography can suggest the presence of specific ductal pathology in approximately two-thirds of cases, but a negative study should not preclude surgical exploration. False negatives can certainly occur, i.e., a relatively large papilloma or malignant tumor that completely occludes the duct and is radiographically undetectable.

When an abnormality is observed, surgery will almost always be required, as there are no defined galactogram characteristics that will reliably distinguish malignant from benign lesions. Similarly, cytologic evaluation of nipple discharge is helpful only when it is clearly abnormal. A normal or acellular result obviously cannot exclude malignancy. Statistically, since neoplastic changes are more often associated with a bloody discharge, all nonopaque fluids should be tested for occult blood. Cytologic examination is most appropriate in bloody or Hematest-positive fluid if the result will affect plans for surgery.

When the duct of origin of a suspicious discharge can be identified, limited excision of that duct, referred to as *microdochectomy* or *ductolobular segmentectomy,* is reasonable to limit the extent of surgery since most patients will be found to have a benign etiology. If there is a positive galactogram, injection of methylene blue through a small duct cannula immediately preoperatively may be helpful for localization, and needle localization directed at an abnormality on the galactogram has also been described. The surgery is usually performed through a circumareolar approach, which allows visual identification of the affected subareolar duct. This is typically ligated and divided just beneath the tip of the nipple, and a wedge of tissue is excised in a retrograde fashion along the tract of the duct. If the discharge is clinically significant and either multifocal in origin or nonfocal despite careful radiographic evaluation, a complete subareolar duct excision can be performed. Thus the nipple discharge symptoms can be eliminated and also a correct diagnosis can be obtained in most patients. In a small number of women, no specific diagnosis is made, but long-term follow-up studies suggest a very minimal risk of missing an underlying carcinoma. Magnetic resonance imaging and other new diagnostic techniques may further decrease the incidence of blind duct excision in the future.

Finally, some patients exhibiting a serous, but Hematest-negative, discharge that is nonfocal and not associated with any radiographic or clinical abnormalities may have symptoms that persist for years in the absence of any definable underlying breast pathology. These are often elderly women in whom the mammogram is relatively easy to monitor and who may have significant coexisting medical problems or other relative contraindications to surgery. If the fluid cytology is repeatedly negative, and the patient is agreeable, careful observation may be reasonable, with biopsy reserved for any sign of clinical or radiographic change.

6. FUTURE DIRECTIONS

Current investigations related to ductal secretions and nipple discharge are primarily focused on improving diagnostic procedures in symptomatic women and the use of nipple aspirate fluid in assessing the presence of breast cancer or future breast cancer risk. More sophisticated use of breast ultrasound as well as magnetic resonance galactography has been used in an attempt to diagnose intraductal lesions more precisely without surgery. When surgery is required, attempts at improved localization for biopsy using a hook wire directed by galactography or ultrasound, or placement of a polypropylene suture through a nipple cannula into the affected duct, have been reported. Fine needle aspiration of intraductal masses identified on galactography and ultrasound may provide improved diagnostic accuracy over nipple fluid cytology and help to select patients who do not require subsequent surgical duct excision. Endoscopy of the mammary duct system with endoscopic biopsy under topical anesthesia has been described, but its use will probably be limited to the largest subareolar ducts. Since most patients with an intrinsic breast source for the nipple discharge prove to have benign disease, these studies may eventually lead to a more precise selection of patients who will actually benefit from surgical intervention.

Nipple aspirate fluid, which can be obtained in most women in an experimental setting, has been evaluated for cytologic characteristics as well as multiple biomarkers including carcinoembryonic antigen, prostate-specific antigen, and lactate dehydrogenase isoenzymes. Atypia identified on cytologic examination of the nipple aspirate appears to correlate well with other known risk factors for breast cancer, and fluid prostate-specific antigen in particular appears promising as a predictor of the presence or absence of premalignant or malignant change. Nipple aspirate fluid evaluation and, more recently, ductal lavage offer noninvasive techniques that can be employed in a serial fashion over time and may eventually provide a method for monitoring breast cellular activity and the success of any intervention to reduce breast cancer risk.

BIBLIOGRAPHY

Bauer RL, Eckhert KH Jr, Nemoto T (1998) Ductal carcinoma in situ-associated nipple discharge: a clinical marker for locally extensive disease. *Ann. Surg. Oncol.* **5,** 452–455.

Bolivar AV, Alvaro RML, Garcia EO (1997) Intraductal placement of a Kopans spring-hookwire guide to localize nonpalpable breast lesions detected by galactography. *Acta Radiol.* **38,** 240–242.

Carter D (1977) Intraductal papillary tumors of the breast—a study of 78 cases. *Cancer* **39,** 1689–1692.

Carty NJ, Mudan SS, Ravichandran D, Royle GT, Taglor I (1994) Prospective study of outcome in women presenting with nipple discharge. *Ann. R. Coll. Surg. Engl.* **76,** 387–389.

Chaudary MA, Millis RR, Davies GC, Hayward JL (1982) Nipple discharge: the diagnostic value of testing for occult blood. *Ann. Surg.* **196,** 651–655.

Chung SY, Lee KW, Park KS, Lee Y, Bae SH (1995) Breast tumors associated with nipple discharge: correlation of findings on galactography and sonography. *Clin. Imaging* **9,** 165–171.

Ciatto S, Bravetti P, Cariaggi P (1986) Significance of nipple discharge clinical patterns in the selection of cases for cytologic examination. *Acta Cytol.* **30,** 17–20.

Dawes LG, Bowen C, Venta LA, Morrow M (1998) Ductography for nipple discharge: no replacement for ductal excision. *Surgery* **124,** 685–691.

Foretova L, Garber JE, Sadowsky NL, et al. (1998) Carcinoembryonic antigen in breast nipple aspirate fluid. *Cancer Epidemiol. Biomarkers Prev.* **7,** 195–198.

Gülay H, Bora S, Kilicturgay S, Hamaloglu E, Goksel HA (1994) Management of nipple discharge. *J. Am. Coll. Surg.* **178,** 471–474.

Haagensen CD (1986) *Diseases of the Breast.* WB Saunders, Philadelphia.

Hittmair AP, Lininger RA, Tavassoli FA (1998) Ductal carcinoma in situ (DCIS) in the male breast. *Cancer* **83,** 2139–2149.

Hou M, Huang CJ, Huang YS, et al. (1998) Evaluation of galactography for nipple discharge. *Clin. Imaging* **22,** 89–94.

Hou MF, Huang TJ, Huang YS, Hsieh JS (1995) A simple method of duct cannulation and localization for galactography before excision in patients with nipple discharge. *Radiology* **195,** 568–569.

Hughes LE, Mansel RE, Webster DJT (eds.) (1989) *Benign Disorders and Disease of the Breast: Concepts and Clinical Management.* Baillière Tindall, London.

Ito Y, Tamaki Y, Nakano Y, et al. (1997) Nonpalpable breast cancer with nipple discharge: how should it be treated? *Anticancer Res.* **17,** 791–894.

Jardines L (1996) Management of nipple discharge. *Am. Surg.* **62,** 119–122.

Kawamoto M (1994) Breast cancer diagnosis by lactate dehydrogenase isoenzymes in nipple discharge. *Cancer* **73,** 1836–1841.

Keller-Wood M, Bland KI (1991) Breast physiology in normal, lactating and diseased states. In: Bland KI, Copeland EM (eds.) *The Breast.* WB Saunders, Philadelphia, pp. 36–45.

King EB and Goodson, WH III (1991) Discharges and secretions of the nipple. In: Bland KI, Copeland EM (eds.) *The Breast.* WB Saunders, Philadelphia, pp. 46–67.

Kleinberg DL, Gordon LN, Frantz AG (1977) Galactorrhea: a study of 235 cases, including 48 with pituitary tumors. *N. Engl. J. Med.* **296,** 589–600.

Kline TS Lash S (1962) Nipple secretion in pregnancy—a cytologic and histologic study. *Am. J. Clin. Pathol.* **37,** 626–632.

Koretz M, Strano S (1998) Bloody nipple discharge after lumpectomy (letter). *Am. J. Radiol.* **170,** 1400.

Lafreniere R (1990) Bloody nipple discharge during pregnancy: a rationale for conservative treatment. *J. Surg. Oncol.* **43,** 228–230.

Makita M, Sakamoto G, Akiyama F, et al. (1991) Duct endoscopy and endoscopic biopsy in the evaluation of nipple discharge. *Breast Cancer Res. Treat.* **18,** 179–188.

Ohuchi N, Abe R, Kasai M (1984) Possible cancerous change of intraductal papillomas of the breast. *Cancer* **54,** 605–611.

Ohuchi N, Furuta A, Mori S (1994) Management of ductal carcinoma in situ with nipple discharge. *Cancer* **74,** 1294–1302.

Petrakis NL (1986) Physiologic, biochemical, and cytologic aspects of nipple aspirate fluid. *Breast Cancer Res. Treat.* **8,** 7–19.

Petrakis NL (1993) Nipple aspirate fluid in epidemiologic studies of breast disease. *Epidemiol. Rev.* **15,** 188–195.

Rongione AJ, Evans BD, Kling KM, McFadden DW (1996) Ductography is a useful technique in evaluation of abnormal nipple discharge. *Am. Surg.* **62,** 785–788.

Sardanelli F, Imperiale A, Zandrino F, et al. (1997) Breast intraductal masses: ultrasound-guided fine needle aspiration after galactography. *Radiology* **204,** 143–148.

Sauter ER, Daly M, Linahan K, et al. (1996) Prostate-specific antigen levels in nipple aspirate fluid correlate with breast cancer risk. *Cancer Epidemiol. Biomarkers Prev.* **5,** 967–970.

Sauter ER, Ross E, Daly M, et al. (1997) Nipple aspirate fluid: a promising non-invasive method to identify cellular markers of breast cancer risk. *Br. J. Cancer* **76,** 494–501.

Seltzer MH, Perloff LJ, Kelley RI, Fitts WT Jr (1970) The significance of age in patients with nipple discharge. *Surg. Gynecol. Obstet.* **131,** 519–522.

Van Zee KJ, Ortega Perez G, Minnard E, Cohen MA (1998) Preoperative galactography increases the diagnostic yield of major duct excision for nipple discharge. *Cancer* **82,** 1974–1880.

Yoshimoto M, Kasumi F, Iwase T, Takahashi K, Tada T, Uchida Y (1997) Magnetic resonance galactography for a patient with nipple discharge. *Breast Cancer Res. Treat.* **42,** 87–90.

19 Sarcoma and Lymphoma of the Breast
Presentation, Diagnosis, and Treatment

Helena Chang, MD, PHD, *and Jane Kakkis,* MD

CONTENTS

BREAST SARCOMAS
BREAST LYMPHOMAS
REFERENCES

1. BREAST SARCOMAS

Sarcomas arise from mesodermal structures. Common morphologic appearance and similar clinical patterns characterize these connective tissue tumors. The etiology is unknown, and most soft tissue sarcomas arise *de novo.* Soft tissue sarcomas expand radially and spread along paths of least resistance. Most develop pseudocapsules that contain tumor cells and therefore cannot be shelled out, as the risk of local recurrence is very high. Sarcomas rarely metastasize to regional lymph nodes. Hematogenous spread is common and occurs early. Pulmonary metastasis is often the first site of disseminated disease. Local recurrence is associated with disseminated disease in one-third of patients. The most important prognostic factors are histologic grade and size of tumor.

Cancers of nonepithelial origin rarely occur in the breast. Breast sarcomas represent less than 1% of all primary malignancies of the breast. The incidence of sarcomas of the breast has been reported to be 18 cases yearly for every 1 million patients evaluated *(1)*. Presentation is usually rapid enlargement of the breast. Various types of sarcomas are reported to arise from the stromal tissues of the breast, including cystosarcoma phylloides, angiosarcoma, liposarcoma, and osteosarcoma, among others *(2)*. The most common is cystosarcoma phylloides. Although the name implies malignancy, only 1 in 10 of these tumors is truly malignant. Outcomes of mammary sarcomas depend on grade of the tumor rather than specific sarcoma type (Table 1) *(3,4)*. Axillary adenopathy is rare and if present is a grave sign signaling disseminated disease *(5–7)*. Death is usually caused by blood-borne metastases, particularly to the lungs.

Diagnosis of these tumors is difficult. Mammographic findings include dense masses with irregular margins and no calcifications, frequently leading to a falsely benign interpretation. Ultrasound is not very helpful in elucidating the nature of the tumor. Fine needle aspirates have been interpreted as benign or nondiagnostic in more than half of patients studied. The rate of misdiagnosis in premenopausal women can approach 74%. There are no biologic markers for these tumors, and the expression of estrogen and progesterone receptors is var-

From: *Current Clinical Oncology:*
Breast Cancer: A Guide to Detection and Multidisciplinary Therapy
Edited by: M. H. Torosian © Humana Press Inc., Totowa, NJ

Table 1
Outcomes Predicted by Histologic Grade
of Breast Sarcomas

Grade	Survival	
	5-year	10-year
Low	75%	63%
Intermediate	55%	40%
High	29%	19%

Data from ref. *4.*

ied. The lack of expression of cytokeratin may help differentiate these tumors from meta-plastic carcinoma histologically.

The rarity of this disease is problematic in determining optimal therapy. Surgical resection with clear margins is the mainstay of therapy. Incisional biopsy provides the necessary tissue for accurate histologic diagnosis for large tumors. For small tumors, excisional biopsy can be performed. Care must be taken to avoid shelling out the tumor from the pseudocapsule during definitive surgery. Mastectomy is often required for large tumors. Postoperative radiation is utilized for high-grade sarcomas or if the adequacy of surgical margins is in question. Adjuvant chemotherapy after complete resection has not been proved beneficial.

1.1. Cystosarcoma Phylloides

Cystosarcoma phylloides is a rare variant of fibroadenoma of the breast. It is a misnomer because the tumor is usually benign and not cystic. It is a rare and distinctive fibroepithelial tumor without a counterpart in any other organ. The classical description (by Johannes Müller) appeared in 1838 *(8)*. This tumor presents as a painless breast mass, most commonly in women aged 30–40 years, although it can occur at any age. Cystosarcoma may arise in a preexisting fibroadenoma and may be the only breast tumor that can become malignant from a previously benign entity *(9,10)*. Although 25% appear histologically malignant, only 10% have metastatic potential. These tumors account for less than 1% of all breast lesions, benign and malignant. Differentiation from a fibroadenoma is based on a greater degree of stromal cellularity, cellular pleomorphism, hyperchromatic nuclei, and a significant number of mitotic figures.

These tumors average 5–10 cm in size at presentation and have a rubbery and firm consistency. Mammography usually reveals a well-circumscribed lesion with one or more borders that may appear indistinct. The cut surface tends to be slimy or mucoid with a bulging appearance. They usually have a lobulated leaf-like appearance, with stromal and epithelial elements seen microscopically. Fibrous tissue and soft fleshy areas alternate. Rarely, there may be areas of cystic degeneration within a solid mass, represented by clear or semisolid bloody fluid-filled cysts. Often malignant areas are focal and can be missed if insufficient tissue is analyzed. Ultrastructural analysis has not been shown to contribute to the differentiation between benign and malignant disease.

Management of benign phylloides tumors consists of wide local excision. Resections should include a 2-cm disease-free margin. Relative breast-to-tumor size is used in consideration of simple mastectomy. Even the benign variant has a high recurrence rate if incompletely excised. A local recurrence rate as high as 20% has been reported *(11,12)*. The tendency for microscopic projections to penetrate the surrounding parenchyma creates diffi-culty in assessing resection margins grossly. Axillary nodal disease is rare, and therefore axillary node dissection is not performed.

1.1.1. MALIGNANT CYSTOSARCOMA PHYLLOIDES

Lee and Pack *(13)* described the first case of metastatic cystosarcoma phylloides in 1931. It is the most common malignancy of the breast not of ductal origin. The malignant variety of cystosarcoma phylloides represents approximately 10–13% of these tumors and is recog-nized by features of a highly anaplastic lesion or by metastatic properties. Malignant histol-ogy correlates with pain, large size (≥7 cm), and advanced age at diagnosis (>52 years). Lymph node metastases are rare, as this tumor primarily metastasizes through the blood. Approximately 20–30% of these patients develop distant disease. Like other sarcomas, it has a predilection to metastasize to the lungs *(14,15)*. Liver and bone are other sites that are fre-quently involved. Cisplatin-based and ifosfamide plus doxorubicin chemotherapy regimens have been used to treat these patients with marginal effects. Osseous metastases are the next most common, and other sites are rarely involved *(16)*.

These tumors present as rapidly growing palpable masses that may be attached to the skin or underlying tissues. Mammography reveals a round, lobular lesion with circumscribed margins; there are usually no spiculations or calcifications. Mammography cannot distin-guish between benign and malignant lesions. Ultrasound may show low-level echoes, cir-cumscribed margins, and occasional cystic regions. Open biopsy is required to obtain a reliable diagnosis. Five histologic features differentiate benign and malignant disease:

1. Number of mitoses per high power field
2. The character of the tumor margin (pushing versus infiltrating)
3. The presence of stromal overgrowth
4. Increased stromal cellularity
5. Degree of cellular atypia

Most authors recommend total mastectomy for local control of malignant cystosarcoma *(17)*. Surrounding tissue may need to be excised to achieve 2-cm clear resection margins. Axillary metastases are rare, and low axillary dissection is reserved for cases with suspicious nodal tissue. Prognosis of metastatic disease is poor. No sustained remissions have been reported with the use of radiation, hormonal therapy, castration therapy, or chemotherapy.

1.2. Radiation-Induced Sarcomas:
Lymphangiosarcoma (Stewart-Treves Syndrome)

Patients who received postoperative radiation in addition to radical mastectomy were prone to develop chronic lymphedema and in certain cases this led to the development of lymphangiosarcoma, also known as Stewart-Treves syndrome. Lymphangiosarcoma typi-cally involves the upper extremity but occasionally originates in the axilla or soft tissues of the chest. The combination of ipsilateral axillary node dissection with radiation of the breast is thought to disrupt collateral lymphatic drainage of the arm and sometimes chest wall, causing lymphedema.

Whereas radiation therapy appears to aggravate the lymphedema after modified radical mastectomy, radiation therapy after segmental excision appears to play a more direct role in the development of lymphangiosarcoma *(18–21)*. Most treatment-related sarcomas are diag-nosed 5–10 years after the initial breast cancer therapy. The current incidence appears to be 2 cases per 5,000 patient-years *(22)*. The development of sarcoma does not appear to be related to the source of radiation or to the dose delivered *(23)*.

The presentation is purplish red nodules, and sometimes these are mistaken for a bacterial cellulitis. The lesions are almost always high grade and spread rapidly to include the arm, shoulder, and chest wall. Disseminated disease occurs shortly after diagnosis.

These tumors are unresponsive to radiation therapy. Resection is indicated in the absence of metastasis. Regional or systemic chemotherapy is frequently included as part of treatment, although the prognosis is dismal. Radical four-quarter amputation has been proposed to manage massive lymphedema and ulcerative complications; however, owing to poor survival, it is rarely employed. Five-year survival is uncommon; most patients die of metastasis within 2 years *(24)*. Survival duration averages 6 months from diagnosis *(25,26)*. The abandonment of radical mastectomy and radiation as therapy for breast cancer has decreased the frequency of these tumors. Avoidance of postoperative radiation after radical or modified radical mastectomy can decrease the risk of this disease, although it is known to occur after breast conservation therapy with axillary dissection and radiation therapy *(27)*.

1.3. Angiosarcoma

Angiosarcoma is the only soft tissue sarcoma with a predilection for the breast. It occurs in mainly in women with a median age of 35 years, although it has been described in patients from age 14 to 82 years *(28)*. Among radiation-induced sarcomas, lymphangiosarcoma is the most common histologic type. Malignant fibrous histiocytoma, fibrosarcomas, and osteogenic sarcoma are less commonly observed. The conserved breast tissue is the most common soft tissue site for its occurence *(22)*. It typically presents as a painless mass or a diffuse enlargement of the breast. The skin overlying the lesion has a characteristic bluish purple discoloration. Size at presentation is variable, ranging from 1.5 to more than 12 cm. Mastectomy with wide skin removal has limited value in patients with localized disease.

These tumors appear spongy, friable, and hemorrhagic. Microscopically, the tumor usually extends beyond grossly apparent limits. Tumor cells are endothelial in origin and express endothelial antigens such as CD34 and factor VIII-related antigen. At the ultrastructural level, Weibel-Palade bodies have been identified. Although some tumors exhibit a weak expression of estrogen receptors, most do not *(29)*.

Metastases are frequent and are found either at the time of primary diagnosis or shortly after. The lungs, liver, skin, and bones are the common sites of disseminated disease *(30)*. The histologic grade is the most reliable prognostic factor for localized disease (Tables 2 and 3.) It is estimated that 90% of patients die within 2 years of diagnosis.

2. BREAST LYMPHOMAS

Primary lymphomas of the breast are rare. Diagnosis requires that patients have not previously had the diagnosis of lymphoma and do not have evidence of concurrent lymphomatous disease in other parts of the body *(33)*. Mean age at diagnosis is 60 years. Cases have been reported to occur during pregnancy and in the postpartum period. The incidence of lymphoma of the breast is estimated to be 0.05–0.5% of the total number of breast malignancies *(34)*. Bilateral breast involvement can occur in up to 15% of cases.

Presentation is with a painless mass with an average size of 4 cm. There tends to be a predominance of right-sided lesions. Ipsilateral axillary nodes are often involved *(35)*. Mammographically, there are differences between nodular and diffuse lymphomas. Nodular lymphomas are seen as distinct masses, and the diffuse variety are seen as parenchymal den-

Table 2
Histologic Grading of Angiosarcomas

Grade	Histologic characteristics
Low (type I)	Irregular anastamosing vascular channels lined by endothelial cells
	Mild nuclear atypia
Intermediate (type II)	Mixed solid and vascular growth patterns
	Intermediate nuclear grade
High (type III)	Hypercellular with solid growth pattern
	Polygonal or spindle-shaped cells
	Marked nuclear atypia
	High mitotic activity (>5 mitotic figures/10 high power field:)
	Inconspicuous vessel formation

Data from ref. *31*.

Table 3
Histologic Grade of Angiosarcoma and Survival

Grade	Median disease-free survival
Low (type I)	>15 yr
High (type III)	15 mo

Data from ref. *32*.

sities with or without skin thickening *(36)*. Adequate open biopsy is necessary for diagnosis with material taken for touch prep, cell surface markers, and electron microscopy. Well-differentiated lymphomas appear microscopically as small, mature lymphocytes. Poorly differentiated lymphomas have marked nuclear pleomorphism and cellular immaturity; occasionally sheets of pure lymphoblasts are seen *(33)*. A uniform population of malignant lymphoid cells can be seen densely infiltrating the lobules and disrupting the surrounding parenchyma. The diffuse histiocytic subtype is seen in approximately half the patients with extranodal lymphoma, most of which are B cell in origin *(37)*.

Treatment of primary breast lymphoma should be coordinated by an experienced hematologist and according to the treatment principles of lymphoma of the same type found elsewhere in the body. Treatment usually involves a combination of radiation and chemotherapy. Some authors advocate total mastectomy and axillary node sampling for large primary lymphomas *(38)*. Other authors have acknowledged that very few patients have undergone mastectomy as part of the treatment of this disease *(34)*. Recurrent local disease and accessible regional nodal disease can be treated with radiotherapy, and systemic or multiregional disease is treated with chemotherapy. Survival rates vary in the literature. Five-year survival rates have been reported in the range of 35–74% *(34,38)*. The absolute survival and disease-free survival rates are similar to those of nodal lymphoma of corresponding histologic factors and stages.

REFERENCES

1. May DS, Stroup NE (1991) The incidence of sarcomas of the breast among women in the U.S, 1973–1986. *Plast. Reconst. Surg.* **87,** 869–878.
2. Page DL, Anderson TJ, Connelly JL, Schnitt SF (1987) Miscellaneous features of carcinoma. In: Page DL, Anderson TJ (eds.) *Diagnostic Histopathology of the Breast.* Churchill Livingstone, Edinburgh pp. 269–299.

3. Costa J, Wesley RA, Glatstein E, et al. (1984) The grading of soft tissue sarcoma. Results of clinicopatho-logic correlation in a series of 163 cases. *Cancer* **53**, 530–541.

4. Russell WO, Cohen J, Enzinger F, et al. (1977) A clinical and pathological staging system for soft tissue sarcomas. *Cancer* **40**, 1562–1570.

5. Gutman H, Pollock RE, Ross MI, et al. (1994) Sarcoma of the breast: implications for extent of therapy; the M.D. Anderson experience. *Surgery* **116**, 505–509.

6. Ciatto S, Bonardi R, Cataliotti L, et al. (1992) Sarcomas of the breast: a multicenter series of 70 cases. *Neoplasma* **39**, 375–379.

7. Smola MG, Ratschek M, Amann W, et al. (1993) The impact of resection margins in the treatment of primary sarcomas of the breast: a clinicopathological study of 8 cases with review of the literature. *Eur. J. Surg. Oncol.* **19**, 61–69.

8. Müller J (1838) *Uber den feineran Bau and die Forman der krankhaften Geschwilste.* G. Reimer, Berlin.

9. Dyer NH, Bridger JE, Taylor RS (1966) Cystosarcoma phylloides. *Br. J. Surg.* **53**, 450–455.

10. Treves N (1964) A study of cystosarcoma phylloides. *Ann. NY Acad. Sci.* **114**, 922–935.

11. Hajdu S, Espinosa MH, Robbins GF (1976) Recurrent cystosarcoma phylloides—a clinicopathologic study of 32 cases. *Cancer* **38**, 1402–1406.

12. McDivitt RW, Stewart FW, Berg JW (1968) Tumors of the breast. In: *Atlas of Tumor Pathology,* 2nd series, Fascicle 2. Armed Forces Institute of Pathology, Washington, DC.

13. Lee B, Pack G (1931) Giant intracanalicular fibroadenomyxoma of the breast. *Am. J. Cancer* **15**, 2583–2595.

14. Hart WR, Bauer RC, Oberman HA (1978) Cystosarcoma phylloides. A clinicopathologic study of 26 hyper-cellular periductal stroma tumors of the breast. *Am. J. Clin. Pathol.* **70**, 211–216.

15. Pietrusz M, Barnes L (1978) Cystosarcoma phylloides. A clinicopathologic analysis of 42 cases. *Cancer* **41**, 1974–1983.

16. Kessinger A, Foley JF, Lemon HM, et al. (1972) Metastatic cystosarcoma phylloides: a case report and review of the literature. *J. Surg. Oncol.* **4**, 131–145.

17. West L, Weiland LH, Clagett OT (1971) Cystosarcoma phylloides. *Ann. Surg.* **173**, 520–528.

18. Givens SS, Ellerbroek NA, Butler JJ, et al. (1989) Angiosarcoma arising in an irradiated breast. A case report and review of the literature. *Cancer* **64**, 2214–2216.

19. Edeiken SR, Russo DP, Knecht J, et al. (1992) Angiosarcoma after tylectomy and radiation therapy for carcinoma of the breast. *Cancer* **102**, 757–763.

20. Moshaluk CA, Merino MJ, Danforth DN, et al. (1992) Low grade angiosarcoma of the skin of the breast: a complication of lumpectomy and radiation therapy for breast carcinoma. *Hum. Pathol.* **23**, 710–714.

21. Slotman BJ, van Hattum AH, Meyers S, et al. (1994) Angiosarcoma of the breast following conserving treatment for breast cancer. *Eur. J. Cancer* **30A**, 416–417.

22. Pendlebury SC, Bilous M, Langlands AO (1995) Sarcomas following radiation therapy for breast cancer: a report of three cases and a review of the literature. *Int. J. Radiat. Oncol. Biol. Phys.* **31**, 405–410.

23. Zucali R, Merson M, Placucci M, et al. (1994) Soft tissue sarcoma of the breast after conservative surgery and irradiation for early mammary cancer. *Radiother. Oncol.* **30**, 271–273.

24. Woodward AH, Ivins JC, Soule EH (1972) Lymphangiosarcoma arising in chronic lymphedematous extremities. *Cancer* **30**, 562–572.

25. Brady MS, Garfein CF, Petrek JA, et al. (1994) Post-treatment sarcoma in breast cancer patients. *Ann. Surg. Oncol.* **I**, 66–72.

26. Janse AJ, van Coevorden F, Peterse H, et al. (1995) Lymphedema-induced lymphangiosarcoma. *Eur. J. Surg. Oncol.* **21**, 155–158.

27. Fineberg S, Rosen PP (1994) Angiosarcoma and atypical cutaneous lesions after radiation therapy for breast carcinoma. *Am. J. Clin. Pathol.* **102**, 757–763.

28. Brentani MM, Pacheco MM, Oshima CTF (1983) Steroid receptors in breast angiosarcoma. *Cancer* **51**, 2105–2111.

29. Lesueur GC, Brown RW, Bhathal PS (1983) Incidence of perilobular hemangioma in the female breast. *Arch. Pathol. Lab. Med.* **107**, 308–310.

30. Steingaszner LC, Enzinger FM, Taylor HB (1965) Hemangiosarcoma of the breast. *Cancer* **18**, 352–361.

31. Rosen PP, Kimmel M, Ernsberger DL (1988) Mammary angiosarcoma. The prognostic significance of the tumor differentiation. *Cancer* **62**, 2145–2151.

32. Donnell RM, Rosen PP, Lieberman PH, et al. (1981) Angiosarcoma and other vascular tumors of the breast. Pathologic analysis as a guide to prognosis. *Am. J. Surg. Pathol.* **5**, 629–642.

33. Wiseman C, Liao KT (1972) Primary lymphoma of the breast. *Cancer* **29**, 1705–1712.

34. Mambo NC, Burke JS, Butler JJ (1977) Primary malignant lymphomas of the breast. *Cancer* **39**, 2033–2040.

35. Dixon JM, Lumsden AB, Krajewski A, et al. (1987) Primary lymphoma of the breast. *Br. J. Surg.* **74,** 214–217.

36. D'Orsi CJ, Feldhaus L, Sonnenfeld M (1983) Unusual lesions of the breast. *Radiol. Clin. North Am.* **21,** 67–80.

37. Bobrow LG, Richards MA, Happerfield LC, et al. (1993) Breast lymphomas: a clinicopathologic review. *Hum. Pathol.* **24,** 274–278.

38. Brustein S, Kimmel M, Lieberman PH, et al. (1987) Malignant lymphoma of the breast: a study of 53 patients. *Ann. Surg.* **205,** 144–149.

III CURRENT CONTROVERSIES AND RESEARCH

20   Breast Conservation Without Radiation Therapy for Carcinoma of the Breast

Gordon F. Schwartz, MD, MBA

CONTENTS

INTRODUCTION
LOBULAR CARCINOMA *IN SITU*
DUCTAL CARCINOMA *IN SITU*
INVASIVE CARCINOMA (DUCTAL OR LOBULAR)
BIBLIOGRAPHY

1. INTRODUCTION

The surgical management of carcinoma of the breast has evolved from the Halstedian radical mastectomy of the last millennium through first more radical (extended) and then less formidable (modified) forms of mastectomy, but still using the same adjective, "radical," in the description of the operation. Dissection of the axilla was truncated from complete dissection of levels I, II, and III, to dissection of levels I and II only. In the last quarter of the last century, following reports of successful clinical trials of radiation therapy as an alternative, mastectomies of all kinds began to be replaced by so-called breast-conserving therapy (BCT), implying local excision of the primary tumor with "clear" margins around it, plus axillary dissection of levels I and II, and then radiation therapy to the entire breast and a boost of radiation to the site of the tumor itself. Despite the obvious difference in the technique and its appearance, the same principles apply for BCT as for mastectomy. Whether removed or radiated, the entire breast is treated, and whether the entire axilla is dissected or merely sampled by sentinel node biopsy, axillary node status is addressed.

Therefore, the first major departure from this treatment occurred as *in situ* carcinoma of the breast became more than a curiosity. Both the lobular and ductal versions of *in situ* carcinoma have become more frequently encountered as their existence became more common knowledge, and ductal carcinoma *in situ* (DCIS) has become almost a household word, not only within the medical community, but within Internet sites devoted to disseminating information about these diseases to the public. Now that we are entering a new millennium, perhaps it is appropriate to ask another question—are there situations in which the previously dogmatic approach to the breast and axilla can be abandoned in favor of lesser procedures?

From: *Current Clinical Oncology:*
Breast Cancer: A Guide to Detection and Multidisciplinary Therapy
Edited by: M. H. Torosian © Humana Press Inc., Totowa, NJ

2. LOBULAR CARCINOMA *IN SITU*

First described in 1941, the term "carcinoma" should not really apply to this disease, since it is not malignant in its own right. As a correction to this misconception, Lattes suggested the term "lobular neoplasia" (LN), but this correction has never replaced lobular carcinoma *in situ* (LCIS) in most texts and pathology reports, at least in the United States. Although initially a source of extreme controversy, it has now been almost universally accepted that LCIS is a marker of risk and not itself malignant in the customary sense of that term. It should be considered a benign pathologic-clinical entity when it occurs by itself, without a coexisting invasive lobular carcinoma. In spite of efforts to effect a name change for this condition, from the pejorative term, "lobular *carcinoma* in situ," to the less awesome "lobular *neoplasia,*" LCIS remains the most commonly used name.

LCIS is an incidental finding in a breast biopsy specimen, the biopsy having been performed for another reason. Unlike DCIS, it does not form a mass, it does not produce nipple discharge, and there are no mammographic findings to signal its presence. It is often multicentric and bilateral, occuring in multiple foci in both breasts. Metastasis does not occur in LCIS. The lesion often involves both the acini of the lobules and the terminal ducts, and within the ducts, its differentiation from DCIS is sometimes difficult. For reasons that remain unexplained, LCIS most often occurs in premenopausal women, or in postmenopausal women who are using estrogen replacement therapy, with or without concurrent progestins.

The early Columbia studies of Haagensen convinced that institution's surgeons to follow rather than treat these patients, so long-term data are available in that patient population. Among the largest series of such patients are those from the Columbia-Presbyterian Medical Center and also from Memorial Sloan-Kettering Cancer Center. Observations at the two institutions were similar, with only a minority of patients developing a subsequent invasive cancer. Their treatment options were initially quite different, however (surveillance alone versus mastectomy, often bilateral), and the differences in treatment were considered to be related to where in New York City the diagnosis was made—West Side (Columbia-Presbyterian) or East Side (Memorial).

That patients with LCIS are at increased risk for invasive breast cancer at some time in the future is not questioned. Major studies have all made this observation, although the reported incidence of subsequent breast cancer varies, from a low of 4% to a high of 35%. In the longest follow-up series, the probability of developing an invasive carcinoma by 10 years after the diagnosis of LCIS was 13%, 26% after 20 years, and 35% by 35 years, roughly 1% par year. Of crucial importance is the observation that after an initial diagnosis of LCIS, both breasts are at the same risk. Therefore, there seems to be no logical reason to perform mastectomy of *only* the breast known to harbor LCIS. The appropriate prophylactic procedure would be *bilateral* total mastectomy.

An understanding of the typical course of the breast cancer that may develop is also crucial to the formulation of a treatment plan when LCIS is encountered. Both breasts, not just the one in which the LCIS was detected, are at approximately the same long-term risk for subsequent breast cancer. This observation suggests that LCIS, if not excised, does not itself progress to invasive cancer. Moreover, such lack of progression may be inferred by the histology of the subsequent breast cancer. In the review by Bodian et al., only 27% of the subsequent breast cancers were invasive lobular carcinomas; the remainder were invasive ductal carcinomas, with several subtypes found. If progression from LCIS to invasive cancer were the rule, it would be expected that the later invasive cancer would be of the same origin. (Although purely invasive lobular carcinoma constitutes only about 10% of all breast cancers, many cancers seem to have both lobular and ductal features in association with each other.)

Despite the reluctance of the medical community to change the name of LCIS to LN or another less pejorative term, the treatment of LCIS has undergone significant evolution as physicians have accepted the concept that what had initially been considered a "real" cancer was in fact a marker of increased risk. Prior to its recognition as a marker, rather than as malignant, *sui generis,* it was most often treated by mastectomy. As this disease became better understood, unilateral mastectomy was abandoned as *treatment,* in favor of surveillance alone. To be sure, there are women for whom the specter of a subsequent invasive breast cancer is too great to endure, and this increased risk of developing a potentially life-threatening cancer leads them to choose mastectomy, with or without reconstruction. However, it must be stressed that mastectomy, in this context, is a prophylactic, not therapeutic, procedure. If chosen, it should be bilateral, since both breasts are at about equal risk. Unilateral mastectomy, even with so-called mirror-image biopsy of the opposite breast, is not a logical choice. If the diagnosis of LCIS is made on the basis of a biopsy of the right breast for an unrelated benign finding, it should be accepted that LCIS might also be present in the left breast as well, given its predilection for bilaterality and multicentricity. Radiation therapy for LCIS is never indicated.

It has been a major undertaking to convince many surgeons that observation alone is appropriate when LCIS is detected. As recently as 1988, surgical oncologists were surveyed about their approach to LCIS, and one-third of the respondents still advocated mastectomy. A slim majority, 54%, advised observation alone. When a similar questionnaire was sent to the same physician groups in 1996, 10% of the respondents still recommended unilateral mastectomy, suggesting their lack of information about this disease.

Patients whose otherwise benign breast biopsies reveal the presence of LCIS should be informed that a marker for increased risk has been detected. They should be aware of the nomenclature and the difference between the incorrect use of the word "carcinoma" in this diagnostic phrase and as it is customarily employed. As mammography has become the mode of diagnosis for DCIS, the differences between DCIS and LCIS should be discussed. Even when DCIS is treated by observation alone, it requires clear surgical margins and is considered a unilateral threat. The multicentricity and bilaterality of LCIS is assumed; it requires no further treatment after its diagnosis. However, the patient should be informed of her two options—either bilateral total mastectomy without or without reconstruction or lifetime observation. If mastectomy is chosen, it must be done with the patient's understanding that it is a prophylactic, not therapeutic, procedure. When acquainted with the risk of subsequent invasive cancer, using an approximation of a 25% risk in the next 25–30 years, the patient's choice depends on her own perceptions of this risk. Is her glass 75% full or 25% empty? Thus far, I have not performed a bilateral mastectomy for a patient with this disease.

Therefore, from the standpoint of breast conservation without radiation therapy, according to the title of this chapter, LCIS more than adequately fits this option. Moreover, LCIS occurring by itself requires no further treatment unless the patient's perceptions of risk are so threatening as to induce her to undergo *bilateral prophylactic* mastectomy. As noted above, radiation therapy is never warranted.

3. DUCTAL CARCINOMA *IN SITU*

Although the initial descriptions of what we currently call DCIS may have been in 1946, it was not until two decades later that the difference between its behavior and that of frankly invasive breast cancer was really considered. Based on our ignorance of the differences between purely *in situ* ductal carcinoma and invasive cancer, as initial experience with mammography was being gained in the late 1960s and early 1970s, these smaller and entirely intraductal cancers were detected with increasing frequency, usually as tiny groups of clustered calcifications, not yet forming an actual mass. Nevertheless, the standard of care remained mastectomy. It was assumed that, despite the absence of invasion in the sections studied, progression to invasive cancer would inevitably occur. This assumption was based, in general, on observations of the coexistence of DCIS with invasive carcinomas, as well as studies of patients who subsequently developed breast cancer after prior biopsies for what was thought to be benign disease, but that on review demonstrated DCIS. This led to the recommendation for mastectomy, albeit with the expectation that the likelihood of the patient dying of breast cancer would be remote.

Only in the late 1970s was it confirmed that untreated DCIS did not necessarily progress to invasive cancer, at least in some patients. That observation has, in part, led to the current controversy about the treatment of this disease, compounded by the increasing incidence of DCIS detected by mammograms. This has occurred as screening mammography for asymptomatic women has been embraced as a major advance in the discovery of earlier malignancies and as notable improvements in mammographic technique, such as magnification films, have detected tiny, subtle changes within the breast. In the past several years, current experience including our own data indicates that as many as one-fourth of nonpalpable breast cancers (those detected by mammography) will prove to be DCIS. As this inevitable progression of DCIS to invasive carcinoma has been challenged, the identification of DCIS at some early stage in its natural history that will obviate the obligatory treatment of the *entire* breast (whether by mastectomy or by irradiation), with a minimum risk to the patient of developing a subsequent, life-threatening cancer, has become a topic of great debate.

If, as is now accepted, DCIS is not always accompanied by invasion and/or does not necessarily progress to this stage, to prescribe lesser treatment for DCIS than for invasive carcinoma implies an obligation to recognize the time at which the identification and excision of DCIS at this one site might constitute adequate treatment. This premise, however, also implies that the eradication of DCIS at one location ensures that the site detected is no greater in significance than what might be a concurrent, as yet undetected, but more important (e.g., invasive) finding at another location within the same breast. Gump et al. first suggested the separation of clinical from subclinical DCIS to permit a more careful comparison of equivalent diseases, and their distinction also has great implications for treatment. DCIS presenting as a palpable mass, as nipple erosion (Paget's carcinoma), or as nipple discharge is not the same as DCIS presenting as an area of calcifications on a screening mammogram or discovered as an incidental finding in a specimen of breast tissue removed for another reason. Haagensen and his contemporaries detected "intraductal" cancer based on clinical findings, i.e., mass, nipple erosion, or nipple discharge; the masses he treated that were so-called intraductal cancers had a mean diameter of almost 2 inches!

Staging systems for breast cancer have not yet addressed the entire spectrum of DCIS, so that all DCIS is considered stage 0, Tis. The subdivision of DCIS into categories for consideration is somewhat arbitrary. Therefore, it is easier to discuss *clinical DCIS* (see below) from the treatment viewpoint than *subclinical DCIS,* detected by mammography or as an incidental finding. If there are patients in whom DCIS is *not* inexorably followed by invasive cancer, as current data indicate, I do not consider most women with *clinical* DCIS currently among that group. Currently, I believe that, except for highly selected patients, patients with clinically detected DCIS should continue to undergo treatment that includes the entire breast (i.e., irradiation or mastectomy) and, in selected patients, the axilla—at least a sentinel node biopsy. Exceptions to this dictum may be made for those patients with small (≤1 cm diameter), palpable, but biologically favorable types of DCIS, e.g., *in situ* papillary carcinoma arising in an intraductal papilloma.

Therefore, using these definitions, the term "palpable DCIS" is almost an oxymoron. As a palpable mass, a carcinoma may be largely intraductal, but it should not be considered noninvasive. The appropriate designation should probably be "no invasion documented in the sections studied." Except in the case of specially selected patients, these allegedly intraductal but palpable lesions are often accompanied by microinvasion, even when not seen, and the appropriate treatment addresses the entire breast and, arguably, the axilla as well. Some of these predominantly intraductal but palpable lesions may achieve considerable size and may be accompanied by clinically involved axillary nodes. They are characterized by their firmness, their fairly well delimited margins, and an abundance of malignant-appearing calcifications on mammography. Patients with these large lesions are usually not candidates for treatment by irradiation because of the difficulty of excising all the calcifications that permeate the ducts contiguous to and even at great distance from the mass itself. The palpable masses called DCIS that radiotherapists currently covet remain small ones, amenable to wide local excision with clear surgical margins.

Since DCIS itself is not a threat to the patient's outcome, it is only those patients who will progress to invasive cancer who theoretically require (prophylactic) treatment. It is now accepted that many patients, perhaps a majority, with DCIS will not ever develop invasive cancer. What is currently unclear is how to make this distinction and recommend appropriate therapy for those who are in jeopardy.

It is generally accepted that the goal of treatment for DCIS is breast conservation, with optimal cosmesis, with a minimum risk of subsequent invasive or *in situ* recurrence. There are some women for whom mastectomy remains the optimal treatment, but most women with DCIS are candidates for breast conservation. Each patient should be apprised of her own situation and each option discussed with her in detail, including local excision and radiation therapy, local excision alone, or mastectomy.

The factors that influence the recommendation for any treatment of the breast are the size of the area of DCIS, its biology, and its margin status. Although no randomized clinical trials have compared total mastectomy with breast conservation, total (simple) mastectomy is the gold standard against which any other treatment must be compared. There are ample data from retrospective studies of the treatment of DCIS and the treatment of invasive cancers to permit this extrapolation. Because, by definition, DCIS lacks the ability to metastasize, systemic failure after mastectomy implies the presence of undiagnosed (clinically occult) invasive carcinoma.

Regardless of the goal of breast conservation, mastectomy is one of the acceptable treatment options for patients with DCIS, irrespective of their eligibility for breast conservation. This statement should not be misconstrued as a recommendation that all, even most, patients with DCIS should undergo mastectomy. A minority of patients with DCIS require mastectomy, probably less than 25% of patients with this diagnosis, but mastectomy could be performed if it were the patient's preference.

Most women with DCIS are candidates for breast conservation. This implies wide local excision of the disease within the breast. All patients for whom breast conservation is anticipated should undergo a postexcision mammogram to ensure that all the suspicious calcifications have been removed. This step may be avoided only if the specimen radiograph performed at the time of initial biopsy shows all the suspicious calcifications to be well within the excised tissue, and the margins are widely clear (≥ 10 mm) microscopically. Even then, no harm is done nor is it redundant to perform a postbiopsy mammogram prior to a final recommendation about treatment. The timing of the postbiopsy mammogram is flexible. Since any residual calcifications must be imaged, the mammogram should not be performed until the patient is comfortable enough to undergo the compression necessary to achieve a technically optimal mammogram. Magnification films of the biopsy site are also advisable. In some patients, this postbiopsy mammogram may not be feasible for 2 or 3 months after the initial biopsy. Patients and physicians should not feel intimidated by any delay necessary to complete this important step, since the treatment of DCIS is not an emergency. In fact, contraction of the surgical biopsy site is an advantage if reexcision is planned; the volume of tissue removed at the second operation is usually less if the procedure is performed later rather than sooner after the initial procedure.

Whether radiation therapy, surveillance alone, or either of these plus tamoxifen, is the optimal treatment when breast conservation is employed is controversial. There are groups of patients with DCIS who fall into each of these categories, but no one has yet defined the selection criteria for each of them precisely enough to make dogmatic recommendations. Clinical trials have shown that local excision and radiation therapy in patients with negative margins provide excellent rates of local control. Patients treated by excision alone have a greater chance of local recurrence. There is evidence that recurrence is decreased with wider surgical margins around the area of DCIS. The available data indicate that the likelihood of developing *invasive* cancer of the breast following treatment by breast conservation with or without radiation therapy is about 1% or less a year following the initial diagnosis and treatment.

Although adding radiation therapy to wide local excision benefits all groups of DCIS patients who are candidates for breast conservation, the magnitude of that benefit may be small enough in some patient subgroups that radiation can be omitted. However, patients who may avoid radiation therapy have not been reproducibly and reliably identified by any clinical trials. There are institutional and individual reports of large series of such patients treated by wide excision alone who also achieve a 1% or less a year risk of invasive recurrence.

For consideration of DCIS treatment with wide excision alone without radiation therapy, patients should meet at least the following criteria:

1. The size of the area of DCIS, whether measured by the pathologist or by measuring the area of calcifications on the mammogram, should be small, preferably less than 2–3 cm in diameter. When size is based on mammographic measurement of calcifications, if the area of calcifications on the mammogram is more quadrangular than round in shape, it should be less than approximately 6 cm^2 in area. Occasionally, marginally larger areas of calcifications may be encountered that can be well excised because the breast is large enough to accommodate the loss of a greater volume of tissue without significant deformity.
2. Margins around any site of DCIS should be 10 mm or greater (see discussion of margins below).
3. The nuclear grade of the DCIS should be low or intermediate, as defined by the 1997 Consensus Conference, although some panelists believe that patients with high nuclear grade

DCIS may also be candidates for local excision alone, if wider margins than 10 mm can be achieved.

4. The aesthetic appearance of the breast following local excision should be appropriate. A well-performed mastectomy may be preferable to local excision that is so large with respect to the volume of the breast that the patient is unhappy with her appearance.

Candidates for breast conservation who do not fit these guidelines are best treated by the addition of radiation therapy after wide local excision. Radiation therapists generally prefer that the size of the area of DCIS be less than 5 cm in its greatest dimension. This is for technical reasons and because of the difficulty in achieving a wide local excision with negative margins and an acceptable cosmetic result when the area is larger. Any grade or subtype of DCIS is appropriate for radiation therapy.

Clear surgical margins are a major criterion for treatment of DCIS by breast conservation, especially if radiation therapy is to be avoided; the wider the margin, the lower the rate of local recurrence. Margin status is of importance because it is the one variable that the physician can control. The biologic character, i.e., nuclear grade and architecture, and the size of the area of DCIS cannot be influenced by treatment. The margins can. A 10-mm margin is the best compromise between removal of so much tissue that the cosmetic result would be less than desirable and the likelihood of local recurrence. When treatment by local excision alone without radiation is to be considered, a clear margin of 10 mm is important. Reexcision to achieve clear margins is appropriate if an initial attempt is unsuccessful. How many attempts at reexcision are acceptable before admitting that clear margins cannot be achieved is not clear, but, at least in theory, whatever might be necessary to clear the margins is acceptable, consistent with the patient's desire for breast conservation and the final aesthetic result. Well-performed mastectomy and reconstruction is, however, preferable to multiple attempts at reexcision that destroy the contour and size of the breast.

Another reason to choose excision alone without radiation therapy for DCIS is the ability to use radiation therapy subsequently when and if recurrence does take place. If invasive cancer is the recurrence, its treatment should be as for any other invasive cancer of the same stage. The prognosis should be excellent, since most of these are detected as new areas of calcifications on follow-up mammograms and are often microinvasive in character (T1mic). However, a small number of these women are destined for metastasis, and this possibility is truly the crux of the treatment dilemma in breast conservation.

When DCIS only is the recurrence, a different question exists. When DCIS *only* (i.e., without invasive cancer) occurs after treatment by local excision alone, the usual treatment is radiation or mastectomy, based on the same selection criteria as for DCIS treatment when it occurs for the first time. However, there are no data extant that address the likelihood of further recurrence, either DCIS or invasive cancer, if this second event is treated by local excision alone. Radiation therapy or mastectomy as a choice would be based on the same criteria as noted at the time of initial diagnosis. Therefore, for the women who underwent local excision only, the choices include reexcision, reexcision and radiation therapy, or mastectomy. Highly motivated women may choose additional attempt(s) at local excision alone, presuming that the recurrence is entirely DCIS, recognizing the lack of information about their long-term outcome. Because radiation therapy to the same area cannot be undertaken safely, the recommendation for the treatment of recurrence in patients who had undergone radiation at the time of the initial diagnosis is mastectomy. When recurrence, whether invasive or noninvasive (DCIS), occurs as the second event after radiation therapy had been used initially, fewer options are available; mastectomy is usually the recommendation.

4. INVASIVE CARCINOMA (DUCTAL OR LOBULAR)

The customary treatment of invasive carcinoma of the breast, whether of ductal or lobular origin, includes treatment of the entire breast and the axilla. Prior to the advent of breast conservation, treatment of the breast mandated mastectomy. Currently, in many, if not most, patients, breast conservation *with* radiation therapy has replaced mastectomy. Wide local excision to gain clear margins, as described above under DCIS, is equally if not even more important in invasive cancer. One might consider the local excision as preparation of the breast for the radiation therapy, minimizing the likelihood of local recurrence, but with the presumption that the radiation therapy is truly the treatment for the cancer.

Axillary dissection had been the standard practice, whether accompanying mastectomy or preceding radiation therapy, until the introduction of sentinel node biopsy. At least for the time being, sentinel node biopsy is replacing or at least preceding axillary dissection in women undergoing breast conservation. Postmastectomy radiation to chest wall and regional node areas is being revisited in patients who have significant axillary node metastasis. However, this selective use of postmastectomy radiation therapy is beyond the scope of this chapter.

Despite the increasing occurrence of noninvasive cancers, most breast carcinomas encountered remain life-threatening (i.e., invasive) and require treatment as their character implies. Previously stated in the introduction to this chapter is the presumption that such treatment includes the entire breast. Therefore, there must be situations in which this dogma can be violated or there would be no reason to proceed further. These may include situations in which the cancer encountered, although invasive in character, has so little likelihood of being elsewhere in the same breast that its local excision may be treatment enough. Additionally, there may be circumstances that render the patient constitutionally inoperable, even though her cancer might be.

When breast cancer is encountered in a patient who has other medical problems of significance, an assessment must be made of the patient's overall health status. The interrelations of the patient's breast cancer and her (or his) expected longevity in general must be addressed. For example, a patient with chronic obstructive pulmonary disease who requires a mobile oxygen canister as she ambulates has a poorer 5-year prognosis from this disease than from a stage I carcinoma of the breast discovered by screening mammography.

In general, although the diagnosis of any breast lesion requires only local anesthesia and may be accomplished on an outpatient basis, contemporary curative procedures such as mastectomy or breast conservation require general anesthesia. Sentinel node biopsy may be an exception to this dictum. Although these procedures may be undertaken under local anesthesia, they are more meticulously performed under general anesthesia. Once the diagnosis of breast cancer has been established, treatment is usually advocated expeditiously, but *breast cancer is not an emergency.* There is more than enough time to evaluate the patient thoroughly, from every standpoint, in order to assess the relative risks of all aspects of therapy. Recommendations for care must be made by collaboration, and the usual team of surgeon, radiation oncologist, and medical oncologist must look to the primary care physician or other specialists as necessary for counsel. Unlike therapeutic decisions, for example, for perforated appendicitis, there are alternative treatments for breast cancer that may have reasonably equivalent outcomes. It is important to evaluate the patent from the perspective of which may be the preferable treatment for each particular patient. This is not the same, for example, as trying to lessen the risks for an operative procedure that must be undertaken irrespective of risk, such as the emergency drainage of an intraabdominal abscess.

Despite the virtually exponential increase in the frequency of detection of noninvasive carcinomas in the past few years thanks to screening mammography, most breast cancers currently treated remain invasive and life-threatening. How then, may the patient and her physicians balance the challenge created by the discovery of an invasive cancer, regardless of size, with the hazards presented by intercurrent major maladies? It is implicit in confronting treatment of any invasive cancer to dismiss the misleading, even tragic, presumption that small and inconsequential are in any way synonymous terms. The term "minimal" is a spurious and inappropriate description for any invasive cancer. Our own data have established convincingly that nonpalpable invasive carcinomas, whether detected as tiny masses or as clusters of calcifications, still may metastasize to axillary nodes. Therefore, concessions to other conditions when these lesions are encountered must be recognized as just that. Patients and their families look to physicians for guidance when these difficult decisions become necessary, and these ethical and philosophical dilemmas embody the art as well as the science of medicine. Nevertheless, the decision to undertake what might be considered "less" treatment is not a unilateral one made by a physician on behalf of his or her patient. Having determined that compromises in care are occasionally, albeit infrequently, indicated, the recommendation to deviate from what would be advocated in another optimal situation should be discussed with the patient herself, or with her legal guardians if she is not competent to comprehend this dialogue. The initial management of invasive carcinomas of the breast, under ideal circumstances, remains "selective," with the relative merits of therapeutic alternatives depending on numerous factors such as clinical stage, histology of the tumor, and even patient preferences. In general, therapy for clinical stages I and II cancer includes treatment of the entire breast and the ipsilateral axilla, either by irradiation (preceded by local excision and some form of axillary dissection, most often levels I and II) or by modified radical mastectomy. Except under special circumstances, these are considered equivalent modes of therapy.

However, in women who are unable to undergo any surgical procedure, for example, a patient with a blood dyscrasia that would contribute to unacceptable blood loss or major problems if transfusions were necessary, the diagnosis of malignancy by aspiration biopsy may precede irradiation alone, accepting a higher risk of local recurrence if the tumor is not excised completely. Irradiation may include the axilla, even the supraclavicular and internal mammary- node-bearing areas, depending on the clinical stage of the disease. Before the current era, patients considered "inoperable" because of internal mammary or subclavicular node metastasis were customarily treated by this technique, with acceptable local control of tumor until they succumbed to systemic disease. Women whose intercurrent disease makes them equivalently inoperable are in an analogous situation. However, irradiation must not be considered trivial because it is not surgical. In addition to its own set of complications, it requires almost religious devotion to daily, enervating trips back and forth to therapy.

An exciting approach that has been debated especially in the British medical literature has been the use of tamoxifen only in elderly women, after either local excision or needle aspiration biopsy. Most of the current controversy addresses the equivalence of this technique to either mastectomy or irradiation. Additionally, the reported trials generally have been indiscriminate with respect to debility. Patients entering the clinical trials have been selected on the basis of age alone (usually >70 years) as the criterion. Chronologic age is an inappropriate criterion if, as suggested, tamoxifen alone does not provide the same (or better) disease-free survival as other modes of therapy. However, tamoxifen alone (usually as a daily dose of 20 mg) is virtually without major acute side effects; most side effects are related to the exacerbation of menopausal symptoms or vaginal discharge. Significant side effects are unusual, although an increase in the observed incidence of endometrial proliferations, including cancer, in women taking tamoxifen for more than 2 years has been reported. Because the choice of tamoxifen as the sole treatment for these patients (other than the local excision of the macroscopic lesion) is based on the pessimistic prognosis of their underlying infirmities, the theoretical long-term development of endometrial carcinoma is a moot point. Parenthetically, although much more likely to demonstrate a striking response if the tumor's estrogen/progesterone receptors are high, the absence of receptors does not imply the lack of tamoxifen effect in these elderly women.

The susceptibility of patients with major intercurrent diseases to complications of cytotoxic chemotherapy makes this undertaking an especially precarious maneuver. It is not a substitute for radiation therapy or mastectomy in the care of local disease in the breast or axilla. Probably, if a patient is well enough to withstand the rigors of cytotoxic chemotherapy she is well enough to undergo at least radiation therapy. Chemotherapy should be undertaken only under the supervision of a well-trained oncologist, and even then, if associated illness has already extracted concessions in the surgical care of the patient, it is likely that a similar compromise might be appropriate in the decision about chemotherapy. It is often forgotten that the treatment is not supposed to be worse than the disease; this shibboleth is even more valid in this group of patients.

A physician involved for the first time with a patient who has breast cancer must not presume the privilege of predicting the outcome of various other chronic problems with which the patient may have been living symbiotically for years. Nevertheless, with the help of the patient's treating physicians, at least the same estimation of prognosis may be offered for these other problems as for the breast cancer that has been diagnosed. Physicians are not therapeutic nihilists, but it is clinical judgment that separates one physician from another. The treatment of breast cancer in this group of patients is one of the few situations in which scrupulous sensitivity to the vagaries of the natural history of the disease and its treatment may be exercised. Because differences in the outcome of therapy for breast cancer are measured in years, rather than weeks or months, subtleties of treatment may be obscured by more acute problems with more vivid consequences. Although tempted to use his or her considerable skills, the surgeon must often yield to less dramatic and daring techniques; the judicious use of more mundane remedies may be the best approach in these unusual circumstances.

BIBLIOGRAPHY

Bodian CA, Perzin KH, Lattes R (1996) Lobular neoplasia. Long term risk of breast cancer and relation to other factors. *Cancer* **78,** 1024–1034.

Gazet J-C, Ford HT, Bland JM, Markopolous CH, Coombes RC, Dixon RC (1988) Prospective randomized trial of tamoxifen versus surgery in elderly patients with breast cancer. *Lancet* **1,** 679–681.

Gazet J-C, Ford HT, Coombes RC, et al. (1994) Prospective randomized trial of tamoxifen vs surgery in elderly patients with breast cancer. *Eur. J. Surg. Oncol.* **20,** 207–214.

Gazet J-C, Markopoulos C, Ford HT, Coombes RC, Bland JM, Dixon RC (1988) Tamoxifen and breast cancer in the elderly [letter]. *Lancet* **1,** 1218.

Gump FE, Kinne DW, Schwartz GF (1998) Current Treatment for Lobular Carcinoma in Situ. *Ann. Surg. Oncol.* **5,** 33–36.

Schwartz GF (1993) Treatment considerations in poor-risk patients. In: Ariel IM, Cahan AC (eds.) *Treatment of Pre-Cancerous Lesions and Early Breast Cancer.* Williams & Wilkins, Baltimore, pp. 295–301.

Schwartz GF (1997) Treatment of sub-clinical ductal carcinoma in situ by local excision and surveillance: a personal experience. In: Silverstein MJ, Lagios MD, Recht A, Pollen DN (eds.) *Ductal Carcinoma In Situ of the Breast.* Williams & Wilkins, Baltimore, pp. 353–360.

Schwartz GF, Finkel GC, Garcia JC, Patchefsky AS (1992) Sub-clinical duct carcinoma in situ of the breast (DCIS): treatment by local excision and surveillance alone. *Cancer* **70,** 2468–2474.

Schwartz GF, Solin LJ, Olivotto IA, Ernster VL, Pressman PI, the Consensus Conference Committee (2000) Consensus Conference on the Treatment of In Situ Ductal Carcinoma of the Breast. *Cancer* **88,** 946–954.

Silverstein MJ, Lagios MD, Oroshen S, et al. (1999) The influence of margin width on local control in patients with ductal carcinoma in situ (DCIS) of the breast. *N. Engl. J. Med.* **340,** 1455–1461.

Silverstein MJ, Poller DN, Craig PH, et al. (1996) A prognostic index for ductal carcinoma in situ of the breast. *Cancer* **77,** 2267–2274.

21

Axillary Node Dissection in Breast Cancer

James F. Pingpank, Jr., MD,
and Elin R. Sigurdson, MD, PHD

CONTENTS

INTRODUCTION
SURGICAL MANAGEMENT OF BREAST CANCER
STAGING BREAST CANCER
THE THERAPEUTIC VALUE OF AN AXILLARY DISSECTION
CONCLUSIONS
REFERENCES

1. INTRODUCTION

Axillary node dissection has been part of standard therapy for early breast cancer for more than a century. Since Fisher proposed that most breast cancers have spread before their detection, there has been controversy surrounding whether axillary node dissection is necessary in the treatment of early breast cancer. A trend toward less radical surgery and the possibility that axillary node involvement represents only a marker for distant disease has led many to believe that sampling the axilla is adequate and that full axillary dissection need not be performed. Reliable identification of the first node draining the tumor (the sentinel node), better pathologic staging of the primary tumor, more aggressive use of chemotherapy, and detection of smaller and smaller lesions have all contributed to the controversy.

The incidence of node-negative breast cancer has increased and with it the number of women who may not need an axillary dissection. With radiation therapy and the widespread application of chemotherapy for even small breast tumors, some have proposed that even the axilla involved with metastatic disease is adequately treated today without dissection. This chapter reviews the role of axillary surgery in staging of breast cancer, methods of predicting node positivity in the axilla, and the therapeutic role of an axillary dissection in managing early breast cancer.

2. SURGICAL MANAGEMENT OF BREAST CANCER

Early in the sixteenth century, Michael Servetus advocated excision of the pectoralis major along with the overlying breast tissue, a practice that continued for two centuries. Le

From: *Current Clinical Oncology:*
Breast Cancer: A Guide to Detection and Multidisciplinary Therapy
Edited by: M. H. Torosian © Humana Press Inc., Totowa, NJ

Dran *(1)* and Petit *(2)* added the removal of the axillary lymph nodes to the operation during the 18th century (based on observation that spread to nodes signaled worsening prognosis). This was contrary to a common contemporary theory that tumor spreads through the blood, rather than through lymphatics *(3,4)*. Halstead *(5)* modified the operation by stressing the importance of *en bloc* removal of all tissues, including the overlying skin, to avoid contamination of the surgical field with cancer cells from transected lymphatics. He argued that the operation was justified based on the high rates of local control achieved (93 versus 30% in prior series). The "Halsted radical" mastectomy became the standard against which all subsequent techniques have been judged. Indeed, for a brief period, Urban and Baker *(6)* employed an extended surgical approach, with the inclusion of internal mammary and supraclavicular lymph nodes in the operative dissection. Ultimately, improved survival and local control did not accompany this more aggressive approach except in medial lesions *(7)*.

In the second half of the 20th century, with the advent of mammography, the diagnosis of earlier stage breast cancer, and improved radiation therapy, interest developed in the use of less radical surgical procedures. The first modification of the Halstead radical mastectomy was preservation of the pectoralis major muscle, as well as preservation of sufficient skin to avoid a skin graft. In 1948, Patey and Dyson *(8)* published their results using the so-called modified radical mastectomy, showing no decrease in tumor control. In the same year, McWhirter *(9)* published similar results with simple mastectomy and postoperative radiation therapy.

The next group of studies examined the issue of breast preservation. The National Surgical Adjuvant Breast and Bowel Project (NSABP)B-06 and Italian (National Cancer Institute, Milan) trials confirmed the efficacy of breast-conserving surgery with adjuvant radiotherapy in the control of localized breast cancer. The NSABP trial examined the role of segmental mastectomy, with or without radiation, versus total mastectomy for breast cancers less than 4 cm in diameter. All patients in this trial underwent axillary dissection. There was no decrease in local control or survival as long as radiation remained part of the treatment *(10)*.

3. STAGING BREAST CANCER

Although the size of the primary breast cancer is important, the presence of tumor in axillary lymph nodes is the most accurate predictor of overall outcome in women without metastatic disease. Sentinel node biopsy will in most cases ascertain whether nodes of the axilla contain cancer. It will not, however, determine the number of lymph nodes involved. Complete staging of the patient is not possible without a thorough node dissection, and proper regional and systemic adjuvant therapy cannot be selected unless the tumor burden in the axilla is known.

Clinical examination of the axilla, computed tomography (CT), magnetic resonance imaging (MRI), and positron emission tomography (PET) scans, and monoclonal antibody imaging cannot accurately predict nodal involvement. The accuracy of nodal staging through sentinel node analysis in larger studies is between 90 and 95%. In single-institution studies, it approaches 100%. Most breast oncologists today believe that few women will benefit from axillary dissection if there is no tumor in the sentinel node(s). Sentinel node identification to ascertain nodal status has been suggested as standard therapy, for patients with early-stage breast cancer.

Some have suggested omitting axillary node dissection from the routine management of breast cancer, basing their recommendations on a presumed unproven therapeutic benefit from axillary lymphadenectomy. Nonetheless, the NSABP and the Italian research groups continue to use axillary node status as an entry and stratification criterion for their studies. The ability to employ the results of prior trials in the current clinical setting is based on a staging system in which axillary node status plays a fundamental role.

There is increasing enthusiasm for treating patients with breast cancers greater than 1 cm in diameter with chemotherapy. Patients with such small breast cancers are increasingly common owing to the increased use of screening mammography. These patients, even when free of node metastases, are increasingly advised to receive adjuvant systemic therapy. Such changes in demographics and treatment practices have raised doubts surrounding the need for axillary node dissections. These doubts have been combined with renewed concerns surrounding the morbidity of axillary dissection *(11,12)*.

A full axillary lymphadenectomy is associated with both cost and morbidity. Costs include those of general anesthesia and drain management. Acute complications include infection, bleeding, and seroma formation. Chronic complications include postmastectomy pain syndrome (from division of the intercostal brachial cutaneous nerves), shoulder dysfunction, numbness, and lymphedema. It is assumed, but not yet proved, that sentinel node biopsy alone will not be followed by significant arm edema.

The risk of measurable lymphedema for an uncomplicated level I–II node dissection is about 8%. This is comparable to the risk of radiation treatment to the axilla and supraclavicular nodes without node dissection. The addition of radiation therapy after axillary node dissection increases the risk of lymphedema. If the supraclavicular fossa is treated after radiation and lymphadenectomy, the risk of significant lymphedema rises to about 25%.

Axillary node evaluation should not be abandoned until it has been established that 1) accurate staging and prognostic information can be obtained through alternate means; 2) a patient is at such low risk for axillary metastasis that axillary dissection imposes unacceptable morbidity; 3) the pathologic features of the primary tumor dictate adjuvant therapy regardless of the state of the axillary lymph nodes; and 4) systemic treatment and radiation therapy will adequately control occult axillary nodal disease. Patients identified as having an extremely low risk of axillary metastases (<5%) will have tumors less than 1 cm with low to intermediate grade features. Although they are unlikely to have node-positive disease, these patients would not routinely receive adjuvant chemotherapy, and thus identification of the 5% with node-positive disease is extremely important and would significantly alter their adjuvant therapy. For this group of patients, the role of sentinel node biopsy is very attractive.

Finally, although the prognostic role of an axillary dissection may be unimportant for some patients with larger primary tumors, it cannot be abandoned until it is clear that there is no therapeutic value of an axillary lymphadenectomy. Before we abandon a century of progress in the management of breast cancer and return to the surgical techniques of the 19th century (of tumor removal only), we must prove that systemic chemotherapy and radiation therapy are comparable to surgical extirpation of gross and microscopic disease in the breast and axilla.

3.1. Using the Primary Tumor to Predict Node Positivity

Over the last decade, there has been much interest in the identification of those patients at decreased risk for axillary and distant metastases, based on primary tumor characteristics. Since the likelihood of node positivity correlates closely with primary tumor size, the identification of a patient group most likely not to need axillary dissection should come from those patients with the smallest T stage. As expected, the subdivision of T1 breast cancer into T1a, T1b, and T1c based on tumor size (<5 mm, 0.5–1.0 cm, and 1.0–2.0 cm, respectively) has been shown to correlate with incidence of axillary metastasis *(13,14)*. In the smallest set of tumors, T1a, there remains a 7–10% risk of axillary disease, with the performing of an axillary node dissection being an independent predictor of disease-free, disease-specific, and overall survival *(15)*. Controversy exists surrounding the subset analysis of T1a lesions with regard to lymphovascular invasion, tumor grade, patient age, and method of tumor detection. The presence of high-grade and (especially) lymphovascular invasion correlates very strongly with increased risk of metastatic disease, up to 49%, but establishing a low-risk group by the absence of these same characteristics has not been possible on a consistent basis *(16,17)*. Although these patients may be able to avoid a node dissection, as they are likely to be node-negative, they would not routinely receive chemotherapy, and thus the accurate identification of nodal status is critical.

Investigators have examined the incidence of axillary metastases based on method of detection of the primary tumor, with patients having mammographically detected tumors still carrying a 10–18% incidence of lymphatic disease *(12,18)*. A recent multivariate analysis of 11,964 patients with breast cancers less than 5 cm and complete axillary node dissection (using tumor size, number of positive nodes, estrogen and progesterone receptor status, DNA ploidy, S-phase fraction, and patient age) was unable to establish a subset of patients with a greater than 95% likelihood of being free of axillary metastases *(19)*.

In women with advanced age or significant coexisting medical disease, axillary dissection in low-risk patients with clinically negative axillae may be safely excluded in many cases *(20)*. These patients will not be fit to receive chemotherapy, and if the patient is followed closely for axillary recurrence, the disease is generally amenable to axillary dissection at that time. The impact of local-regional recurrence on life expectancy will be minimal in a group of patients with a short life expectancy. However, in most patients, adjuvant therapy decisions continue to be made on the status of the axilla, and not on the histopathology of the primary tumor.

3.2. Using Radiologic Techniques to Predict Node Positivity

The increased use of mammography in the early detection of breast cancer, coupled with increasing imaging technology, has led to examination of a broad range of radiographic techniques for axillary examination. Dependent on tumor size, 20–50% of patients with invasive cancer can be predicted to have histologically proven lymph node metastases. Physical examination alone has historically been inaccurate, with false-negative rates between 25 and 40% *(21)*, whereas only 70% of patients with palpable lymph nodes will be shown to have metastatic disease *(22)*. Mammographic analysis of axillary lymph nodes is remarkably inaccurate, with only the most clinically obvious nodes being apparent on exam. In a recently reported series from Duke University, only 20 of 94 patients with axillary lymph nodes visible on mammogram were found to have metastatic disease. Associated findings of homogeneously dense, nonfatty lymph nodes, nodes greater than 33 mm, ill-defined, spiculated margins, or intranodal microcalcifications were significantly associated with the presence of malignancy *(23)*. CT scan has proved superior to physical exam alone, with a positive predictive value of 83% and a negative predictive value of 88% *(24)*. Other series, however, have reported specificity and sensitivity as low as 50 and 75%, respectively, with a negative predictive value of only 20% *(25)*. MRI has shown a high sensitivity (100%) but low specificity (73%) in the detection of axillary lymph node metastases in a small group of patients *(26)*. Finally, the use of PET based on 6-fluoro-deoxyglucose metabolism, has proved effective in up to 40% of patients without clinical evidence of disease, with sensitivity and specificity of 79–100% and 66–97%, respectively *(27,28)*. PET scan does not accurately stage patients with axillary micrometastases.

3.3. Using the Sentinel Node to Predict Node Positivity

The concept of ordered, predictable patterns of spread of cancer has been advocated since Halstead first proposed the radical mastectomy and has been reinforced by survival data that point to axillary lymph node status as the greatest predictor of survival in breast cancer. Indeed, for a brief period, formal axillary dissection was replaced by axillary node sampling, in which a smaller amount of axillary tissue was removed in order to limit the complications of complete lymphadenectomy. This approach did not lead to a significant reduction in morbidity but did result in the reduction of accurate disease staging. Recent data from Iyer et al. (29) reveal that the accuracy of the pathologic status of the axilla depends on the number of nodes examined and thus the extent of axillary dissection.

The concept of a sentinel node was first proposed by Cabanas (30) in the treatment of penile cancer and has been subsequently adopted for the staging of melanoma (31) and breast cancer (32,33). Biologically, the sentinel node represents that node through which the lymphatic drainage passes in transit between a specific area of the breast and the remainder of the lymph node basin. The technical approach to sentinel lymphadenectomy involves the injection of vital blue dye and/or radiolabeled technetium sulphur colloid into the breast tissue surrounding the lesion, and allowing the lymphatic drainage to concentrate the marker in the initial node. Various modifications have yielded good success, with one to three nodes extracted in a limited, directed procedure. A recent multicenter study examined the validity of this approach in 443 patients under the care of 11 different surgeons. All patients underwent subsequent axillary dissection (levels I and II), and the pathologic status of the node was compared with the remainder of the axilla. In 93% of the patients, a sentinel node(s) was identified, and this node(s) accurately represented the metastatic status of the remainder of the axilla in 97% of patients. The specificity and sensitivity of the procedure were 89% and 100%, respectively, with a positive predictive value of 100% (34). The false-negative rate was 11%. Clearly, this technique can spare many patients with low likelihood of axillary disease the anesthetic and surgical complications of full axillary dissection, although some argue that a false-negative rate of 11% is too high. Current studies indicate false-negative rates with this technique range from 2 to 4%.

Subsequently, a group of patients at extremely low risk of metastases (and most suitable to sentinel node biopsy) has been evaluated by examining both patient and tumor characteristics. When one sets a standard of 5% risk of lymph node involvement, those patients with mammographically detected ductal carcinoma in situ, microinvasive tumors, and pure tubular carcinomas less than 1 cm can be safely excluded from axillary dissection. These patients have chances of axillary metastases of less than 1%, less than 5%, and 5%, respectively (35), and sentinel node biopsy could obviate the need for node dissection in over 95% of patients.

Although it is not clear who should be offered a sentinel node biopsy, most studies attempt to define patients with less than a 25–30% risk of node positivity. Clinical trials generally accept patients with tumors less than 3–4 cm, without evidence of lymphovascular invasion. Most exclude patients with large cavities in which the location of the primary tumor within the large cavity is not clear. Although the notion is unproved, it is felt that the accuracy of the sentinel node in these cases would be less accurate.

An additional benefit of this technology is improved pathologic staging, through serial sectioning, and the use of immunohistochemistry and polymerase chain reaction to identify microscopic metastases. Ultimately, those patients with positive sentinel nodes undergo completion axillary dissection, to stage the extent of metastatic disease fully and remove all gross and microscopic regional disease.

4. THE THERAPEUTIC VALUE OF AN AXILLARY DISSECTION

The NSABP undertook a series of randomized trials beginning during the early 1970s to examine surgical and nonsurgical approaches to the local (breast) and regional (axillary lymph nodes) control of breast cancer. The NSABP B-04 trial compared radical mastectomy with total (simple) mastectomy with or without postoperative radiation. Only patients who subsequently developed clinical disease in the axilla were supposed to undergo axillary dissection *(36)*. The results of this trial, reported at 10-year follow-up, reveal no statistically significant differences in disease-free (local or distant) or overall survival between any of the three, clinically node-negative, treatment arms. The same was true for those patients with clinically apparent axillary disease who were randomized between radical mastectomy and total mastectomy with radiation therapy *(37)*. Review of the data revealed that many of the patients randomized to no axillary dissection did indeed have nodes removed, and 11 was the mean number of nodes removed in this group. For those patients without any axillary dissection, a 21.2% recurrence rate was observed. This rate drops to 12.0 and 0.3% with 1–6 nodes and more than 10 nodes, respectively *(38)*. Additional analysis of the group of patients assigned to total mastectomy alone in that same trial shows a median time to axillary recurrence of 14.8 months (range 3–134.5), with 85% of those patients having systemic metastasis within 17.2 months (mean) of salvage axillary dissection. This represents a 15.4% rate of systemic failure, higher than either group with clinically palpable axillary involvement at the time of mastectomy *(37,39)*. Therefore, it is difficult to interpret these data. Harris, in a review of the study, noted that the group undergoing axillary dissection did indeed have an improved survival, and that if the study had had 2000 patients, the study would be positive in favor of axillary dissection.

Several series have reported axillary recurrence rates in clinically negative axillae not dissected ranging from 16 to 37% (Table 1) *(37, 40–42)*. Although the impact of elective axillary dissection on local recurrence is clear, controversy exists surrounding its impact on survival. Since the initial publication, the results of the NSABP B-04 trial have been extensively analyzed, with much of the criticism centered on the conclusion regarding the impact of axillary dissection. Gardner and Feldman *(43)* argue that there is insufficient statistical power in this trial to assess the impact of axillary node dissection on survival adequately in node-negative patients. Additionally, if a survival advantage did exist, it may be masked by the presence of axillary nodes in 35% of the control group specimens *(44)*.

The Breast Carcinoma Collaborative Group of the Institut Curie reported on a prospective, randomized trial of 658 patients with early breast cancer who received lumpectomy and radiation therapy with or without axillary dissection. The radiation therapy was identical in both arms and treated both the breast and the axilla. As all patients had lumpectomies, there was no contamination with removal of nodes in patients randomized to no node dissection, as occurred in the NSABP study. At 54-month follow-up, breast recurrence was the same in both arms. Regional failure in the axilla, despite full-dose radiation therapy, was more than two times greater in the undissected arm. This resulted in a demonstrated survival advantage of 96.6 versus 92.6% (p = 0.014), along with decreased distant disease, in those patients undergoing axillary dissection *(45)*.

A metaanalysis of six randomized controlled trials, consisting of almost 3000 patients, showed axillary node dissection to be associated with a 5.4% survival advantage *(46)*. With clinical trials under way designed to show a 3–5% improvement in overall survival, contamination of the study by new surgical techniques in which the axilla is not dissected could significantly alter study results. As noted by the author, in contrast to present practice, the

Table 1
Impact of Axillary Node Dissection on Survival[a]

Trial	No. of patients	Follow-up (yr)	Survival improvement (%)	p-value
Copenhagen	425	10	4	NS
Guy's I	370	10	8	NS
South-East Scotland	498	10	9.5	0.04
NSABP B-04	727	10	4	NS
Guy's II	258	10	16	0.01
Institut Curie	658	5	4	0.03

[a] The impact of node dissection in the clinically negative axillae remains unclear. A survival benefit was seen in three large randomized trials, but not in others. Many patients not undergoing formal node dissection had large numbers of nodes in the lateral breast specimen, and great variability existed in the number of nodes removed in the axillary dissection group. NSABP, National Surgical Adjuvant Breast and Bowel Project.

number of patients receiving adjuvant therapy was minimal, which would complicate direct translation into present practice.

When patients with locally advanced breast cancer at high risk for axillary metastases are examined, a nihilistic approach has been advocated. Arguments are based on the need for aggressive adjuvant therapy regardless of axillary pathology. This criteria may well prove invalid, as recent data from the M.D. Anderson Cancer Center examining the effect of neoadjuvant chemotherapy on axillary node metastases reveal a 23% rate of conversion from cytologically documented lymph node-positive disease to a pathologically negative axilla in patients undergoing neoadjuvant chemotherapy for breast cancer. In comparison, patients achieving complete axillary conversion had statistically significant increases in both disease-free (87%) and overall survival (87%) at 5 years, versus patients with complete axillary response (58 and 51%, respectively) (47). The ultimate fate of residual axillary disease and its impact on the development of subsequent systemic metastases will be unclear until a comparison between patients undergoing postinduction axillary dissection and salvage procedures is undertaken.

Two randomized trials recently reported on the impact of radiation therapy to the chest wall in premenopausal women with one to three positive nodes following modified radical mastectomy. Prior to these studies, postmastectomy radiation therapy had been reserved for patients with T3 tumors or four or more positive nodes in the axilla. The group receiving postmastectomy radiation therapy had an improvement in survival, through improved regional control of the axilla. When examined further the numbers of lymph nodes removed in these studies were fewer than 10, and a high nodal failure rate resulted in the control arm. These studies clearly demonstrated the impact of local-regional failure on overall survival. They both also demonstrated that systemic chemotherapy in clinically node-negative women with minimal pathologic nodal disease did not control the axilla.

These data provide sufficient compelling evidence for the therapeutic benefit of treating the involved axilla (either by complete surgical extirpation or possibly by radiation therapy after nodal sampling). As this benefit appears to be at least 5%, it is clear that axillary node dissection cannot yet be abandoned in node-positive patients. Furthermore, studies searching for small benefits from adjuvant chemotherapy must carefully control for surgical variability in axillary dissection and axillary sampling to avoid its significant impact on outcome.

5. CONCLUSIONS

Currently, the presence of tumor in the axilla remains the single greatest predictor of overall outcome for patients with early-stage breast cancer and is used to determine adjuvant therapy. Although many investigators have attempted to find alternate means of establishing prognosis, none have proved more accurate than lymph node status. Current evidence suggests that patients with axillary metastases derive therapeutic benefit from the removal of all nodal disease. This, along with recent reports indicating less than expected complications from axillary dissection *(48),* argues for the continued need for this procedure.

Axillary sentinel lymphadenectomy appears to be highly accurate in experienced hands in identifying the node-negative patient. Early studies demonstrate minimal morbidity. With training and experience, this is expected to become the standard of care for breast cancer patients in the United States. There are no data to support abandoning axillary dissection in node-positive patients, and this is the subject of clinical trials in the United States and Europe. Long-term follow-up (5–10 years) will be necessary to determine the impact of local-regional failure on overall survival.

REFERENCES

1. le Dran F (1757) Memoire avec un precis de plusieurs observations sur le cancer. *Mem. Acad. R. Chir. Paris* **3,** 1–56.
2. Petit JL (1837) *Oeuvres Completes,* section VII. R. Chapoulard, Limoges, pp. 438–445.
3. Robinson JO (1985) Treatment of breast cancer through the ages. *Am. J. Surg.* **151,** 317–333.
4. Wagner FB, Martin RG, Bland KI (1998) History of the therapy of breast disease. In: Bland KI, Copeland EM (eds.) *The Breast: Comprehensive Management of Benign and Malignant Diseases,* 2nd ed. WB Saunders, Philadelphia.
5. Halstead WS (1894–1895) The results of operations for cure of cancer of the breast performed at the Johns Hopkins Hospital from June 1889 to January 1894. *Johns Hopkins Hosp. Rep.* **4,** 297–350.
6. Urban JA, Baker HW (1952) Radical mastectomy in continuity with en-bloc resection of the internal mammary lymph node chain. *Cancer* **5,** 992–1008.
7. Nemoto T, Vana J, Bedwani RN, et al. (1980) Management and survival of female breast cancer: results of a national survey by the American College of Surgeons. *Cancer* **45,** 2917–2924.
8. Patey DH, Dyson WH (1948) The prognosis of carcinoma of the breast in relation to the type of operation performed. *Br. J. Cancer* **2,** 7–13.
9. McWhirter R (1948) The value of simple mastectomy and radiotherapy in the treatment of cancer of the breast. *Br. J. Radiol.* **21,** 599–610.
10. Fisher B, Bauer M, Margolese R, et al. (1985) Five-year results of a randomized clinical trial comparing total mastectomy and segmental mastectomy with or without radiation in the treatment of breast cancer. *N. Engl. J. Med.* **312,** 665–673.
11. Cady B, Stone MD, Schuler JG, et al. (1996) The new era in breast cancer: invasion, size, and nodal involvement dramatically decreasing as a result of mammographic screening. *Arch. Surg.* **131,** 301–308.
12. Silverstein MJ, Gierson ED, Waisman JR, et al. (1994) Axillary lymph node dissection for T1a breast carcinoma. Is it indicated? *Cancer* **73,** 664–667.
13. Fein DA, Fowble BA, Hanlon AL, et al. (1997) Identification of women with T1–T2 breast cancer at low risk of positive axillary nodes. *J. Surg. Oncol.* **65,** 34–39.
14. Barth A, Craig PH, Silverstein MJ (1997) Predictors of axillary lymph node metastases in patients with T1 breast carcinoma. *Cancer* **79,** 1918–1922.
15. White RE, Vezeridis MP, Konstadoulakis M, et al. (1996) Therapeutic options and results for the management of minimally invasive carcinoma of the breast: influence of axillary dissection for treatment of T1a and T1b lesions. *J. Am. Coll. Surg.* **183,** 575–582.
16. Port EP, Tan LK, Borgen PI, Van Zee KJ (1998) Incidence of axillary lymph node metastases in T1a and T1b breast carcinoma. *Ann. Surg. Oncol.* **5,** 23–27.

17. McGee JM, Youmans R, Clingan F, et al. (1996) The value of axillary dissection in T1a breast cancer. *Am. J. Surg.* **72,** 501–505.

18. Olivotto IA, Jackson JS, Mates D, et al. (1998) Prediction of axillary lymph node involvement of women with invasive breast cancer. *Cancer* **83,** 948–955.

19. Ravdin PM, DeLaurentiis M, Vendely T, Clark GM (1994) Prediction of axillary node status in breast cancer patients by use of prognostic indicators. *J. Natl. Cancer Inst.* **86,** 1771–1775.

20. Fiegelson BJ, Acosta JA, Feigelson HS, et al. (1996) T1 breast carcinoma in women 70 years of age and older may not require axillary lymph node dissection. *Am. J. Surg.* **172,** 487–490.

21. Danforth D, Findlay P, McDonald H, et al. (1986) Complete axillary lymph node dissection for stage I–II carcinoma of the breast. *J. Clin. Oncol.* **4,** 655–662.

22. Fisher ER, Sass R, Fisher B, et al. (1984) Pathologic findings from the National Surgical Adjuvant Project for breast cancers. *Cancer* **53,** 712–723.

23. Walsh R, Kornguth PJ, Soo MS, et al. (1996) Axillary lymph nodes: mammographic, pathologic, and clinical correlation. *AJR* **168,** 33–38.

24. Hata Y, Ogawa Y, Nishioka A (1996) Evaluation of thin section CT scanning in the prone position of metastatic axillary lymph nodes for breast cancer. *Nippon Igaku Hoshasen Gakki Zasshi* **56,** 1027–1031.

25. Isaacs RJ, Ford JM, Allan SG, et al. (1993) Role of computed tomography in the staging of primary breast cancer. *Br. J. Surg.* **80,** 1137.

26. Heiberg EV, Perman WH, Herrmann VM, et al. (1996) Dynamic sequential 3D gadolinium-enhanced MRI of the whole breast. *Magn. Reson. Imaging* **14,** 337–348.

27. Nieweg OE, Kim EE, Wong WH, et al. (1993) Positron emission tomography with fluorine-18-deoxyglucose in the detection and staging of breast cancer. *Cancer* **71,** 3920–3925.

28. Schnider K, Scharl A, Pietryzk U, et al: (1996) Qualitative [18F] FDG positron emission tomography in breast cancer: clinical relevance and practicability. *Eur. J. Nucl. Med.* **23,** 618–623.

29. Iyer R, Hanlon AL, Fowble B, et al. Accuracy of the extent of axillary nodal positivity related to primary tumor size, number of involved, and number of nodes examined. *Int. J. Radiat. Oncol. Biol. Phys.* **47,** 1177–1183.

30. Cabanas R (1977) An approach to the treatment of penile carcinoma. *Cancer* **39,** 456–466.

31. Morton DL, Wen DR, Wong JH, et al. (1992) Technical details of intraoperative lymphatic mapping of early stage melanoma. *Arch. Surg.* **127,** 392–399.

32. Krag DN, Weaver DL, Alex JC, et al. (1993) Surgical resection and radiolocalization of the sentinel lymph node in breast cancer using a gamma probe. *Surg. Oncol.* **2,** 33–340.

33. Giuliano AE, Kirgan DM, Guenther JM, et al. (1994) Lymphatic mapping and sentinel lymphadenectomy for breast cancer. *Ann. Surg.* **220,** 391–401.

34. Krag D, Weaver D, Ashikaga T, et al. (1998) The sentinel node in breast cancer: a multicenter validation study. *N. Engl. J. Med.* **339,** 941–946.

35. Morrow M (1996) Axillary dissection: when and how radical? *Semin. Surg. Oncol.* **12,** 321–327.

36. Fisher B, Wolmark N, Redmond C, et al. (1981) Findings of the NSABP Protocol No. B-04: Comparison of radical mastectomy with alternative treatments. II. The clinical and biologic significance of medial-central breast cancers. *Cancer* **48,** 1863–1872.

37. Fisher B, Redmond C, Fisher E, et al. (1985) Ten-year results of a randomized clinical trial comparing radical mastectomy and total mastectomy with or without radiation. *N. Engl. J. Med.* **312,** 674–681.

38. Fisher B, Wolmark N, Bauer M, et al. (1981) The accuracy of clinical nodal staging and of limited axillary dissection as a determinant of histologic nodal status in carcinoma of the breast. *Surg. Gynecol. Obstet.* **152,** 765–772.

39. Deckers PJ (1991) Axillary dissection in breast cancer; when, why, how, much, and for how long? Another operation soon to be extinct? *J. Surg. Oncol.* **48,** 217–219.

40. Lythoge J, Palmer M (1982) Manchester regional breast study—5 and 10 year results. *Br. J. Surg.* **69,** 639–636.

41. Crile G (1964) Results of simplified treatment of breast cancer. *Surg. Gynecol. Obstet.* 517–523.

42. Forrest A, Stewart H, Steele R, et al. (1982) Simple mastectomy and axillary node sampling in the management of primary breast cancer. *Ann. Surg.* **196,** 371–378.

43. Gardner B, Feldman J (1993) Are positive axillary nodes in breast cancer markers for incurable disease? *Ann. Surg.* **218,** 270–278.

44. Harris J, Osteen R (1985) Patients with early breast cancer benefit from effective axillary treatment. *Breast Cancer Res. Treat.* **5,** 17–21.

45. Cabanes PA, Salmon RJ, Vilcoq JR, et al. (1992) Value of axillary dissection in addition to lumpectomy and radiotherapy in early breast cancer. *Lancet* **339,** 1245–48.

46. Orr RK (1999) The impact of prophylactic axillary node dissection on breast cancer survival—Bayesian meta-analysis. *Ann. Surg. Oncol.* **6,** 109–116.

47. Kuerer HM, Sahin AA, Hunt KK, et al. (1999) Incidence and impact of documented eradication of breast cancer axillary lymph node metastases before surgery in patients treated with neoadjuvant chemotherapy. *Ann. Surg.* **230,** 72–78.

48. Roses DF, Brooks AD, Harris MN, et al. (1999) Complications of level I and II axillary dissection in the treatment of carcinoma of the breast. *Ann. Surg.* **230,** 194–201.

22 Internal Mammary Lymph Nodes
Management and Other Controversies

James C. Watson, MD*, and John P. Hoffman,* MD

CONTENTS

INTRODUCTION
LYMPHATIC DRAINAGE TO THE INTERNAL MAMMARY CHAIN
PREDICTORS OF INTERNAL MAMMARY LYMPH NODE METASTASES
PROGNOSIS OF INTERNAL MAMMARY LYMPH NODE METASTASES
TREATMENT OF THE INTERNAL MAMMARY CHAIN
INTERNAL MAMMARY LYMPH NODE BIOPSY
CONCLUSIONS
BIBLIOGRAPHY

1. INTRODUCTION

Identification of metastases to the axillary lymph nodes is a well-recognized prognosticator in patients with invasive breast cancer. Knowledge of axillary lymph node status has long influenced whether adjuvant therapy is offered to these patients in an attempt to decrease the rate of recurrence and prolong survival. The value of staging and treatment of the internal mammary lymph nodes, on the other hand, has remained controversial for more than 100 years. Although evolutionary changes have been made in the treatment of this disease during the last century, the principle of excision of lymphatics draining a solid tumor has remained a fundamental concept in surgical oncology. Halsted first devised the radical mastectomy as an operation designed to remove the breast, as well as the axillary lymph nodes at risk for harboring metastatic tumor. Ironically, even though the internal mammary lymphatics were recognized as a possible route for breast cancer cell dissemination during the conception of this operation, neither of the classical radical mastectomies described by Halsted or Meyer were designed to encompass possible internal mammary node (IMN) metastases.

W. Handley, utilizing radium wires prior to 1927, is credited with being the first to treat IMN metastases. He also proposed surgical removal of IMNs at the time of radical mastectomy as early as the 1930s. However, at that time the frequency of involvement in clinically early cases of breast cancer was not fully appreciated. It was not until 1949 that the true incidence of IMN metastases in breast cancer patients was determined by R. Handley and Thackery when IMN biopsies performed during 50 radical mastectomies revealed metastases in 38% of patients. During the next two decades, dissection of the IMNs became increasingly popular, and retrospective evaluation of several studies seemed to

From: *Current Clinical Oncology:*
Breast Cancer: A Guide to Detection and Multidisciplinary Therapy
Edited by: M. H. Torosian © Humana Press Inc., Totowa, NJ

show a survival advantage with the addition of this procedure to the classic radical mastectomy. This position was supported by Turner-Warwick, who, in 1959, showed that the internal mammary lymphatics provide the primary drainage for approximately one-fourth of the lymph from the breast. His work confirmed that the chain of IMNs was susceptible to metastases from medially located cancers in a fashion similar to that for axillary nodes from lateral tumors. Nonetheless, the utility of treating IMNs remained unproved, and several randomized clinical trials were begun as early as 1962 comparing radical mastectomy plus IMN dissection [extended radical mastectomy, ERM] with radical mastectomy. The initial 5-year follow-up from the earliest of these studies suggested an advantage of ERM over radical mastectomy for patients with central or medial tumors. However, the results of 10-year follow-up failed to demonstrate any superiority, except in local-regional recurrence, in which parasternal recurrences occurred almost exclusively in the radical mastectomy group.

Other studies were designed to address the relationship between defined, randomized variations in the extent of surgery and survival after at least 10 years. Generally their statistical power was compromised owing to the low incidence of isolated internal mammary node metastases, but most survival data gleaned from these studies tended to favor the larger procedure (ERM). However, by this time clinical trials conducted simultaneously by the National Surgical Adjuvant Breast and Bowel Project (NSABP) and others redirected surgical philosophy toward treatment strategies based on breast conservation coupled with adjuvant therapy. Because doubt had been cast on the Halstedian principles of tumor spread in this disease and therefore interest in IMN significance and the extended radical surgery devised to treat them subsided. Recently, however, the rapid and widespread incorporation of sentinel lymph node technology to assess regional metastasis in breast cancer patients has reawakened interest in the implications of IMN metastases and the potential benefit of their treatment.

Certain factors must be considered in estimating the benefits of treatment of IMNs: 1) the incidence and location of IMN metastases and the clinical correlates of such involvement; 2) the incidence of lymph node failure in the absence of treatment; 3) the ability of radiotherapy or surgery, either alone or in combination, to prevent such failure; 4) whether surgery or radiotherapy given to the IMNs ultimately has a clinically significant impact on disease-free or overall survival; and 5) the morbidity of substernal failure and whether it can be treated effectively when it occurs. This chapter addresses these issues as well as the utility of emerging sentinel lymph node technology in assessing the internal mammary chain and how this technique may impact patients with breast carcinoma. Finally, our technique of internal mammary lymph node biopsy and the criteria for which it is currently performed are outlined.

2. LYMPHATIC DRAINAGE TO THE INTERNAL MAMMARY CHAIN

As much as 25% of the lymph from the breast is estimated to flow to the internal mammary chain, and injection studies with radiolabeled colloid have demonstrated that drainage to IMNs may be observed following injection of any quadrant of the breast. Lymphatic flow in the breast proceeds unidirectionally from the superficial to the deep plexus and from the subareolar plexus through the lymphatic vessels of the lactiferous ducts to the perilobular and deep subcutaneous plexus. Flow from the deep subcutaneous and intramammary lymphatic vessels then moves centrifugally toward the axillary and internal mammary nodes.

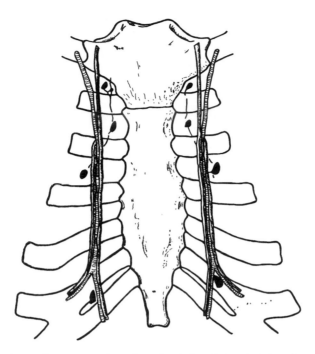

Fig. 1. Anatomy of the internal mammary lymph node chain relative to internal mammary vessels. (From Stibbe, E. (1918) The internal mammary lymphatic glands. *J. Anat.* **52**, 257–264. Reprinted with permission of Cambridge University Press).

The lymph nodes of the internal mammary chain lie in the intercostal spaces (ICS) in the parasternal region. They lie close to the internal mammary vessels in extrapleural fat and are distributed in the ICS, as shown in Figure 1. From the second ICS downward, the IMNs are separated from the pleura by a thin layer of fascia in the same plane as the transverse thoracic muscle (Fig. 2). The nodes lie medial to the internal mammary vessels in the first and second intercostal spaces in 88 and 76% of cases, respectively, and lateral to the vessels in the third ICS in 79% of cases. The number of lymph nodes described in the internal mammary chain varies. Autopsy studies by Stibbe identified the prevalence of nodes in each ICS as follows: first space, 97%; second space, 98%; third space, 82%; fourth space, 9%; fifth space, 12%; and sixth space, 62%. Noguchi and colleagues noted that most IMN metastases were found in the first three ICS. However, locations of metastases were not dominated by a single ICS position. Li and Shen found that most IMN metastases (132/215 patients, 61%) were found in single nodes when the first four ICS were dissected in unselected patients. However, this same series noted that 17/215 or 8% of IMN-positive patients had metastases in as many as three ICS.

3. PREDICTORS OF INTERNAL MAMMARY LYMPH NODE METASTASES

Internal mammary nodal metastases are present at the time of diagnosis in approximately 20% of all patients with operable breast cancers. "Clinical staging" of IMNs is not considered possible owing to their intrathoracic location, as well as their uncommon clinical presentation. Furthermore, the size of the typical IMN harboring a breast cancer metastasis usually approximates 5 mm or less, which is below the resolution of most current radi-

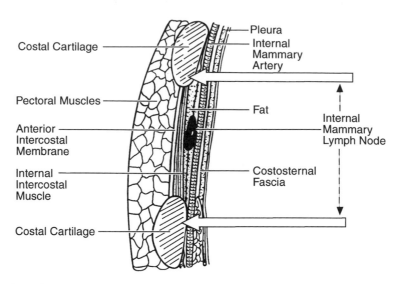

Fig. 2. Lateral view of intenal mammary lymph node position. Dashed line between open arrows represents range in which lymph node may be found. (Adapted from Stibbe, E. (1918) The internal mammary lymphatic glands. *J. Anat.* **52,** 257–264. Reprinted with permission of Cambridge University Press).

ographic imaging technology. However, correlates of IMN involvement have been identified through retrospective analysis of several large series in which IMNs were histologically assessed following either biopsy through intercostal incisions (Handley's technique) or various ERM procedures in which the internal mammary chain was dissected. Table 1 represents a partial list of the more than 20 separate series in the literature documenting the incidence of IMN metastases. Studies employing Handley's biopsy technique preclude a complete analysis of the IMNs, suggesting the possibility that IMN involvement might be underestimated. Conversely, some later series utilized patient selection criteria associated with an increased incidence of IMN metastases and may overrepresent IMN involvement. Interpretation of these studies thus requires knowledge of the method used to obtain IMNs for histologic inspection as well as initial patient selection criteria to determine true predictors of IMN metastases.

3.1. Axillary Node Involvement

The most consistent finding in IMN involvement in any study is its relation to axillary node involvement (Table 1). Overall, axillary lymph node involvement is more likely to occur than IMN involvement. In series in which both axillary and internal mammary lymph nodes have been histologically assessed, axillary node metastases are found in roughly 50% of cases, whereas IMN involvement is seen in approximately 20%. These studies universally agree that axillary involvement influences the likelihood of IMN involvement. When axillary nodes are negative in unselected series, IMN involvement is uncommon (4.3–11.1%). However, when axillary nodes test positive, IMN involvement increases to 27.9–40.9%. Furthermore, the greater the extent of axillary node involvement, the greater the likelihood of IMN involvement. This was demonstrated by Noguchi and colleagues, who determined by multivariate analysis that the number of involved axillary lymph nodes was a significant prognostic criteria for IMN involvement (4.8, 20.0, and 51.7% incidence of IMN involvement with

Table 1
Regional Nodal Involvement in Patients with Operable Breast Cancer

Author	No. of patients	Surgical treatment	Frequency (%)				IM involvement by Ax status (%)	
			Ax– IM–	Ax+ IM–	Ax– IM+	Ax+ IM+	Ax–	Ax+
Unselected patients								
Handley, 1975	500	RM + IM Bx	37	35	4.6	23.4	11.1	40.1
Donegan, 1977	105	RM + IM Bx	42.9	38.1	1.9	17.1	4.3	31
Veronesi and Zingo, 1967	700[a]	ERM	45.9	29.1	4.9	20.1	9.6	40.9
Lacour et al., 1983	703	ERM	42	38.5	4.6	14.9	9.8	27.9
Li and Shen, 1984	1242	ERM	46.5	35.7	2.4	15.4	4.9	30.1
Noguchi et al., 1993	142	ERM[b]	55.6	26.8	2.8	14.8	4.8	35.6
Selected patients[c]								
Deemarski and Seleznev, 1984	478	ERM	43.3	25.5	9.0	22.2	17.2	46.5
Cody and Urban, 1995	195	ERM	50.3	24.6	11.3	13.8	18.3	36

Ax, axillary nodes; IM, internal mammary nodes; +, positive; –, negative; Bx, biopsy; ERM, extended radical mastectomy with IM dissection of first four intercostal spaces; RM, radical mastectomy.

[a] 285 patients selected for extended radical mastectomy based on primary tumor location (inner quadrants).

[b] Sixteen patients underwent IM Bx only.

[c] All patients had larger, more centrally/medially located primary tumors in an effort to maximize the IM involvement.

0, 1–3, and >3 axillary node metastases, respectively). In addition, Urban and Eqeli reported an increasing risk of IMN metastases with higher levels of axillary nodal involvement.

Overall, review of any of these studies reveals that the incidence of positive IMNs is strongly associated with the pathologic status of the axilla. An explanation for this observation has been offered by Deemarski and Seleznev. They believed that the increased IMN involvement seen with positive axillary nodes might actually originate through retrograde lymphatic flow after metastatic tumor deposits within the axillary lymph nodes blocked the main outflow of lymph. This hypothesis, however, would not account for the small incidence of isolated IMN metastases seen in all series.

3.2. Primary Tumor Location

Location of the primary tumor within the breast may also influence the likelihood of IMN involvement. Interpreting this influence as a predictive factor for IMN involvement can be difficult because patients in the reported series were often selected to undergo ERM based solely on tumor location. Nonetheless, several studies have indicated that IMNs are more commonly involved when tumors are located in the central or medial portion of the breast than when they are in the lateral portion (Table 2). R. Handley was the first to note that IMN involvement was more common for inner quadrant or central primaries than for outer quadrant primaries. He noted a more than twofold differential between the frequency of IMN metastases associated with central-medial lesions compared with lateral lesions (29% versus 13.9%, respectively). Other investigators have also identified a significant relationship between tumor location and IMN involvement in unselected series and, like Handley, have found that IMN involvement is more common for medial or central tumors (Table 2).

In both Handley's and other series, axillary involvement remained more common than IMN involvement, even in patients with inner or central tumors. In a metaanalysis of 17 reports of either extended radical mastectomy or IMN biopsy, Morrow and Foster identified a 7.6% incidence of IMN metastatic disease without concurrent axillary nodal disease in a subgroup of nearly 2000 patients with medial tumors. The incidence of isolated IMN metastases in patients with lateral tumors was 2.9%. It is noteworthy that the frequency of isolated IMN metastases increases to 17.2–18.3% in at least two studies focusing solely on patients with larger and more medially located tumors (Table 1), thus suggesting the ability to select for patients with higher likelihood of harboring IMN metastases based on primary tumor location.

3.3. Primary Tumor Size

Analogous to its relation to axillary involvement, there is good evidence that the size of the primary tumor in the breast also influences the likelihood of IMN involvement. Table 3 describes the incidence of IMN metastases related to the maximum diameter of the primary tumor in three series of unselected patients. The larger the primary tumor, the greater the risk for IMN involvement. Tumors greater than 5.0 cm in greatest dimension (T3) exhibit a 36.7–55.6% incidence of IMN positivity regardless of tumor location within the breast. Many of these studies were performed during an era prior to the recommendation of routine breast exam and utilization of screening mammography. Thus, there tended to be a higher proportion of large tumors than characteristically seen today. However, these studies still reveal that IMN metastases can be identified in even the smallest tumors. When patients were selected to undergo ERM based on a central-medial location of their tumor, Deemarski and Seleznev identifed IMN metastases in 15 of 98 patients (15.3%) with a T1 tumor. Iso-

Table 2
Frequency (%) of Internal Mammary Lymph Node Metastases by Tumor Location
and Axillary Status in Series of Unselected Patients

Author	Surgical treatment	No. of cases	Medial/ central	Lateral	Total
Total					
Handley, 1975	RM + IM Bx	1000	29.9	13.9	22.3
Lacour et al., 1976	ERM	1391	24.1	16.2	19.7
Li and Shen, 1984	ERM	1168	22.0	14.1	17.9
Veronesi and Valagussa, 1981	ERM	342	24.1	17.8	20.5
Axilla negative					
Handley, 1975		465	10.6	4.3	7.7
Lacour et al., 1976		605	10.4	7.9	9.1
Li and Shen, 1984		569	7.9	2.1	4.9
Veronesi and Valagussa, 1981		161	10.3	8.6	9.3
Axilla positive					
Handley, 1975		535	48.1	21.5	35.0
Lacour et al., 1976		786	36.2	21.9	27.9
Li and Shen, 1984		599	35.8	25.2	30.2
Veronesi and Valagussa, 1981		181	36.4	26.0	30.4

IM, internal mammary nodes; Bx, biopsy; RM, radical mastectomy; ERM, extended radical mastectomy with IM dissection of first four intercostal spaces.

Table 3
Internal Mammary Node Involvement by Tumor Size

Author	No. of patients	Surgical treatment	Tumor size (cm)	Total cases[c]	No. with IM metastases	Frequency (%) of IM involvement
Noguchi et al., 1993	142[a]	ERM	≤2.0	59	2	3.4
			2.1–5.0	65	13	20.0
			≥5.1	18	10	55.6
Handley, 1975	1000	RM + IM Bx	<2.5	476	68	14.3
			2.5–5.0	419	109	26.0
			5.1–7.5	93	41	44.1
			>7.5	12	7	58.3
Veronesi and Zingo, 1967	700[b]	ERM	<1	23	2	8.7
			1.1–3	329	57	17.8
			3.1–5	252	78	30.9
			5.1–8	79	29	36.7
			>8	17	9	52.9

IM, internal mammary nodes; Bx, biopsy; RM, radical mastectomy; ERM, extended radical mastectomy with IM dissection of first four intercostal spaces.

[a] Sixteen patients underwent IM Bx only.

[b] Two hundred eighty five patients were selected for ERM based on primary tumor location (inner quadrants).

[c] Total cases with IM involvement.

lated IMN metastases were identified by Lacour in colleagues in 7% of the 453 patients with T1 and T2 disease.

3.4. Patient Age

Age of the patient also appears to be an important factor with respect to the frequency of IMN metastases. Various age distributions have been evaluated in different series, but all typically agree that the younger the patient, the more likely is the risk of IMN involvement. In the trial conducted by the National Cancer Institute of Milan, patients younger than 40 years had a nearly twofold greater incidence of IMN metastases compared with patients older than 50 (27.6% versus 15.6%, respectively; $p = 0.01$). Noguchi and colleagues also determined that patient age was a significant prognostic criteria for IMN metastases by multivariate analysis (45.5, 17.1, and 13.1% incidence of IMN involvement for patients ≤ 35, 36–50, and >50 years of age, respectively).

3.5. Histologic Type

The impact of the histologic features of the primary tumor on the risk of IMN involvement has not been extensively studied. The distribution of internal mammary node metastases according to the histologic type of primary has been evaluated in only two studies. Veronesi and colleagues showed that there was little difference in histologic types associated with IMN metastases and the characteristic distribution of breast cancer. As expected, a higher incidence of IMN positivity was seen in infiltrating ductal and lobular carcinomas (19.4 and 19.1%, respectively); uncommon well-differentiated types (papillary, tubular, gelatinous, and medullary carcinomas) were associated with a lower incidence. Examination with respect to biologic variables by Noguchi and co-workers identified solid-tubular (24.4%) and scirrhous (18.5%) as the most common histologic subtypes of infiltrating ductal breast cancer associated with internal mammary metastases. Again, however, there was not a significant association between histologic type and incidence of IMN involvement.

3.6. Other Biologic Characteristics

Very little is known regarding how other biologic characteristics of breast cancers may affect the risk of IMN involvement. Veronesi and colleagues evaluated estrogen receptor status in only 127 patients from a much larger series, but the presence or absence of such receptors in the primary tumor was not associated with IMN status. Noguchi and colleagues analyzed IMN incidence based on DNA ploidy status of the primary tumor. They found that DNA aneuploidy was associated significantly with IMN metastases ($p = 0.002$). In addition, by adding DNA ploidy to patient age, axillary node involvement, and tumor size, this group achieved a diagnostic accuracy of 82%, a sensitivity of 84%, and a specificity of 82% in identifying IMN metastases. However, no other investigator has reported ploidy status as a prognostic criteria for IMN involvement.

4. PROGNOSIS OF INTERNAL MAMMARY LYMPH NODE METASTASES

IMN metastases have historically been considered a grave prognostic sign, indicative of advanced disease, but it is controversial whether IMN involvement actually worsens the prognosis. Donegan reported on a series of 113 patients treated by radical mastectomy and internal mammary node biopsy only, in an attempt to determine the influence of untreated IMN metastases. Twenty-five patients (22%) had histologically documented internal mammary metastases; of these, 20 received no further treatment and 5 received adjuvant chest wall (but not internal mammary) irradiation. Only 1 of these 25 patients with untreated internal mammary metastases survived for 10 years (4%), and even this patient subsequently died of disseminated cancer. Deemarski and Seleznev concurred that IMN involvement carried a poor prognosis in certain instances. Following ERM, they reported that 10-year survival after treatment for a single IMN metastasis was significantly worse than for a single axillary metastasis (46.2% versus 61.1%, respectively). However, most studies demonstrate that 10-year disease-free survivals for axillary node-negative/internal mammary node-positive patients are quite comparable to those of axillary node-positive/internal mammary node-negative patients.

In Table 4, Donegan's results with untreated internal mammary metastases are compared with results obtained when such metastases are treated by ERM. As expected, patients without lymph node metastases have the best survival rates. Those with only axillary or IMN metastases have similar survival rates, as evidenced by the study of Veronesi and colleagues (Fig. 3). When only internal mammary metastases are present, 10-year survival rates for treated patients range from 45 to 61%. When both the axillary and the IMNs were involved, the survival rates were the worst (9.5–39% 10-year survival). Additionally, the location and number of IMN metastases is also prognostic. According to the large series of Li and Shen, those patients with metastases to the first or second ICS had lower survival rates than those with metastases to the third or fourth ICS. When there was metastasis to one or two ICS, the survival rates were similar. However, when there are metastases to three or more ICS, the survival rates were the lowest (21% 10-year survival). It may be concluded from these studies that it is the number of regional lymph nodes (whether axillary or internal mammary) containing metastases that provides the most important prognostic index, not the anatomic location of the nodes.

5. TREATMENT OF THE INTERNAL MAMMARY CHAIN

5.1. Surgical Dissection

Primary surgical treatment for operable breast cancer has changed dramatically during the last 40 years. The Halsted radical mastectomy, along with the extended variations of this classic operation, has yielded to modified radical mastectomy and breast-conserving approaches combining surgery and radiotherapy, based on the results of multiple randomized trials. Criticism of prophylactic treatment of the IMN chain by surgical dissection has been attributed to rarity of the clinical appearance of IMN metastases compared with the expected frequency of IMN nodal involvement. In a randomized series, Veronesi and Valagussa followed patients given radical mastectomy to determine the rate of subsequent clinical appearance of IMN metastases compared with the incidence of histologically proven IMN metastases identified by extended radical mastectomy. Patients in the two groups received no postoperative chemo- or radiotherapy and were comparable in age, menopausal status, quadrant distribution, and frequency of axillary metastases. In this series, clinically apparent parasternal relapses occurred only in patients who underwent radical mastectomy. However, the incidence of parasternal recurrence in this group was surprisingly low, 3.7% at a median follow-up in excess of 10 years, compared with a 20.5% incidence of histologically proven IMN metastases identified in patients undergoing extended radical mastectomy.

Regardless of the discrepancy between histologically proven IMN metastases and the rate of clinically apparent parasternal relapses, the results of several randomized and retrospective studies suggest that patients who have breast cancer in the central or medical quadrants

Table 4
Reported 10-Year Survival Rates (%) According to Status of Axillary and Internal Mammary Nodes

Author	No. of patients	Surgical treatment	Adjuvant radiotherapy	Adjuvant chemotherapy	Nodal status			
					Ax– IM–	Ax+ IM–	Ax– IM+	Ax+ IM+
Donegan, 1977	113	RM +IM Bx	5/113	—	40	21	0	6
Veronesi and Zingo, 1967	183	ERM	—	—	67.1	28.7	50	9.5
Urban and Egeli, 1986	815	ERM	Yes	—	82	63	56	38
Li and Shen, 1984	1242	ERM	—	—	84.5	44	61	27
Deemarski and Seleznev, 1984	325	ERM	—	Yes	77.4	57	45	39

Ax, axillary nodes; ERM, extended radical mastectomy; IM, internal mammary nodes; MRM, modified radical mastectomy; RM, radical mastectomy; +, positive; –, negative.

Adapted from Hundahl and Urban, 1998.

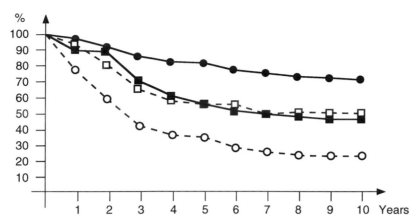

Fig. 3. Ten-year disease-free survival in patients without regional lymph node metastases (●), with axillary node metastases only (■), with internal mammary node metastases only (□), and with both regional node groups involved (○); p = 10⁻⁹. (From Veronesi, U., Cascinelli, N., Greco, M., et al. (1985) Prognosis of breast cancer patients after mastectomy and dissection of internal mammary nodes. *Ann. Surg.* **202,** 702–707. Reprinted with permission of Lippincott, Williams & Wilkins).

have better 5-year survival rates after ERM (Table 5). In the randomized trial of Meier and colleagues, patients with central or medial tumors who underwent ERM had a significant improvement in 10-year survival compared with radical mastectomy only ($p = 0.039$). Patients with lateral tumors, however, derived no apparent benefit from ERM. In a comparison of similar nonrandomized groups reported by Deemarski and Seleznev, dissection of the internal mammary chain in patients with primary breast cancer of central or medial origin improved the 10-year results by 31.9% in those who had metastases in both axillary and internal mammary lymph nodes. In the case of isolated IMN metastases, ERM resulted in a 10-year disease-free recurrence rate of 46.2%. Li and Shen concurred that surgical treatment of the IMNs improved both disease-free and overall survival. They compared 705 patients treated by the classic radical mastectomy with 1049 patients treated by ERM and demonstrated better 5-, 10-, and 20-year survival rates for ERM, regardless of the site of the primary tumor. From these data, it appears that extended operations to include the internal mammary chain are theoretically and practically sound in patients harboring or at significant risk of harboring IMN metastases.

5.2. Irradiation

Indications for irradiation of the internal mammary chain are controversial. The incidence of toxicity from treatment (mainly pneumonitis and cardiotoxicity), although minimized with modern radiotherapeutic techniques, may be greater than the low risk of clinically evident recurrence in the IMNs. Two randomized trials support the routine use of perioperative IMN radiotherapy after demonstrating a survival advantage in treated patients. However, two later metaanalyses of all randomized trials of postmastectomy radiation, most including IMN irradiation, determined that no 10-year survival advantage existed, and instead showed a significant increase in non-breast cancer mortality in irradiated patients. Cuzick and colleagues reported data on causes of death from nine early trials of postmastectomy radiation in women surviving at least 10 years from trial entry. The cardiac-related causes of death were significantly increased in patients randomized to

Table 5

Results of Prospective, Randomized Trials of Radical Mastectomy Versus Extended Radical Mastectomy in Patients with Central or Medial Tumors

| Author | No. of patients | Tumor size | Ax status | Adjuvant therapy | | F/U (yr) | Survival (%) | | p-value |
				Radiat.	Chemo.		RM	ERM	
Meir et al., 1989	70	T1–T2	±	No	Yes	10	60	86	0.025
Lacour et al., 1976	192	T1–T2	+	No	No	5	52	71	0.01
Veronesi and Valagussa, 1981	286	T1–T3a	±	No	No	10	56	62	NS
Lacour et al., 1983	70	T1–T2	+	No	No	15	28	53	0.05

Ax, axillary nodes; F/U, length of follow-up; RM, radical mastectomy; ERM, extended radical mastectomy; +, positive; –, negative.

Adapted from Hundahl and Urban, 1998.

receive radiotherapy ($p < 0.001$). The Early Breast Cancer Trialists' Collaborative Group reported data on non-breast cancer death from 28 trials of postmastectomy radiation involving over 13,000 women. In this report, the overall rate of death from non-breast cancer causes was again increased for patients who received irradiation (odds ratio = 1.24 ± 0.08, $p = 0.002$ for irradiated patients).

Furthermore, when irradiated patient subgroups from these trials were analyzed based on IMN treatment, the odds ratio for excess non-breast cancer death significantly increased for patients who received IMN irradiation compared with those who did not. These differences persisted throughout follow-up exceeding 10 years. Long-term results from two prospective randomized clinical trials of irradiation versus no treatment of the regional lymph nodes (IMN included) after mastectomy confirmed a significant increase in non-breast cancer mortality in irradiated patients owing to an increase in cardiovascular death. From the Oslo II trial, Host and colleagues reported that the mortality from non-breast cancer causes at 15 years was 22% versus 11% in stage I patients treated with radiation therapy compared with nonirradiated patients ($p = 0.02$). The only significant difference in cause of death was from acute myocardial infarction. The Manchester II trial also demonstrated a decrease in non-breast cancer-specific survival after 15 years following postmastectomy regional lymph node irradiation. Again, this difference was determined to be owing to cardiovascular death after irradiation.

It is possible that age at diagnosis may impact on cardiac toxicity following irradiation to the IMN chain. Increased non-breast cancer mortality following irradiation was more apparent in women 60 years of age or older at randomization (15.3% versus 11.1% for untreated) compared with women under 50 (2.5% versus 2.0% for untreated) in the Early Breast Cancer Trialists' Collaborative Group metaanalysis. In addition, Ragaz and colleagues reported only one cardiac event in 164 premenopausal patients randomized to post-mastectomy radiation that included the IMN chain. Longer follow-up will be needed to determine whether premenopausal women are relatively protected from these complications or if the interval to cardiac events is simply prolonged beyond the 10–15 years observed in postmenopausal women.

Currently two trials involving prophylactic IMN irradiation using modern techniques that will exclude excess cardiac irradiation are under way. The European Organization for Research and Treatment of Cancer (EORTC) is conducting a trial in which stage I–III patients with positive axillary nodes regardless of primary tumor location or central/medial tumors with negative axillary nodes are randomized to radiotherapy to the breast (following breast conservation) or chest wall (following mastectomy) with or without inclusion of the IMNs and supraclavicular nodes. The National Cancer Institute of Canada is conducting a similar trial in patients with factors predictive of increased risk for IMN metastastases who need radiotherapy following breast-conserving surgery. Until data from these trials are mature, prophylactic irradiation to the internal mammary chain must be viewed as controversial.

5.3. Treatment of Substernal Failure

As noted previously, clinically evident parasternal recurrence occurs much less often than is predicted by the incidence of histologically proven IMN involvement in many series. When present, it generally manifests clinically as a firm, fixed, mound-like mass projecting from the medial aspect of an ICS. Radiation therapy can sometimes control a parasternal recurrence adequately. However, in certain patients, the parasternal recurrence may be the first evidence of recurrent/metastatic disease and may be a source of distant metastases.

Sanger reported that the parasternal recurrence in four of seven patients responded to radiation therapy, but that five of these ultimately died of disseminated disease. Shah and Urban first reported the technique and results of full-thickness chest wall resection with immediate plastic reconstruction. In the largest series to date, Noguchi and colleagues reported on 11 patients who developed parasternal recurrence. The time interval from initial operation to parasternal recurrence was 9 months to 19 years (mean 6 years and 7 months). The recurrent tumors were located in the first ICS in one case, the second ICS in two cases, the third ICS in six cases, and the fourth ICS in three cases. In five (45%) of these patients, distant metastasis was found at the time of the parasternal recurrence. One patient refused further surgery. The remaining five patients underwent radical resection of the parasternal portion of the chest wall, including complete dissection of the IMNs, supraclavicular lymph nodes, or both. Four of these remained disease-free at 19–52 months.

6. INTERNAL MAMMARY LYMPH NODE BIOPSY

The controversial clinical utility of staging the IMNs when the axilla is positive and the low rate of IMN metastases in the absence of axillary nodal involvement preclude the universal application of internal mammary chain dissection or even biopsy in patients with operable breast cancer. Several investigators have attempted to identify the most probable location of metastatic IMNs so that limited biopsies (as opposed to complete parasternal dissections) could be utilized. Analysis of large retrospective studies in which the IMNs have been either biopsied or dissected form the basis for their recommendations. Veronesi advocated a biopsy of the IMN in only the first ICS in selected high-risk patients. To determine the most common location of metastatic IMNs, Noguchi and colleagues reviewed 21 patients with IMN metastases who underwent dissection of the first four ICS. They concluded that biopsy of only the first ICS did not provide adequate data on IMN status, as metastatic incidence was only 90%, but that biopsy of both the first and second ICS identified IMN metastases with 100% sensitivity. Recommendations for limited internal mammary biopsies were contradicted by Li and Shen after more than 20% of the 205 patients who underwent dissection of the first four ICS had IMN metastases that would not have been identified by sampling of only the first two ICS.

Several authors of the previously cited studies have advocated IMN biopsy in selected patients at the time of extirpative operation if there is no histologic evidence of axillary node metastasis on frozen section examination. At our institution, rather than relying on frozen section to rule out metastases in axillary lymph nodes, we now use sentinel lymph node technology as a means of identifying the internal mammary sentinel lymph node (IMSLN). We use the following criteria for determining the best candidates for IMSLN biopsy. The patient must be clinically staged as axillary node-negative. The patient's age and general health must permit systemic adjuvant therapy. The patient must have perioperative lymphoscintigraphy demonstrating lymphatic drainage to the IMNs; and either (1) a primary tumor located in the central or medial portion of the breast, or (2) a lateral tumor 2 cm or more in diameter.

Radioisotope that is used to localize axillary sentinel lymph nodes will also drain to the IMSLNs. At our institution perioperative lymphoscintigraphy demonstrates lymphatic drainage to the IMNs in approximately one-third of the patients regardless of primary tumor site (unpublished data). We modify our sentinel lymph node technique in selected patients in order to assess IMN status. Patients without clinical suspicion of axillary nodal metastasis following axillary assessment (either sentinel lymph node biopsy or complete axillary dissection) and meeting the criteria noted above undergo IMSLN biopsy if a "suspicious" or "hot" ICS is identified by the gamma probe. Often the scatter from a medial or large primary tumor must first be eliminated (by excision or lead shielding of the primary tumor) in order to use the gamma probe to identify the appropriate ICS.

Biopsy of an IMN may be obtained through the incision used to extirpate the primary tumor (i.e., lumpectomy or mastectomy) or through a separate incision. Most lumpectomy incisions in the medial aspect of the breast may be retracted to gain exposure to any of the first four ICS. The intercostal musculature may be approached most easily by splitting the muscle fibers of the pectoralis major. An alternative technique, described by Haagensen, is detaching the pectoralis major from the sternum and costal cartilages of the ICS to be explored. The areolar tissue and nodes around the internal mammary vessels are carefully teased away from the internal mammary vessels and the pleura. Electrocautery is usually adequate for hemostasis as long as the internal mammary vessels are not entered. IMN biopsies can be accomplished with a minimum of morbidity and only a small increase in operating time. The most common complication is pneumothorax, which routinely responds to simple aspiration unless there is an injury to the underlying lung. Internal mammary SLNs are pathologically evaluated in the same manner as axillary SLNs: hematoxylin and eosin staining of serial step-sections every 2–3 mm throughout the lymph node followed, if necessary, by immunolabeling for cytokeratin.

7. CONCLUSIONS

Tissue preservation supplemented with radiation as well as chemotherapy or hormone therapy has replaced more radical surgery in the management of breast carcinoma. Although the internal mammary lymph nodes are a well-documented site of metastasis, current clinical management stratifies patients only according to axillary status. However, IMN metastases, present in approximately 20% of unselected patients, serve as a prognosticator second only to axillary node status. Ignoring the internal mammary chain thus creates a heterogeneous group of axillary node-negative patients in whom outcome will be adversely affected by unrecognized IMN involvement. It is true that axillary nodal status is the best predictor of IMN metastases and that IMN status may be of little concern if systemic adjuvant therapy is already planned. However, in a selected group of axillary node-negative breast cancer patients, knowledge of IMN status may be of increasing clinical relevance.

Only 80% of stage I breast cancers are currently cured by local therapy alone. Node-negative patients represent an ever-increasing proportion of breast cancer patients as earlier diagnoses continue to be made. As the proportion of axillary node-negative breast cancer patients has increased, so has the intensity of the search for other prognostic factors to define high-risk patients who might benefit from systemic adjuvant treatment. Unidentified IMN metastases may account for treatment failures owing to initial inadequate staging of these patients. Multiple studies have demonstrated that even small primary tumors may be associated with IMN involvement. In selected series the incidence of isolated IMN involvement may be as high as 17.2–18.3% (Table 4). These patients obviously would benefit from more intensive adjuvant therapy, but the key is to identify this subset as early as possible.

With widespread acceptance of sentinel lymph node technology and increased utilization of lymphoscintigraphy, clinicians are once again confronted with the recognition that lymph does not universally flow from breast cancer to the axilla. Sentinel lymph node technology can improve the accuracy of diagnosing "truly node-negative" breast cancer patients as a result of more rigorous and sensitive histopathologic evaluation of axillary lymph nodes.

Sentinel lymph node technology also offers an opportunity for complete and accurate staging of breast cancer patients beyond its current utility in assessing the axilla. Axillary nodal status remains the major prognosticator of IMN metastases, but several clinical factors are indicative of an increased likelihood of IMN involvement. Selecting patients based on their age as well as location and size of their primary tumor can identify this increased risk. Sentinel lymph node technology may be used in selected breast cancer patients to assess the internal mammary chain with minimal morbidity. With the application of this new technology, further clinical research is warranted to determine the significance of IMN metastases in patients with breast cancer.

BIBLIOGRAPHY

Cody H III, Urban J (1995) Internal mammary status: a major prognosticator in axillary node-negative breast cancer. *Ann. Surg. Oncol.* **2,** 32–37.

Cuzick J, Stewart H, Ritqvist L, et al. (1994) Cause-specific mortality in long-term survivors of breast cancer who participated in trials of radiotherapy. *J. Clin. Oncol.* **12,** 447–453.

Deemarski LY, Seleznev IK (1984) Extended radical operations on breast cancer of medial or central location. *Surgery* **96,** 73–77.

Donegan W (1977) The influence of untreated internal mammary metastases upon the course of mammary cancer. *Cancer* **39,** 533–538.

Early Breast Cancer Trialists' Collaborative Group (1995) Effects of radiotherapy and surgery in early breast cancer. *N. Engl. J. Med.* **333,** 1444–1455.

Ege G (1983) Lymphoscintigraphy—techniques and applications in the management of breast carcinoma. *Semin. Nucl. Med.* **13,** 26–34.

Fisher B, Redmond C, Fisher E, et al. (1985) Ten-year results of a randomized clinical trial comparing radical mastectomy and total mastectomy with or without radiation. *N. Engl. J. Med.* **14,** 674–681.

Haagenson C (1971) *Disease of the Breast,* 2nd ed. WB Saunders, Philadelphia, pp. 413–426.

Halsted W (1891) The treatment of wounds with especial reference to the value of the blood clot in the management of dead space. V. Operations for carcinoma of the breast. *Johns Hopkins Hosp. Rep.* **2,** 189–194.

Handley R (1975) Cancer of the breast. *Am. Surg.* **41,** 667–670.

Handley R, Thackery A (1949) The internal mammary lymph chain in carcinoma of the breast: study of 50 cases. *Lancet* **2,** 276–278.

Handley W (1927) Parasternal invasion of the thorax in breast cancer and its suppression by the use of radium tubes as an operative precaution. *Surg. Gyneolc. Obstet.* **45,** 721–728.

Host H, Brennhovd I, Loeb M (1986) Postoperative radiotherapy in breast cancer: long-term results from the Oslo study. *Int. J. Radiat. Oncol. Biol. Phys.* **12,** 727–732.

Hundahl S, Urban J (1998) Extended radical mastectomy. In: Bland K, Copeland E (eds.) *The Breast: Comprehensive Management of Benign and Malignant Diseases.* WB Saunders, Philadelphia, pp. 871–880.

Jones J, Ribeiro G (1989) Mortality patterns over 34 years of breast cancer patients in a clinical trial of post-operative radiotherapy. *Clin. Radiol.* **40,** 204–208.

Lacour J, Bucalossi P, Caceres E, et al. (1976) Radical mastectomy versus radical mastectomy plus internal mammary dissection: five-year results of an international cooperative study. *Cancer* **37,** 206–214.

Lacour J, Le M, Caceres E, Koszarowski T, Veronesi U, Hill C (1983) Radical mastectomy versus radical mastectomy plus internal mammary dissection. *Cancer* **51,** 1941–1943.

Li K, Shen Z-Z (1984) An analysis of 1,242 cases of extended radical mastectomy. *Breast* **10,** 10–19.

Meier P, Ferguson D, Karrison T (1989) A controlled trial of extended radical versus radical mastectomy: ten-year results. *Cancer* **63,** 188–195.

Morrow M, Foster Jr R (1981) Staging of breast cancer: a new rationale for internal mammary node biopsy. *Arch. Surg.* **116,** 748–751.

Noguchi M, Ohta N, Koyasaki N, Taniya T, Miyazaki I, Mizukami Y (1991) Reappraisal of internal mammary node metastases as a prognostic factor in patients with breast cancer. *Cancer* **68,** 1918–1925.

Noguchi M, Ohta N, Thomas M, Kitagawa H, Miyazaki I (1993) Risk of internal mammary lymph node metastases and its prognostic value in breast cancer patients. *J. Surg. Oncol.* **52,** 26–30.

Noguchi M, Tanaka S, Fuji H, Takikawa Y, Miyazaki I (1985) The surgical management of parasternal recurrence of breast cancer. *Int. Surg.* **70,** 211–214.

Ragaz J, Jackson S, Le N, et al. (1997) Adjuvant radiotherapy and chemotherapy in node-positive premenopausal women with breast cancer. *N. Engl. J. Med.* **337,** 956–962.

Rosen P, Groshen S, Saigo P, et al. (1989) A long-term follow-up study of survival in stage I (T1N0M0) and stage II (T1N1M0) breast carcinoma. *J. Clin. Oncol.* **7,** 355–366.

Sanger G (1963) An aspect of internal mammary metastases from carcinoma of the breast. *Ann. Surg.* **157,** 180–185.

Shah J, Urban J (1975) Full thickness chest wall resection for recurrent breast carcinoma involving the bony chest wall. *Cancer* **35,** 567–573.

Stibbe E (1918) The internal mammary lymphatic glands. *J. Anat.* **52,** 257–264.

Turner-Warwick R (1959) The lymphatics of the breast. *Br. J. Surg.* **46,** 574–582.

Urban J, Egeli R (1986) Extended radical mastectomy. In: Strombeck JO, Rosato FE (eds.) *Surgery of the Breast.* Thieme, New York, pp. 138–147.

Veronesi U, Cascinelli N, Greco M, et al. (1985) Prognosis of breast cancer patients after mastectomy and dissection of internal mammary nodes. *Ann. Surg.* **202,** 702–707.

Veronesi U, Valagussa P (1981) Inefficacy of internal mammary nodes dissection in breast cancer surgery. *Cancer* **47,** 170–175.

Veronesi U, Zingo L (1967) Extended mastectomy for cancer of the breast. *Cancer* **20,** 677–681.

Wallgren A, Arner O, Bergstrom J, et al. (1986) Radiation therapy in operable breast cancer: results from the Stockholm trial on adjuvant radiotherapy. *Int. J. Radiat. Oncol. Biol. Phys.* **12,** 533–537.

23 High-Dose Chemotherapy and Autologous Stem Cell Transplantation for Breast Cancer

Edward A. Stadtmauer, MD

CONTENTS

INTRODUCTION
METASTATIC BREAST CANCER
HIGH-RISK PRIMARY BREAST CANCER
REFERENCES

1. INTRODUCTION

The combination of surgery, radiation therapy, chemotherapy, and hormonal therapy has led to the cure of over 50% of patients with low stage breast cancer *(1)*. Despite this success, however, most patients with locally advanced and metastatic disease will ultimately progress and succumb despite conventional dose therapy. By the mid-1980s, a strong relationship of dose to response, particularly for alkylating agents in breast cancer, had been demonstrated. The major dose-limiting toxicity was myelosuppression, and techniques of bone marrow and blood-derived stem cell harvesting, storage, and infusion allowed for the ready utilization of hematopoietic stem cells as support and rescue after high-dose therapy. The use of myeloid hematopoietic growth factors enhanced the collection of stem cells and marrow recovery after stem cell transplantation and allowed for rapid and reliable trilineage engraftment after high-dose chemotherapy.

The use of high-dose chemotherapy and autologous stem cell transplantation has risen rapidly over the past 20 years, outstripping allogeneic transplantation because of the lack of need for a donor and the decreased toxicity. The approach has been utilized for the treatment of hematologic malignancies such as Hodgkin's and non-Hodgkin's lymphoma, acute myeloid and lymphoid leukemia, and multiple myeloma. The most rapid growth however, has been for solid tumors, particularly metastatic and high-risk breast cancer, ovarian cancer, germ cell cancer, and selected brain tumors. Currently breast cancer is the number one disease indication for stem cell transplantation of any kind; more than 10,000 procedures have been conducted in North America over the past decade *(2)*. This chapter reviews the outcomes of this procedure in high-risk primary and metastatic breast cancer.

From: *Current Clinical Oncology:*
Breast Cancer: A Guide to Detection and Multidisciplinary Therapy
Edited by: M. H. Torosian © Humana Press Inc., Totowa, NJ

Table 1
Early Pilot Trials of High-Dose Chemotherapy and Stem Cell Transplant in Metastatic Breast Cancer

Author	No. of patients	HDC (%)	RR (mo)	OS (%)	PFS (%)	Toxic death
Peters et al., 1988 (3)	22	CBP	73	10.1	14	23
Williams et al., 1989 (4,6)	27	CT	86	15.1	7	14
Kennedy et al., 1991 (8)	30	CT	100	22	10	0
Antman et al., 1992 (5)	29	CTCb	100	24	17	3

HDC, high-dose chemotherapy; RR, response rate; OS, overall survival; PFS, progression-free survival; Toxic death, death within 100 days of stem cell infusion; CBP, cyclophosphamide, carmustine, and cisplatinum; CT, cyclophosphamide and thiotepa; CTCb, cyclophosphamide, thiotepa, and carboplatin.

2. METASTATIC BREAST CANCER

2.1. History

In the late 1980s, promising preliminary studies of high-dose chemotherapy and stem cell transplant for metastatic breast cancer were reported (3–6). During the early 1980s, phase I and II trials of single-agent and combination chemotherapy for patients with relapsed and refractory metastatic breast cancer were performed (7–14). Response rates of approximately 70% were observed, with 20–30% of the patients achieving complete remission. The average duration of response was approximately 6 months, with an average median survival of approximately 8 months and few, if any, long-term relapse-free survivors. This response rate was higher than would be expected from conventional dose chemotherapy; however, the median duration of response was similar to that achieved with conventional dose therapy.

Because of the high frequency of response in patients with relapsed and refractory breast cancer, Peters and colleagues (3) explored the use of a single course of high-dose therapy with stem cell transplantation as the initial therapy for first relapse from primary disease. Patients in these series were generally young, premenopausal, and estrogen receptor-negative, with measurable visceral disease. This trial and numerous others thereafter suggest that a single course of high-dose chemotherapy produces up to an 80% response rate and up to a 40% complete response rate in metastatic breast cancer. (Table 1) The updated report from Peters et al. (3) suggests that with a minimum follow-up of 11 years, 3 of 22 (14%) patients remain continuously disease-free.

By its very nature, a trial of high-dose chemotherapy and stem cell rescue as the initial therapy of metastatic disease would include a highly selected patient population. These patients would have to be well enough to undergo high-dose therapy and have adequate bone marrow for stem cell selection. Most trials have therefore utilized a course of conventional dose induction chemotherapy to reduce tumor burden, improve performance status, and decrease the chance of stem cell tumor contamination. A number of trials of this design also suggested an approximately 80% response rate, with 10–30% of patients relapse-free at 2 years. The mortality of these early trials, however, was substantial, ranging from 3 to 30% within the first 100 days of transplantation. The survival benefits however, were perceived to be superior to those of historical controls. Registry data reported to the Autologous Bone Marrow Transplant Registry (ABMTR) corroborated these results (2).

Interest in high-dose therapy and stem cell rescue increased, and demands on insurers for coverage increased rapidly. The most common high-dose chemotherapy treatment scenario had become a course of four to six cycles of conventional dose induction chemotherapy, usually cyclophosphamide, doxorubicin, and 5-fluorouracil (CAF) or doxorubicin and cyclophosphamide (AC), and then assessment for response. Patients achieving complete or partial response then proceeded to stem cell collection followed by a single course of high-dose chemotherapy utilizing primarily one of three regimens (cyclophosphamide, etoposide [VP16], and prednisone [CVP], cyclophosphamide, thiotepa, and carboplatin [CTCb], or cyclophosphamide and thiotepa [CT]) and stem cell rescue. Trials comparing high-dose therapy and stem cell transplant with conventional dose therapy were developed and initiated in the early 1990s. The results of a number of these trials have recently been reported.

2.2. Comparison Trials of Induction Therapy Followed by a Single High-Dose Course

In 1990, the Philadelphia Bone Marrow Transplant Group (PBT) (Fox Chase, Hahnemann, Temple, and University of Pennsylvania) developed a randomized trial for chemotherapy untreated metastatic breast cancer. The North Central Cancer Treatment Group (NCCTG), the Eastern Cooperative Oncology Group (ECOG), and the Southwest Oncology Group (SWOG), joined the trial, which was designated high priority by the National Cancer Institute. The trial, PBT-1, met its accrual goal and was closed in December 1998; the results were reported in May of 1999 (18).

PBT-1 was designed to compare the time to progression and overall survival and toxicity of high-dose chemotherapy and stem cell transplantation with a prolonged course of maintenance chemotherapy for women with metastatic breast cancer responding to first-line chemotherapy. Eligibility required locally recurrent or distant metastatic disease, pre- or postmenopausal status, age 60 years or less, no prior chemotherapy for metastatic disease, prior adjuvant chemotherapy more than 6 months before entry, at least one prior hormonal treatment if estrogen receptor-positive unless life-threatening visceral disease present, and performance status of zero or one. Patients then received induction chemotherapy with CAF for four to six cycles or cyclophosphamide, methotrexate, and 5-fluorouracil (CMF) with optional prednisone if the prior doxorubicin dose was 400 mg/m^2 or more. Patients achieving stable or progressive disease were taken off the study, and patients achieving complete or partial response went on to further therapy. To be eligible for randomization, patients could not have had bone marrow involvement with tumor, and normal hematopoietic, cardiac, pulmonary, and hepatic function was required. Additionally, therapy was to begin within 8 weeks of the last chemotherapy.

Eligible patients were randomized to autologous stem cell transplantation or to CMF maintenance chemotherapy for up to 2 years. Patients discontinued CMF early at time of progressive disease, or toxicity, or removal of informed consent. Patients undergoing stem cell transplant underwent bone marrow harvest and granulocyte/macrophage colony-stimulating factor (GM-CSF)-stimulated peripheral stem cell harvest, followed by high-dose CTCb therapy with stem cell transplant and GM-CSF-stimulated marrow recovery. In 1995, the trial was amended to allow for G-CSF-stimulated stem cell harvest as the sole source of stem cells.

Five hundred fifty-three patients were enrolled in the trial; 296 achieved response and were therefore potentially eligible for randomization, and 199 proceeded to randomization. Of the 199 patients, 110 were assigned to transplant and 89 to maintenance therapy; of these, 15 (7.5%) were ineligible (9 autologous bone marrow transplant [ABMT] and 6 CMF), leaving 184 eligible randomized patients (101 ABMT and 83 CMF). With a median follow-up of the entire group of 37 months, there was no difference in median survival between transplant and maintenance therapy (24 months versus 26 months) or 3-year survival 32% versus 38% ($p = 0.23$). Patients in complete remission at time of randomization fared better in both overall survival and time to progression than patients in partial response. There was also no difference in time to progression between ABMT and maintenance chemotherapy, with a median time to progression of 9.6 months versus 9.0 months and a 3-year progression-free survival of 6% versus 12% ($p = 0.31$). No significant benefit for transplant was observed in any stratified subgroup including response, hormone receptor status, age 42 years or less versus more than 42 years, or dominant metastatic site visceral or other.

A surprising finding was the low conversion rate of patients in partial response at time of randomization to complete response with high-dose chemotherapy. One hundred thirty-nine patients were in partial response at time of randomization, and 11 (8%) were converted to complete remission after consolidation therapy; 5 were converted by transplant, and 6 were converted by CMF. Another surprising finding was the low lethal toxicity of transplant on this trial. No lethal toxicity was observed on the CMF arm, and only one patient died on the transplant arm of venoocclusive disease. Nonlethal severe toxicities, however, were increased on the transplant arm, including hematologic toxicity, infection, nausea, vomiting, and diarrhea, as well as cardiac, pulmonary, and hepatic toxicities. Mucositis, however, was not substantially increased. Overall, of the 184 eligible patients randomized, 20 refused randomized assignment, and this was well balanced in both groups. This study demonstrated that high-dose chemotherapy with stem cell rescue did not confer incremental improvement in overall survival or time to progression to CMF, but there were no substantial differences in lethal toxicity, although nonlethal grade serious toxicities were greater in the transplant arm. Alternatively, one could conclude that one cycle of high-dose therapy was equivalent to up to 24 months of CMF.

A similar, smaller trial has been conducted in France *(19)*. Patients with chemotherapy-naive metastatic breast cancer were treated with induction chemotherapy for six cycles, and a partial or complete response was required. Patients then went on to two to four additional cycles of induction chemotherapy, or cyclophosphamide plus G-CSF-stimulated stem cell harvest followed by high-dose cyclophosphamide, melphalan, and mitoxantrone (CMA) with stem cell transplantation. Thirty-two patients were assigned transplant and 29 conventional dose therapy. At 2 years, there was a trend toward improved survival in the transplant arm, but by 5 years no significant difference in the two arms was observed.

The Cancer and Leukemia Group B (CALGB) has conducted a retrospective database comparison utilizing historical data from CALGB metastatic breast cancer trials and compared this database with high-dose chemotherapy and stem cell transplant for metastatic breast cancer as reported to the ABMTR *(20)*. To be eligible, patients on the CALGB trials had to receive CAF induction chemotherapy, and although the induction chemotherapy was not reported in the ABMTR trials, a response was required. In the CALGB trials, the control arm was further courses of CAF with or without other chemotherapy regimens, whereas the experimental arm contained all transplants for metastatic breast cancer reported to the ABMTR from 1989 to 1995. Most patients had received a cyclophosphamide and thiotepa regimen with or without carboplatinum. All patients were younger than 65 years. The overall survival curves of these two groups were not significantly different. Combined analysis of these three comparison trials suggests that the use of cyclophosphamide-containing induction chemotherapy followed by high-dose chemotherapy and stem cell transplant for responding patients has not substantially improved survival for metastatic breast cancer.

Few patients in complete remission were transplanted on these comparative trials. Peters et al. *(21)* have made a preliminary report of a randomized trial examining the use of high-dose chemotherapy and stem cell transplant as consolidation treatment in patients who achieved a complete remission after intensive induction therapy. Four hundred twenty-three patients with hormone-insensitive measurable metastatic breast cancer who had not received any prior chemotherapy received two to four cycles of doxorubicin, 5-fluorouracil, and methotrexate (AFM) induction therapy. Twenty-five percent achieved complete remission (106 patients), and 98 of them were randomized to either immediate consolidation with CBP and stem cell transplantation I versus observation. The randomization was balanced both for pretreatment patient characteristics and for site and extent of the disease. The disease-free survival was significantly improved in the patients who received high-dose chemotherapy up front; with a median follow-up of 3.9 years, the event-free survival at 5 years is 25% for the high-dose arm versus 8% for the observation arm.

As a second part of this trial, patients assigned to the observation arm went on to high-dose chemotherapy and stem cell transplant at time of progression. Patients receiving transplant at time of first progression had superior overall survival to patients transplanted initially, with a median overall survival of 2.25 versus 3.56 years. These results suggest that induction chemotherapy just prior to transplantation may not be the optimal treatment design.

Most recently, a report from the ABMTR analyzed the factors associated with disease progression or death in a total of 1188 consecutive women age 18–70 years receiving autologous transplant or metastatic locally recurrent breast cancer with a median follow-up of $29^1/_2$ months (22). Nine factors were associated with a significantly increased risk of treatment failure, including age older than 45 years, Karnofsky performance score less than 90%, hormone receptor-negative status, prior use of adjuvant chemotherapy, initial disease-free interval after adjuvant chemotherapy less than 18 months, liver metastases, central nervous system metastases, three or more sites of metastatic disease, and less than complete response to standard dose chemotherapy. Tamoxifen treatment post transplant was associated with a reduced risk of treatment failure in women with hormone receptor-positive tumors. Women with no risk factors had a 3-year probability of progression-free survival of 43%, whereas women with more than three risk factors had a 3-year probability of progression-free survival of 4%. The 3-year probability of progression-free survival for the entire group was 13%. The group of patients with no risk factors ($n = 38$) accounted for only 3% of the entire population that was reported, whereas 84% of the patients registered had two or more risk factors and experienced outcomes similar to those seen in phase II and III trials.

2.3. Up-Front Transplantation and Tandem Transplantation

A number of trials utilizing cycles of high-dose chemotherapy in metastatic breast cancer have now been reported (23). One trial has been discredited owing to falsification of data (22). In another trial, investigators from the Dana-Farber Cancer institute have reported on 67 women with metastatic breast cancer receiving the sequence of high-dose melphalan followed by CTCb with stem cell transplantation (23). Patients initially received three or four cycles of doxorubicin and 5-fluorouracil, followed by G-CSF-stimulated peripheral stem cell harvest. Patients received melphalan 140–180 mg/m² with stem cell support followed by CTCb with stem cell transplantation and then went on to radiotherapy, surgery, and hormonal therapy if they were estrogen receptor-positive. Forty-four percent were progression-free a median of 16 months after high-dose therapy. The median progression-free survival, and overall survival were 11 and 20 months, respectively. These were not substantially improved from a historical cohort of single stem cell transplant.

The authors considered possible reasons for this outcome in this group of patients. Acquired drug resistance is likely to have played a role in the failure of high-dose chemotherapy. It is conceivable that induction chemotherapy could produce enough tumor cytoreduction to result in clinical response but that the minimal residual tumor could be induced into a state of drug resistance. This is suggested by the failure to significantly convert patients in partial remission into complete remission after the high-dose therapy (approximately 15% in this series). The sequence of dose-intensive therapy may play an additional role. Tumor cells surviving high-dose melphalan may be particularly resistant to the agents in CTCb, and therefore that sequence of events may not lead to optimal outcome. The same authors have recently reported on a group of 58 patients receiving two courses of induction chemotherapy with 90 mg/m² of doxorubicin, followed by tandem transplant in the opposite sequence with CTCb initially, and then a melphalan and paclitaxel combination *(25)*. Preliminary results show that 78% achieve complete or near complete response, with 60% event-free at 2 years.

A multiinstitutional trial sought to investigate the role of induction chemotherapy as part of tandem sequential high-dose chemotherapy for metastatic breast cancer *(26)*. Sixty-three patients were treated with four cycles of doxorubicin 50 mg/m² and docetaxel 75 mg/m², followed by a course of cyclophosphamide 5 g/m², VP-16 1.5 g/m² and cisplatinum 120 mg/m², with G-CSF-stimulated stem cell harvesting followed by a CTCb transplant. Patients went on to long-term anastrozole. Additionally, a group of 36 patients received the same sequential high-dose chemotherapy without the four cycles of induction therapy. A comparison of these two groups demonstrated a significantly greater complete response rate in the induction therapy group (42% versus 11%), as well as an improved progression-free survival. There was a 2.3-fold increase in risk of disease progression in the noninduction therapy group. At least this one study suggests a benefit for induction chemotherapy for metastatic breast cancer.

2.4. Conclusions and Future Directions for High-Dose Therapy and Stem Cell Transplantation in Metastatic Breast Cancer

After almost two decades of clinical research investigating high-dose therapy and stem cell transplantation for metastatic breast cancer, the body of data, particularly in comparative trials and large registry analyses, has reached a critical mass to aid in clinical decision making. Unfortunately, there is no evidence as yet that induction chemotherapy followed by a single course of high-dose chemotherapy with stem cell transplant improves the outcome for women with metastatic breast cancer, in particular relapse-free survival and overall survival (Table 2). A phase III trial in Canada was recently completed with similar conclusions *(26a)*. Toxicity, however, has been reduced substantially over the last decade, and a single course of high-dose therapy is at least equivalent to multiple cycles of conventional dose chemotherapy. Quality of life and economic analyses and end points remain to be determined, but these must be considered secondary to survival.

However, there are clues in the data to suggest the possibility of improved design of treatment protocols (Table 3):

1. Cycles of high-dose therapy appear to be superior to single courses of high-dose therapy.
2. Induction chemotherapy may induce chemotherapy resistance, and improved forms of induction therapy designed to prevent resistance may result in superior outcomes.
3. The role of infusion of contaminated tumor cells in the relapse of patients after high-dose chemotherapy and stem cell infusion remains to be determined, and improved processing and purging techniques may have a small, but positive impact on outcome.

Table 2

Randomized Trials of High-Dose Chemotherapy in Metastatic Breast Cancer

Trial (ref.)	No. of patients		Patient Assignment		Toxic death		PR → CR (%)	EFS (%)		OS (%)		P-value
	Total	Randomized	ABMT	Control	ABMT	Control		ABMT	Control	ABMT	Control	
Philadelphia (18)	553	199	110	89	1	0	11	6[a]	12[a]	32[a]	38	NS
Duke CR (21)	425	98	49	49	7.5%	0	—	24[b]	8[b]	40[b]	46[b]	<0.0001
French (19)	61	61	32	29	0	0	—	49[a]	21[a]	55[a]	28[a]	0.06
								9[b]	9[b]	30[b]	18.5[b]	NS
Canada (26a)	379	224	112	112	7	0	—	41[c]	28[c]	31[d]	36[d]	0.014
Philadelphia (18)	553	36	20	16	1	0	—	16[a]	25[a]	42[a]	49[a]	NS

ABMT, autologous bone marrow transplant; PR, partial response; CR, complete response; EFS, event-free survival; OS, overall survival.

[a] At 3 yr.

[b] At 5 yr.

[c] At 1 yr.

[d] At 2 yr.

Table 3
Future Directions

Cycles of high-dose therapy
Better induction therapy
Stem cell processing and purging
Posttransplant minimal disease therapy
Better selection of patients

4. Posttransplant therapy with tamoxifen for hormone receptor-positive patients is clearly a benefit after transplant, and other posttransplant therapies (such as cycles of conventional dose chemotherapy, immunotherapies, antiangiogenesis therapies and others), when combined with the maximal cytoreduction of high-dose therapy, may also improve these results.
5. The randomized trials so far presented emphasize the treatment of patients with a number of risk factors for treatment failure; perhaps a trial for younger patients in complete remission with few sites of metastatic disease may be indicated.

The preponderance of evidence suggests that high-dose chemotherapy and stem cell transplant (at least in the way utilized over the last two decades) has not made a substantial impact on treatment for metastatic breast cancer. A collaboration of physicians, patients, and insurers that will design and quickly complete phase I and II trials to investigate these newer approaches, followed by sincere use of the data derived are to design phase III randomized comparison trials (if the data is compelling enough), will ensure optimal care for our patients with metastatic breast cancer.

3. HIGH-RISK PRIMARY BREAST CANCER

3.1. History

High-risk primary breast cancer is disease limited to the breast and axillary lymph nodes that carries with it a less than 40% chance of 5-year relapse-free survival despite surgery, adjuvant and neoadjuvant chemotherapy, and chest wall irradiation. The largest category of these patients who have been treated with high-dose chemotherapy and stem cell transplant are those with 10 or more positive axillary lymph nodes, although trials have included patients with locally advanced (stage IIIB) and inflammatory breast cancer.

During the late 1980s and early 1990s, a number of phase II trials adding a single course of high-dose chemotherapy with stem cell rescue to the base of surgery, chemotherapy, and radiation therapy were performed. These studies generally show that approximately 70% of the patients are progression-free at 2–3 years. The largest study with the longest follow-up was reported by Peters and colleagues (27) and included 85 patients with 10 or more involved axillary lymph nodes. Patients were treated with four cycles of CAF, followed by a high-dose combination of cyclophosphamide, cisplatinum, and carmustine, with stem cell infusion, involved field radiation therapy, and long-term tamoxifen. The event-free survival, which includes all relapses and treatment-related mortality for the treated patients at a median follow-up of 6.9 years, was 62%. The overall survival was 68%. This and other trials compared favorably with historical data, and a number of randomized comparison trials have been reported.

3.2. Comparison Trials of Adjuvant Therapy Followed
by a Single Course of High-Dose Chemotherapy

In 1990, the CALGB developed a randomized trial for newly diagnosed high-risk breast cancer. The preliminary results were reported in May 1999 *(28)*. This study was designed to compare the overall survival and event-free survival and toxicity of high-dose chemotherapy and stem cell transplantation with intermediate-dose chemotherapy without stem cell transplantation. As such, no control arm was present, although the study was a clear comparison of greater dose intensity with lesser dose intensity. Eligibility required stage II or IIIA breast cancer with pathologic identification of 10 or more axillary nodes, less than 8 weeks from definitive surgery, no evidence of metastatic breast cancer, normal organ function, and age 60 years or younger. Patients then received induction chemotherapy with CAF for four cycles. They were then randomized to autologous stem cell transplantation with high-dose cyclophosphamide, cisplatinum, and carmustine (CPB), followed by radiation and long-term tamoxifen, or an intermediate dose of CPB without stem cell transplantation, followed by radiation and tamoxifen. Patients receiving intermediate-dose CPB (cyclophosphamide 900 mg/m^2, cisplatinum 90 mg/m^2, carmustine 90 mg/m^2,) were offered high-dose CPB (cyclophosphamide 5,625 mg/m^2, cisplatinum 165 mg/m^2, carmustine 600 mg/m^2) and stem cell transplant at time of relapse.

Eight-hundred eighty four patients were enrolled in the trial, and 785 went on to randomization, with 394 patients randomized to high-dose chemotherapy and 391 patients randomized to intermediate-dose CPB. With a median of 3.6 years of follow-up, there was no difference in survival (78% versus 80%) and no difference in event-free survival (68% versus 64%). There was, however, a substantial decrease in the relapse rate with high-dose CPB (21.6% versus 32.2%, or 34% fewer relapses). This decrease in relapse rate was offset, however, by treatment-related mortality: there were 31 deaths (7.4%) in the high-dose CPB arm versus zero deaths in the intermediate-dose arm. Causes of mortality were infection, pulmonary toxicity, pulmonary hemorrhage, hemolytic uremic syndrome, and venoocclusive disease of the liver. Of note, a learning curve with the CPB regimen was noted, with a substantially decreased mortality from large centers with significant experience. The preliminary conclusions from this trial were that both arms demonstrated results superior to those of historical controls and that an insufficient number of events had occurred for definitive conclusions to be drawn. An estimated 2 years more of follow-up will be needed.

The Netherlands Cancer Institute reported in 1998 on 97 women who had indirect evidence for extensive axillary node metastases by a positive infraclavicular lymph node biopsy and who received three courses of neoadjuvant 5-fluorouracil, epirubicin, and cyclophosphamide (FEC) weekly for 3 weeks, followed by surgery *(30)*. Patients were then randomly assigned a fourth course of FEC followed by radiation and tamoxifen or a single course of high-dose chemotherapy (cyclophosphamide 6 g/m^2, thiotepa 480 mg/m^2, and carboplatinum 1600 mg/m^2) followed by stem cell rescue after a fourth course of FEC. Ninety-seven patients were enrolled, with 40 assigned conventional dose therapy and 41 assigned high-dose therapy. No patients died from regimen-related toxicity, with a median follow-up of 4 years. The 4-year overall and relapse-free survivals were not significantly different in either group and were 75% and 54%, respectively *(31)*.

Based on the randomized phase II trial, the Dutch working party on autotransplantation in solid tumors reported on a larger Phase III trial of the same design as the Netherlands Cancer Institute report of 1998 *(31a)*. They enrolled 885 patients and have conducted, as planned, a

Table 4
Randomized Trials of High-Dose Chemotherapy in High-Risk Breast Cancer

Trial and reference	No. of patients	Toxic death (%) ABMT	Control	EFS (%) ABMT	Control	OS (%) ABMT	Control	P-value
CALGB Intergroup (28)	783	7.4	0	68[a]	64[a]	79[a]	79[a]	NS
Scandinavian (33)	525	0.7	0	68[b]	62[b]	79[b]	76[b]	NS
Netherlands (30)	81	0	0	70[c]	65[c]	82[c]	75[c]	NS
M.D. Anderson (32)	78	2.5	0	48[c]	55[c]	60[c]	68[c]	NS

ABMT, autologous bone marrow transplant; EFS, event-free survival; OS, overall survival.

[a] At 3 yr.

[b] At 2 yr.

[c] At 4 yr.

subgroup analysis of the first 284. 141 patients were assigned conventional dose therapy, and 143 were assigned high-dose therapy. The treatment-related mortality for the high-dose arm was 1%. The 3-yr overall survival was significantly different, with an advantage for high-dose therapy of 77% versus 62% (p = 0.009). The 3-yr recurrence-free survival was also improved for high-dose therapy, 89% versus 79% (p = 0.039). A more definitive analysis of the entire group is slated for July, 2002.

A small phase II trial from the Dana Farber institute included 50 women with locally unresectable and inflammatory breast cancer. Patients received four 2-week cycles of doxorubicin 90 mg/m^2, followed by STAMP V with stem cell infusion, radiotherapy, and tamoxifen. The 30-month disease-free survival was estimated at 64%, comparable to the results of other high-risk primary breast cancer transplant protocols (23).

3.3. Conclusions and Future Directions for High-Dose Therapy and Stem Cell Transplantation in High-Risk Breast Cancer

Unlike the data for metastatic breast cancer, the information from randomized trials for high-risk breast cancer is premature and inconclusive (Table 4). All trials are either small or have not yet reached maturity of data to make definitive conclusions. Additionally, no study yet reported compares standard therapy with high-dose therapy.

The ECOG initiated a trial in 1990 for patients with 10 or more involved axillary lymph nodes. All patients received six cycles of conventional dose CAF chemotherapy, adjuvant radiation, and long-term tamoxifen. At the time of registration, patients were randomized either to no other therapy or to a single course of high-dose cyclophosphamide 6 g/m^2 and thiotepa 800 mg/m^2 with stem cell infusion. This is the only true comparison of standard dose therapy with high-dose chemotherapy; the results will not be available for another 2 years. Additionally, the group of patients with moderately high-risk breast cancer, those with four to nine involved axillary lymph nodes, or those with inflammatory breast cancer remain to be studied. The SWOG has completed a randomized trial for women with four to nine involved lymph nodes to compare sequential high-dose therapy without stem cell rescue using the Memorial ATC regimen versus a single course of either CBP or CTCb high-dose chemotherapy with stem cell rescue. This important trial did not meet its accrual goal, but still enrolled over 600 patients. No randomized trial in inflammatory breast cancer has yet been initiated. The incidence of this disease is so low that accrual to a randomized trial would probably not be sufficient for completion.

Compilation of data in the high-risk breast cancer setting suggests that high-dose therapy and stem cell transplant remains promising. Patients should continue to enroll in well-designed clinical trials; final therapeutic decision making will require long-term follow-up.

REFERENCES

1. Henderson IC (1990) Basic principles in the use of adjuvant therapy. *Semin. Oncol.* **17**, 40–44.
2. (1990) *ABMTR Newslett.* **5**, 5.
3. Peters WP, Shpall EJ, Jones RB, et al. (1988) High-dose combination alkylating agents with bone marrow support as initial treatment for metastatic breast cancer. *J. Clin. Oncol.* **6**, 1368–1376.
4. Williams, SF, Mick R, Desser R, et al. (1989) High dose consolidation therapy with autologous stem cell rescue in stage IV breast cancer. *J. Clin. Oncol.* **7**, 1824–1830.
5. Antman K, Ayash L, Elias A, et al. (1992) A phase II study of high dose cyclophosphamide, thiotepa, and carboplatin with autologous marrow support in women with measurable advanced breast cancer responding to standard-dose therapy. *J. Clin. Oncol.* **10**, 102–110.
6. Williams SF, Gilewski T, Mick R, et al. (1992) High-dose consolidation therapy with autologous stem cell rescue in stage IV breast cancer: follow-up report. *J. Clin. Oncol.* **10**, 1743–1747.
7. Moonneier JA, Williams SF, Kamminer LS, et al. (1990) High dose trialkylator chemotherapy with autologous stem cell rescue in patients with refractory malignances. *J. Natl. Cancer. Inst.* **82**, 29–34.
8. Kennedy MJ, Beveridge RA, Rowley SD, et al. (1991) High-dose chemotherapy with reinfusion of purged autologous bone marrow following dose intense induction as initial therapy for metastatic breast cancer. *J. Natl. Cancer. Inst.* **83**, 920–926.
9. Eddy DM (1992) Review article. High-dose chemotherapy with autologous bone marrow transplantation for the treatment of metastatic breast cancer. *J. Clin. Oncol.* **10**, 657–670.
10. Klumpp TR, Mangan KF, Glenn LD (1993) Phase II pilot study of high-dose busulfan and CY followed by autologous BM or peripheral blood stem cell transplantation in patients with advanced chemosensitive breast cancer. *Bone Marrow Transplant.* **11**, 337–339.
11. Lazarus HM, Gray R, Ciobanu N, et al. (1994) A phase I trial of high-dose melphalan, high-dose etoposide, and autologous bone marrow reinfusion in solid tumors: an Eastern Cooperative Oncology Group (ECOG) study. *Bone Marrow Transplant.* **14**, 443–448.
12. Weaver CH, Bensinger WI, Appelbaum FR, et al. (1994) Phase I study of high-dose busulfan, melphalan, and thiotepa with autologous stem cell support in patients with refractory malignancies. *Bone Marrow Transplant.* **14**, 813–819.
13. Vaughan WP, Reed EC, Edwards B, et al. (1994) High-dose cyclophosphamide, thiotepa and hydroxyurea with autologous hematopoietic stem cell rescue: an effective consolidation chemotherapy regimen for early metastatic breast cancer. *Bone Marrow Transplant.* **13**, 619–624.
14. Fields KK, Elfenbein GJ, Lazarus HM, et al. (1995) Maximum tolerated doses of ifosfamide, carboplatin, and etoposide given over six days followed by autologous stem cell rescue: toxicity profile. *J. Clin. Oncol.* **13**, 323–332.
15. Spitzer TR, Cirenza E, McAfee S, et al. (1995) Phase I-II trial of high-dose cyclophosphamide, carboplatin and autologous bone marrow or peripheral blood stem cell rescue. *Bone Marrow Transplant.* **15**, 537–542.
16. Gisselbrecht C, Extra JM, Lotz JP, et al. (1996) Cyclophosphamide/mitoxantrone/melphalan (CMA) regimen prior to autologous bone marrow transplantation (ABMT) in metastatic breast cancer. *Bone Marrow Transplant.* **18**, 857–863.
17. Stemmer SM, Cagnoni PJ, Shpall EJ, et al. (1996) High-dose paclitaxel, cyclophosphamide, and cisplatin with autologous hematopoietic progenitor-cell support: a phase I trial. *J. Clin. Oncol.* **14**, 1463–1472.
18. Stadtmauer EA, O'Neill A, Goldstein LJ, et al. (2000) Conventional-dose chemotherapy compared with high-dose chemotherapy plus autologous hematopoietic stem-cell transplantation for metastatic breast cancer. Philadelphia Bone Marrow Transplant Group. *N. Engl. J. Med.* **342**, 1069–1076.
19. Lotz JP, Cure H, Janvier M, et al. (1999) High-dose chemotherapy with hematopoietic stem cells transplantation for metastatic breast cancer: results of the French protocol Pegase 04. *Proc. Am. Soc. Clin. Oncol.* **18**, 43A.

20. Berry DA, Broadwater G, Perry MC, et al. (2002) High-dose vs standard chemotherapy in metastatic breast cancer: comparison of Cancer and Leukemia Group B trials with data from the Autologous Blood and Marrow Transplant Registry. *J. Clin. Oncol.* **20,** 743–750.

21. Peters W, Jones R, Vredenburgh J, et al. (1996) A large prospective randomized trial of high-dose combination alkylating agents (CPB) with autologous cellular support as consolidation for patients with metastatic breast cancer achieving complete remission after intensive doxorubicin-based induction therapy (AFM). *Proc. Am. Soc. Clin. Oncol.* **15,** 121.

22. Rowlings PA, Williams SF, Antman KH, et al. (1999) Factors correlated with progression-free survival after high-dose chemotherapy and hematopoietic stem cell transplantation for metastatic breast cancer. *JAMA* **282,** 1335–1343.

23. Ayash LJ, Elias A, Schwartz G, et al. (1996) Double dose-intensive chemotherapy with autologous stem-cell support for metastatic breast cancer: no improvement in progression-free survival by the sequence of high-dose melphalan followed by cyclophosphamide, thiotepa and carboplatin. *J. Clin. Oncol.* **14,** 2984–2992.

24. Bezwoda W, Seymour L, Dansey R (1995) High-dose chemotherapy with hematopoietic rescue as primary treatment for metastatic breast cancer: a randomized trial. *J. Clin. Oncol.* **13,** 2483–2489.

25. Elias AD, Richardson P, Avigan D, et al. (1999) Phase I development of double cycle stem cell supported high dose chemotherapy (HDC) for metastatic breast cancer (BC): the DFCI/BIDMC experience. *Proc. ASCO.* **18,** 123a.

26. Pecora AL, Lazarus HM, Stadtmauer EA, et al. (2001) Effect of induction chemotherapy and tandem cycles of high-dose chemotherapy on outcomes in autologous stem cell transplant for metastatic breast cancer. *Bone Marrow Transplant* **27,** 1245–1253.

26a. Crump M (2001) A randomized trial of high-dose chemotherapy with autologous peripheral blood stem cell support compared to standard therapy in women with metastatic breast cancer. *Proc. Am. Soc. Clin. Oncol.* **20,** Abstr. 82.

27. Peters WP, Ross M, Vredenburgh JJ, et al. (1993) High-dose chemotherapy and autologous bone marrow transplant support as consolidation after standard-dose adjuvant therapy for high-risk primary breast cancer. *J. Clin. Oncol.* **11,** 1132–1143.

28. Peters WP, Rosner G, Vredenburgh J, et al. (1999) A prospective, randomized comparison of two doses of combination alkylating agents as consolidation after CAF in high-risk primary breast cancer involving ten or more axillary lymph nodes. *Proc. Am. Soc. Clin. Oncol.* **18,** 1A.

29. Bezwoda WR (1998) Primary high-dose chemotherapy for metastatic breast cancer: update and analysis of prognostic factors. *Proc. Am. Soc. Clin. Oncol.* **17,** 115A.

30. Rodenhuis S, Richel KJ, Wall E, et al. (1998) Randomized trial of high-dose chemotherapy and hematopoietic progenitor cell support in operable breast cancer with extensive axillary lymph node involvement. *Lancet* **352,** 515–521.

31. Ayash LJ, Elias A, Ibrahim J, et al. (1998) High-dose multimodality therapy with autologous stem-cell support for Stage IIIB breast carcinoma. *J. Clin. Oncol.* **16,** 1000–1007.

31a. Rodenhuis S (2001) Randomized phase III study of high-dose chemotherapy in operable breast cancer with 4 or more axillary lymph nodes. *Proc. Am. Soc. Clin. Oncol.* **19,** Abstr. 286.

32. Hortobagyi GN, Buzdar AU, Theriault RL, et al. (2000) Randomized trial of hig-dose chemotherapy and blood cell autografts for high-risk primary breast carcinoma. *J. Natl. Cancer. Inst.* **92,** 225–233.

33. Bergh J, Wiklund T. Erikstein B, et al. (2000) Tailored fluorouracil, epirubicin, and cyclophosphamide compared with marrow-supported high-dose chemotherapy as adjuvant treatment for high-risk breast cancer: a randomised trial. Scandinavian Breast Group 9401 study. *Lancet* **356,** 1384–1391.

24 Immunotherapy and Gene Therapy for Breast Cancer

Daniela Santoli, PhD, and Sophie Visonneau, PhD

CONTENTS

INTRODUCTION
GROWTH FACTOR RECEPTOR INHIBITION
ANTIANGIOGENIC THERAPY
GENE THERAPY
ADOPTIVE IMMUNOTHERAPY
CONCLUSIONS
REFERENCES

1. INTRODUCTION

To this day, surgery, chemotherapy, hormonal therapy, and radiation therapy remain the main forms of treatment for breast cancer. Although these approaches reduce the risk of death and can induce complete remissions in most patients, many tumors will recur as metastatic lesions. In recent years, novel therapies have been developed that work independently or in conjunction with conventional treatments to minimize side effects and enhance therapeutic efficacy. At least two areas have emerged in which the biology of breast cancer is most likely to have a therapeutic impact. The first area involves growth factors and their receptors, the second revolves around neoangiogenesis. In addition, cell- and gene-based approaches are being evaluated in the clinic that have either a direct tumoricidal function or act by stimulating the immune system against the patient's own tumor cells. This chapter reviews the current status of these new therapies and some of the new products that are being evaluated for clinical toxicity and preliminary efficacy.

2. GROWTH FACTOR RECEPTOR INHIBITION

At least three classes of specific tyrosine kinase receptors play an important role in the biology of breast cancer: the epidermal growth factor receptor (EGFR), c-*erb* B-2 or (HER-2/*neu*), c-*erb* B-3, c-*erb* B-4, and the fibroblastic growth factor receptors (FGFR). Members of this receptor family are characterized by an external ligand receptor domain, a transmembrane portion, and an internal domain containing a tyrosine kinase responsible for initiation of intracellular signaling of the receptor. The extracellular domain represents an obvious therapeutic target, particularly given the frequent overexpression of cell membrane receptor

From: *Current Clinical Oncology:*
Breast Cancer: A Guide to Detection and Multidisciplinary Therapy
Edited by: M. H. Torosian © Humana Press Inc., Totowa, NJ

sites (for EGF and heregulin) by breast cancers. The external domain can be targeted in several fashions. First, agents blocking or preventing ligand binding (e.g., monoclonal antibodies [MAbs]) may be used in a way analogous to the use of tamoxifen for the estrogen receptor. Second, using either ligand or antibody directed against the extracellular domain, linked toxins may be brought into contact with and internalized by the cancer cell *(1)*. Such toxins include classic chemotherapeutic agents, cell poisons such as ricin or diptheria toxins, and radionucleotides. Third, the external domain may be used to attract immune effector cells, as recently examined in phase I trials, through the use of bispecific antibodies recognizing both breast cancer cells and monocyte/macrophage cells *(2)*. Agents with the ability to affect the internal (tyrosine kinase) domain of members of the EGF family have been recently identified and shown to have in vitro activity against breast cancer cells *(3)*. Several phase I/II trials are currently examining such agents in combination with other drugs in women with advanced disease.

Recently, HER-2/neu has become the target of a new therapy evaluated in a multicenter setting. This receptor is overexpressed in 20–30% of breast tumors. A MAb against neu has been selected for its high affinity for the receptor, lack of crossreactivity with other tyrosine kinase receptors, and ability to inhibit the growth of a cell line overexpressing neu *(4)*. A number of objective responses have been recorded in phase II trials of this MAb in patients with advanced breast cancer who were pretreated with a median number of three chemotherapy regimens *(4)*. In addition, an ongoing international multicenter trial is currently investigating whether a conventional first-line regimen of doxorubicin/cyclophosphamide for metastatic disease can be rendered more effective by concomitant administration of the MAb in patients whose tumors overexpress the neu protein. In particular, the use of naked MAb directed against HER-2/*neu* (c-*erb* B-2) induced a response in approx 12% of patients with advanced breast cancer *(4)*. Pegram et al. *(5)* used an anti-HER-2/neu MAb in combination with cisplatin in patients with advanced breast cancer, with objective response being seen in 25% of patients. Another phase I study was conducted by Valone et al. *(2)* using a bispecific MAb for HER-2/neu and monocyte/macrophage cells in breast cancer patients. As these trials have seen responses in patients refractory to multiple chemotherapy regimens, it will be interesting to examine this approach in less heavily pretreated patients.

3. ANTIANGIOGENIC THERAPY

As first demonstrated by Folkman's group nearly a decade ago, the growth of tumors larger than 1 mm in diameter requires angiogenesis, the development of a new blood supply, from preexisting vasculature *(6)*. This applies to both the primary and secondary lesions. In human tumors, the number of dividing endothelial cells may be 50 times greater than in normal tissue. These vessels are leaky, have upregulated vascular growth factor receptors and cell adhesion molecules, and are in a procoagulant state. Thus, they provide a new therapeutic target with many factors differently expressed between tumor and normal endothelium.

Many immunohistochemical studies have suggested that robust new blood vessel formation is associated with impaired prognosis in early-stage breast cancer. New blood vessel formation therefore represents a promising new therapeutic target for this disease. About 20 angiogenesis inhibitors are currently being tested in early phase I or II clinical trials. Some are entering phase III testing. The five strategies described below are currently being used to design antiangiogenesis agents.

3.1. Blockade of Angiogenic Peptides

New blood vessel formation requires stimulation of vascular endothelial cells through the release of angiogenic peptides, such as FGF and vascular endothelial growth factor (VEGF). Prevention of this stimulation has been demonstrated to prevent angiogenesis and tumor growth in experimental model systems *(7)*. Several agents are capable of preventing binding of basic FGF to its receptor, including pentosan polysulfate, which directly binds FGF, and suramin, which inhibits receptor binding. Thymidine phosphorylase, an enzyme that produces an angiogenic sugar from thymidine, is a novel class of angiogenesis inducer that is upregulated by hypoxia and is overexpressed early in breast cancer. High expression is associated with a good response to cyclophosphamide, methotrexate, and 5-fluorouracil (CMF) chemotherapy, possibly by preventing thymidine salvage. VEGF may function via upregulation of nitric oxide production, which is also angiogenic. A range of proteases expressed by endothelial cells or stroma have an important role in angiogenesis, particularly urokinase. Interferon-α (IFN-α) is another drug that blocks activators of angiogenesis.

3.2. Inhibition of Proliferating Endothelial Cells

Vascular endothelial cells are normally quiescent in adults. Proliferating vascular endothelial cells can be targeted either through the use of MAbs or through the use of agents such as the antibiotic TNP-470 (AGM-1470), a synthetic fumagillin analog that is currently entering phase I and II clinical trials *(8)*. Thalidomide, squalanine, combretastatin A-4, and endostatin are other examples of drugs that inhibit endothelial cells directly.

3.3. Inhibition of Vessel Basement Membrane Turnover

New blood vessel growth is dependent on the enzyme systems required for basement membrane dissolution, in particular, metalloproteinases (MMPs). Inhibition of these MMPs by chemical means has been demonstrated to inhibit angiogenesis *(9,10)*. Marimastat, one of the drugs that blocks the ability of the endothelial cells to break down the surrounding matrix, is being evaluated in a randomized phase III trial in patients with metastatic breast cancer who have responding or stable disease after induction chemotherapy.

3.4. Attacks on Extracellular Matrix Proteins

Cell adhesion molecules of the integrin family ($\alpha_v\beta_3$ and $\alpha_v\beta_5$ integrins) are upregulated on proliferating tumor vessels, and inhibition of their function causes apoptosis of growing endothelial cells. Antibodies blocking attachment of vascular endothelium to such protein inhibits angiogenesis *(11)*. Vitaxin, a drug that inhibits endothelial-specific integrin/survival signaling is being tested clinically.

3.5. Stimulation of Natural Angiogenesis Inhibitors

It is now recognized that angiogenesis is regulated by a balance between proangiogenic and antiangiogenic factors and that loss of inhibitors may be an early stage in tumor progression. Inhibitors include thrombospondin, several cytokines (interleukin [IL]-4 and IL-12), and proteolytic breakdown products of several proteins; in particular, prolactin, EGF, plasminogen, and collagen XVIII can be degraded to produce inhibitory proteins.

New generations of antiangiogenic drugs, such as endostatin and angiostatin, induce regression of tumor vasculature and complete arrest of tumor growth without the development of drug resistance. These drugs are now entering phase I testing.

3.6. Summary

Antiangiogenesis strategies will be an important component of anticancer therapy in the near future and will produce new challenges for clinical trial design. Surrogate markers and monitoring of tumor vascularity may be useful adjuncts in assessing antiangiogenic effects. Furthermore, combinations of antiangiogenic drugs inhibiting different targets may be more effective than single agents. Preclinical studies have shown marked synergy of conventional chemotherapy agents with a range of antiangiogenic agents and have provided the rationale for combining them in clinical trials. Several strategies need to be evaluated for combination therapies, including administration of the antiangiogenesis agent continuously during chemotherapy, or only between courses. Then there is the question of maintenance therapy. This should be answered in randomized trials that compare responses to therapy to see whether remission duration can be prolonged with continuous antiangiogenesis therapy. The outcome of these types of trials will help determine how to use such approaches in the adjuvant setting.

4. GENE THERAPY

Development of gene therapy technologies is approaching clinical realization for the treatment of neoplastic diseases, including breast cancer. Two general strategies are being evaluated: 1) approaches that alter the metabolic or signaling pathways within the breast cancer cells; and 2) approaches designed to enhance the patient's immune response to the tumor cells.

4.1. Therapeutic Genes that Alter the Metabolic or Signaling Pathways in Breast Cancer Cells

All breast cancer cells contain molecular genetic abnormalities that contribute to tumor cell growth. Many of these genetic changes occur sporadically or at such low frequencies that they cannot be used as targets of gene-based therapies. However, a few molecular alterations, such as HER-2/*neu* and *p53,* occur with sufficient frequency that they could become useful therapeutic targets in a significant portion of breast cancer patients. The overexpression of HER-2/neu in 20–30% of breast cancer patients is associated with a worse prognosis by contributing to increased metastases and decreased sensitivity to chemotherapy. Several therapeutic approaches are being developed to target HER-2/*neu* genetically (reviewed in ref. *12*): in one approach, an antibody to HER-2/neu was synthesized within the tumor cell itself; in another system, an adenovirus vector was modified to encode a single-chain MAb that would bind HER-2/neu. Human breast cancers that overexpressed HER-2/*neu* were growth-arrested in vitro, whereas breast cancer cells that expressed little HER-2/neu were much less affected by this treatment. Alternatively, rather than inhibiting the HER-2/neu protein function after it is made, it is possible to block the synthesis of this protein altogether. The adenovirus E1A transcription factor (necessary for adenovirus replication) has been shown to block HER-2/neu expression by inhibiting expression of the HER-2/*neu* gene in breast cancer cells infected with adenovirus (reviewed in ref. *12*). This, in turn, sensitizes the cells to the cytotoxic effects of paclitaxel. This not only confirms the previous association of HER-2/neu overexpression with chemoresistance but also suggests that novel therapies can be based on the combined use of gene therapy and chemotherapy.

Mutations in the *p53* tumor suppressor gene represent the other most common molecular abnormality. Restoring normal *p53* function in breast cancer cells has been shown to decrease tumorigenicity by leading to cell cycle arrest and induction of apoptosis *(13).* Intravenously administered recombinant adenovirus expressing p53 substantially reduced the number of lung metastases and total tumor burden in a murine model of metastatic breast cancer *(14)*. From this and previous studies, it is apparent that intravenous dosing of adenovirus vectors (the current vector of choice for *p53*) induces significant liver injury. However, according to recent data, the newer generation adenovirus vectors, which have deletions of both the E4 and E1 adenovirus genes, have much less hepatotoxicity *(15)*. Application of these new adenovirus vectors to *p53*-based therapies could probably offer substantial improvements to therapeutic strategies. In addition to the direct effects on cell cycle, overexpression of the normal *p53* gene has been shown to restore sensitivity to doxorubicin *(16)*. Because overexpression of *p53* leads to an overall reduction in tumor blood vessels, the influence of the gene transfer extends far beyond the confines of the tumor cell that expresses the therapeutic gene. The enforced expression of *p53* has been shown to upregulate thrombospondin synthesis, which, in turn, is a negative regulator of tumor angiogenesis (see above). The contribution of this antiangiogenic effect to the overall therapy may turn out to be important because, with the current technology, it is not possible to effect gene transfer in all tumor cells. Understanding the mechanism(s) by which *p53* inhibits tumor growth will lead to improvement in cancer therapy.

Systemic antitumor effects may be achieved with tumor suppressor gene therapy by coadministering a cytokine gene. Putzer et al. *(17)* compared the effectiveness of *p53* and *IL-2* gene therapies either alone or in combination using adenovirus vectors. Whereas adenovirus delivery of *p53* or *IL-2* alone produced only transient delays in tumor growth, a single injection of a combination of the two vectors resulted in tumor regressions in 65% of the treated mice. In this immunocompetent transgenic mouse mammary adenocarcinoma model, half of the treated mice remained tumor-free. These mice developed systemic immunity to the tumors, as demonstrated by rechallenge experiments and in vitro measures of tumor-specific cytolytic T-lymphocyte activity.

4.2. Genetic Enhancement of the Immune Response to Breast Cancer

The enhancement of T-cell functions has become a major goal for immunotherapy against malignancies. T cells are highly specific in recognizing antigenic peptides. This is ideal for an anticancer reagent that is expected to recognize and destroy tumor cells, but not normal cells. Once activated, T cells differentiate into long-lived memory cells that recirculate continuously. This enables T cells to detect and destroy metastases that arise at distant sites at an early stage. Tumor-infiltrating lymphocytes (TILs) have been expanded ex vivo prior to readministration to cancer patients in combination with rhIL-2. This form of passive (and transient) immunization has been applied to patients with a variety of tumors, including breast cancer *(18)* (see below).

Rather than readministrating tumor-reactive T cells, active immunization can be used to enhance T-cell functions and potentially provide a longer period of therapy. Different vaccination strategies using DNA (encoding for a tumor antigen), purified protein, peptide, whole tumor cells, or tumor lysates have been developed for the treatment of breast cancer and other tumors *(19)*. Genetically modified tumor cells have been used to induce a cellular antitumor immune response. The rationale of using whole tumor cells as a vaccine is that they express the entire repertoire of antigens that would not be present when a defined tumor antigen is used. Thus, the knowledge of specific antigens is not required for the development of a vaccination strategy.

A recent approach that has been implemented in a variety of murine tumor models and in several clinical studies uses tumor cells that have been modified with gene-encoding cytokines. In these studies, the tumor-secreted cytokines are thought to upregulate locally either the stimulator or the effector arm of the immune system, depending on the cytokine gene used, thereby enhancing normal in vivo tumor surveillance systems. In mouse models, retroviral vectors have been used to transduce the genes for IL-2, granulocyte/macrophage colony-stimulating factor (GM-CSF), IL-4, and other cytokines into mouse tumor cell lines that have subsequently been used to immunize naive or tumor-bearing mice. Similar approaches have been tested in a mammary adenocarcinoma mouse model in which mice were challenged with the syngeneic adenocarcinoma cell line TSA-pc. Ten to 30% of mice injected with tumor cells modified with a variety of cytokine genes were protected even when administered 30 days after the initial tumor inoculum.

A growing number of cytokines and related soluble immune stimulatory factors have been systemically administered to bolster the immune response in patients. The principal problems encountered in the cytokine clinical trials have arisen from the systemic toxicity. Gene transfer strategies may overcome this by the local expression of cytokines within the tumor microenvironment. The gene-modified cells can then be introduced with the tumor cells as an irradiated vaccine (20). This approach allows the technique of gene delivery to be standardized in fibroblasts and is more reproducible than gene modification of tumor cells. Nonetheless, isolation and ex vivo modification of fibroblasts are cumbersome and expensive procedures and not amenable to use in most clinical practices. In vivo gene transfer overcomes this problem and can be readily implemented using adenovirus vectors (21). For example, an adenovirus expressing tumor necrosis factor-α (TNF-α) has been used in murine models of breast cancer to induce complete regression of spontaneous mammary tumors (22). Although the vector was injected into the tumor, systemic levels of TNF-α were achieved and resulted in significant toxicity. Similarly, a recombinant adenovirus expressing a human IFN consensus gene has been shown to induce regression of human breast cancers grown in immunodeficient mice (23).

In an alternative active immunotherapy strategy, the genes encoding some of the tumor antigens that have been definitely associated with breast cancer (such as HER-2 [c-*erb* B2], *p53,* and certain modified mucins) have been incorporated into vaccinia vectors for in vivo immunization. Vaccinia virus (VV) recombinants have been created expressing both the secreted and the membrane forms of epithelial tumor antigen (ETA); immunization of rats with vectors expressing the transmembrane form of ETA prevented tumor development in 82% of the animals inoculated with the tumor (24). In later studies, similar VV vectors containing the mucin Muc1 cDNA were used to immunize mice. These mice produced antibodies that recognized the mucin 20-amino acid tandem repeat, and 30% of them were protected from challenge with Muc1-expressing tumors (25). In addition, Muc1 synthetic peptide vaccines have been shown to inhibit the growth of Muc1-transfected tumor cells for prolonged survival of tumor-bearing mice (26). Similar immunization strategies are under clinical investigation using vector-based and mucin tandem repeat-based vaccines. Optimization of such strategies will be important to maximize therapeutic benefit and to implement adoptive immunotherapy protocols efficiently.

4.3. Gene Therapy in Autologous Transplantation

Several therapeutic strategies for breast cancer have been proposed that involve the transfer of specific genes into hematopoietic stem cells or precursors. One of the major therapeutic strategies targeting gene transfer into CD34+ cells involves the use of the multidrug-resistance (MDR) gene, which codes for the P-glycoprotein transmembrane pump. Production of P-glycoprotein confers resistance to many chemotherapeutic drugs, such as anthracyclines, vinca alkaloids, etoposide, and paclitaxel *(27)*, which have hematopoietic toxicities. Successful expression of a transgenic MDR gene in stem cells and progenitors is hypothesized to increase their resistance to these agents, allowing increased dosages with decreased side effects. In preclinical studies, the MDR gene has been successfully incorporated into retroviral vectors and transduced into mouse cells. Mice transplanted with BM cells carrying the MDR1 transgene became resistant to the myelosuppressive effects of doxorubicin, daunomycin, paclitaxel, vinblastine, vincristine, etoposide, and actinomycin D for up to 17 months post transplant *(28)*. Based on these encouraging results, two clinical protocols involving autologous transplantation in breast cancer patients have been approved for transduction of the MDR1 gene into CD34$^+$ cells in order to monitor MDR1 transduction efficiency, transgene expression, and subsequent resistance of the transduced cells to paclitaxel.

4.4. Summary

Several gene therapy clinical trials are under way for a variety of cancers, but only a few have been initiated for breast cancer. The heterogeneity of breast cancer biology and the secretion of immunosuppressive factors are two examples of the difficulties faced in breast cancer gene therapy. Nevertheless, recent improvements in our understanding of the cellular and molecular biology of breast cancer have revealed several potentially clinically useful gene therapy approaches, thus offering an alternative form of treatment that may be useful in combination with conventional therapies.

5. ADOPTIVE IMMUNOTHERAPY

In the last decade, there have been major advances in the understanding of the immune system and the identification and cloning of tumor-associated antigens (TAAs). This has opened new avenues for cancer immunotherapy. Immunotherapy offers a promising alternative to conventional therapy because the systemic nature of the immune response can access disseminated disease and its specificity may limit undesirable side effects.

5.1. Adoptive Cell Therapy with Nonspecific Effectors

One avenue of adoptive immunotherapy is based on the transfer of autologous, i.e., patient-derived, effector cells, such as lymphokine-activated killer (LAK) cells or TILs. Both types of effectors have been expanded ex vivo and reinjected in the patients in combination with IL-2 for treatment of several types of tumors *(29,30)*.

5.1.1. THERAPY WITH TILS

In breast cancer, TILs have been reported to be associated with a better prognosis *(31)*. It is not known, however, whether these TILs are directed at specific antigens or whether they represent a nonspecific infiltrate in response to cellular damage. In a National Cancer Institute study, the TIL cells characterized from 19 breast cancer patients were, on average, 73% CD3$^+$ and 21% CD8$^+$. Only 1 of 15 cultures tested showed lytic activity against autologous tumor. Three of 11 TIL preparations specifically secreted TNF-α, IFN-γ, and GM-CSF when exposed to autologous tumor and not when cocultured with allogeneic breast tumor. Despite these in vitro studies, very few breast cancer patients have been treated with TIL, and in those treated, there have been no resposes. One significant obstacle to the widespread use of breast TIL is the low number of T cells that can be recovered from the relatively small breast tumors. TIL cytotoxicity can be enhanced in vitro by stimulation with IL-2, suggesting that the differential expression of cytokines by tumor cells or TILs may impair the antitumor immune response in vivo. In mRNA detection assays (using reverse-transcriptase polymerase chain reaction and *in situ* hybridization), TILs from breast cancers did not secrete IL-2 or IL-4 *(32)*, suggesting a downregulation of cellular immunity. Moreover, IL-10, which has been detected in primary breast cancers, is associated with the induction of T-cell anergy *(33)* (as a result of inhibition of T-cell proliferation and function) as well as reduced IL-2 production and antigen presentation *(34)*.

5.1.2. IL-2/LAK Cell Therapy

Two phase II trials of high-dose IL-2/LAK therapy were performed in patients with either advanced breast carcinoma or advanced cancer arising in other sites *(35)*. Most of the patients had failed prior chemotherapy. Patients received high-dose IL-2 (600,000 IU/kg) on days 1–5 and 11–15. Leukophoresis was performed for collection and ex vivo expansion of LAK cells on days 7–10, and the LAK cells were reinfused on days 11, 12, and 14. The studies were designed to determine whether treatment with IL-2/LAK would result in at least a 40% response rate, a level of activity that was believed to be sufficient to justify the toxicity and cost of IL-2/LAK therapy. Of all patients, one with adenocarcinoma of the breast had a partial response of 17 weeks' duration, and 2 had minor tumor regression (adenocarcinoma of the lung and spindle cell sarcoma of the lung). It was concluded that high-dose IL-2/LAK is not likely to be associated with a response rate exceeding 40% for patients with carcinomas arising in the breast, pancreas, ovary, and lung (non-small cell carcinoma) *(35)*.

5.1.3. Allogeneic Cell Therapy

Transfer of allogeneic effectors appears to be an effective treatment for patients relapsing after allogeneic bone marrow transplantation (ABMT), since tumor cells resisting chemoradiotherapy may still respond to immunocompetent allogeneic lymphocytes. Substantial evidence supports the conclusion that donor T cells mediate a potent graft-versus-tumor (GVT) reaction *(36,37)*. For instance, up to 80% of patients who relapse with chronic myelogenous leukemia after ABMT will achieve a complete remission after infusions of unmodified HLA-matched donor leukocytes *(38)*. A complete remission represents an approximate 6-log reduction in tumor burden, highlighting the potency of the GVT effect. Outside the setting of allogeneic transplantation, HLA-matched donor leukocytes have been administered as primary therapy and may induce a direct GVT reaction for some patients with hematologic malignancies who have not had a prior allogeneic stem cell transplant *(39)*. Furthermore, donor cells may engraft and possibly induce a direct GVT reaction in some patients after non-myeloablative chemotherapy *(39–41)*. These methods of adoptive immunotherapy utilize closely HLA-matched donor T cells. Sustained engraftment may not be required for GVT induction, or detectable levels of donor cells may be unnecessary for a response. In studies of human allogeneic adoptive immunotherapy, complete response has been noted even when residual donor cells were undetectable *(39)*. This implies either that the GVT effect occurs before donor cell rejection or that small numbers of donor cells, below the limit of detection by molecular analysis, may be sufficient to generate an antitumor reaction.

GVT potential may not be limited to hematologic malignancies, and preliminary data suggest that breast cancer may be an appropriate target for GVT induction *(41)*. Furthermore, a clinically significant GVT effect has been suggested after HLA-matched sibling allogeneic stem cell transplantation for patients with metastatic breast cancer *(42,43)*. Or et al. *(44)* have recently investigated possible GVT effects in six patients with metastatic breast cancer; such effects would be comparable to the graft-versus-leukemia phenomenon occurring after

ABMT in hematologic malignancies. The patients were cytoreduced with high-dose chemotherapy and autologous stem cell transplantation and were treated on an ambulatory basis by adoptive transfer of HLA-matched donor peripheral blood lymphocytes (PBLs) activated in vivo with rhIL-2. If no graft-versus-host disease (GVHD) developed, allogeneic cell therapy was augmented with infusion of donor PBLs, preactivated in vitro with rhIL-2. Treatment was well tolerated, with low therapy-related toxicity in all patients. Two patients developed signs and symptoms compatible with GVHD grade I–II, one of whom showed no evidence of disease more than 34 months later. In the remaining patients, progression-free survival following allogeneic cell therapy ranged between 7 and 13 months.

5.1.4. TALL-104 Cells: A Novel Cell Therapy Approach to Cancer

Our laboratory has developed a novel and potent adoptive cell therapy approach to cancer based on the transfer of an IL-2-dependent human leukemic T-cell line (CD3/T-cell receptor [TCR]$\alpha\beta^+$CD8$^+$CD4$^-$CD56$^+$CD16$^-$) named TALL-104 *(45–57)*. TALL-104 cells display uniquely potent MHC-nonrestricted cytotoxic and cytostatic activities against tumors across species, without affecting cells from normal tissues. Unlike patient-derived LAK cells and TILs, TALL-104 cells represent a universal donor system and provide an unlimited and reliable source of tumoricidal cells with stable cytotoxic activity, which is ideal for adoptive immunotherapy approaches. Although dependent on IL-2 for expression of cytotoxicity and long-term survival in vitro, TALL-104 cells can exert antitumor effects in vivo without the concomitant administration of IL-2, thus eliminating the potential toxicity of this cytokine *(46–53)*. TALL-104 cells induce necrotic tumor cell death via a perforin-dependent secretory pathway and can also kill targets through the release of cytotoxic mediators, such as TNF-α, TNF-β, IFN-γ, or transforming growth factor-β (TGF-β). Several tumor targets are killed by apoptosis. Adoptively transferred γ-irradiated (nonproliferating) TALL-104 cells were able to induce 70–80% regression of established metastases in 100% of immunodeficient mice bearing human hematopoietic and nonhematopoietic tumors *(45–52)*. Remarkable antitumor effects were also seen in immunocompetent mice bearing syngeneic leukemia *(50)*; importantly, TALL-104 cell transfer in these animals was followed by the development of host antitumor immunity, which was demonstrated by tumor rechallenge experiments *(50)*.

Breast tumors are particularly sensitive to the lytic activity of TALL-104 in vitro. Our laboratory has studied the efficacy of TALL-104 cell therapy in mice implanted with human breast tumors and in pet dogs and cats with spontaneous mammary carcinomas. Because of the encouraging results obtained in these preclinical studies, we have proceeded to perform a phase I clinical trial in women with metastatic breast cancer. Results of these studies are summarized below.

5.1.4.1. TALL-104 Therapy of a Metastatic Breast Cancer Xenograft in Severe Combined Immunodeficient (SCID) Mice.

Tumor fragments from a surgical specimen of a patient with infiltrating ductal carcinoma were implanted subcutaneously in the flank region of SCID mice *(51)*. All animals developed a local tumor mass that metastasized to subaxillary and inguinal lymph nodes, bones, lungs, liver, kidneys, ovaries, and brain, very closely mimicking the human disease. Multiple intraperitoneal transfers of γ-irradiated TALL-104 cells administered in an *advanced disease stage* resulted in a significant or total regression of established metastasis, with no obvious macroscopic changes in the primary tumor mass *(51)*. Although no significant differences could be found between the primary tumor mass of the treated mice and that of the control survivor mice at a macroscopic level, the histologic appearance of the tumors was consistently and strikingly different, with necrosis observed only in the TALL-104-treated group. Unlike the primary tumor mass, metastatic disease was significantly lower in the TALL-104-treated group than in the control group. In addition, whereas 100% of the control mice had macroscopic metastases, histologic analysis performed on the TALL-104-treated mice revealed only the presence of micrometastases in the lungs, liver, and kidneys of 50% of the animals; the other 50% were virtually free of systemic disease.

In a *minimal disease* setting, TALL-104 cell therapy administered intraperitoneally daily for 2 weeks, followed by two weekly injections, completely arrested local tumor growth and prevented systemic spread into local lymph nodes and distant organs. Histologic analysis confirmed the absence of malignant cells both in the tissues surrounding the initial area of engraftment and in lymph node regions. No lung metastases could be detected in any of the treated mice. Polymerase chain reaction (PCR) analysis confirmed the absence of breast cancer cells in the peripheral blood and bone marrow of the treated animals.

Finally, in a more relevant clinical setting (i.e., after *surgical removal of the primary tumor*), TALL-104 cell treatment inhibited regrowth of breast tumor cells at the primary site and the metastatic spread to lymph nodes by 15 and 4.5%, respectively, compared with the controls animals. At necropsy, no macroscopic metastases were detected in any of the TALL-104-treated mice, and only a few micrometastases were seen histologically in their lungs, kidneys, and spinal cord. PCR analysis showed infiltration of the peripheral blood (but not of the bone marrow) in 50% of the animals *(51)*.

The biodistribution of ^{51}Cr-labeled TALL-104 cells was investigated in this tumor model system *(51,54)*. Upon intraperitoneal injection, TALL-104 cell homing in major thoracic and abdominal organs was similar to that observed in healthy mice. It is noteworthy that levels of radioactivity observed in metastatic lymph nodes were consistently two to six times higher than those in the primary tumor masses. Moreover, in mice that showed an imbalanced tumor load in kidneys and ovaries, radioactivity levels were two to three times higher in the organs with more tumor involvement than in the less affected contralateral organs, suggesting a preferential accumulation of the effector cells to tumor sites.

Another metastatic breast cancer xenograft model was established in severe combined immunodeficiency (SCID) mice upon subcutaneous injection of the human breast cancer cell line MDA-MB231. These cells grew locally, giving rise to subcutaneous tumor masses, and spread distantly to lungs, spleen, liver, and kidneys. In this model, biodistribution studies of ^{111}In-labeled TALL-104 cells injected intravenously showed a different migration pattern than the one observed in healthy mice. In particular, the lung clearance of TALL-104 cells was significantly delayed. In paired organs, such as kidneys, there was a selective accumulation of labeled cells into the side where a higher tumor infiltration occurred. Similar studies in immunocompetent BALB/c mice bearing syngeneic 66.1 mammary tumors indicated a selective trapping of TALL-104 cells into pulmonary and lymph node metastases *(54)*.

5.1.4.2. Adoptive Therapy of Canine and Feline Mammary Carcinoma Using TALL-104 Cells. Spontaneously arising tumors in domestic animals share several common features with human cancer in regard to incidence, histologic features, biologic behavior, and response to therapy, thus constituting ideal models to study novel translational forms of cancer therapy not immediately acceptable for use in humans.

Metastatic mammary tumors *in dogs* are poorly responsive to chemotherapy; the prognosis following mastectomy for invasive adenocarcinoma is poor, and, to date, therapeutic studies using hormonal and/or immunotherapy have lacked efficacy. Four dogs diagnosed with anaplastic adenocarcinoma metastatic to lungs (L.H.), highly malignant lobular carci-

Table 1
Canine Mammary Tumors[a]

Dog's initials	Time of first TALL-104 therapy after surgery	Duration of TALL-104 therapy[b] (months)	DFI from start of TALL-104 (months)	Site of relapse	Outcome (from start of TALL-104)
L.H.	—	3	n.a.	n.a.	PR (2 mo) SD (2.5 mo)[c] Died of disease
B.T.[d]	1.5 mo	8.5	n.a.	n.a.	CR (16 mo) Died of unrelated causes
W.P.	10 d	28	19 42	Local LN	Alive with disease
G.M.	2 mo	22	13.5 30.5	Local LN	Died of disease (32 mo)

n.a., not applicable; CR, complete response; PR, partial response; SD, stable disease; DFI, disease-free interval; LN, lymph nodes.

[a] Metastatic mammary tumors in dogs are poorly responsive to chemotherapy, with 80% recurring within 6 months.

[b] Lethally irradiated TALL-104 cells were given systemically for 5 consecutive days at 10^8/kg, followed by monthly boosts for 1–2 days.

[c] L.H. had advanced metastatic disease in the lung: a 50% reduction of the major lung lesion (partial response) as well as stabilization of other lung lesions were seen within 2 weeks from start of TALL-104 therapy.

[d] B.T. went into complete remission after TALL-104 therapy.

noma metastatic to lymph nodes with extensive invasion of the subcutis and vessels (B.T.), tubular adenocarcinoma metastatic to lymph nodes (W.P.), and papillary cystadenocarcinoma metastatic to lymph nodes (G.M.), were entered in the TALL-104 study shortly after removal of their primary tumor mass (Table 1).

Dogs B.T., W.P., and G.M., which showed no evidence of chest metastatic disease at the time of enrollment in the TALL-104 study, underwent surgical removal of the metastatic lymph nodes before cell therapy. Dog L.H. received irradiated TALL-104 cells (10^8 cells/kg) systemically every other day for 2 weeks followed by 12 more injections over a 3-month period; the other dogs were treated daily for 5 days followed by 8 monthly boosts for 2 days each. After 2 weeks of cell treatment, L.H. achieved a partial response consisting of 50% reduction of the largest lung metastases for 2 months; stabilization of the other lung lesions for 10 weeks after initiation of cell treatment was also seen, accompanied by the development of tumor-specific immune responses (57). Upon halting cell therapy, the dog developed new lung lesions within 10 weeks and died 18 months later of slowly progressive disease. Despite its very poor prognosis at the time of diagnosis, B.T. went into complete remission and died 16 months later from causes unrelated to cancer (57). Dogs G.M. and W.P. relapsed locally at 13 and 19 months, respectively, after start of cell therapy; importantly, chest X-rays revealed no lung metastases in these dogs although the monthly boosts had been discontinued 5 and 11 months before local recurrence. After surgical removal of the relapsed tumor, followed by another cycle of cell therapy and monthly boosts, these two dogs were disease-free 30 and 39 months from initiation of cell therapy before developing new lymph node metastases. G.M. died of metastatic disease at 32 months, and W.P. is still alive with disease at almost 4 years from the start of TALL-104 cell therapy (Table 1).

In felines with metastatic mammary carcinoma, surgery in conjunction with chemotherapy (doxorubicin) induces initial short-term partial or complete responses in 50% of the animals; however, the prognosis is generally poor, with median survival of 10 months. Fourteen cats with spontaneous mammary tumors at high risk of relapse after surgical removal of the primary tumor mass and/or lymph nodes were entered in the TALL-104 study. All cats had previous mastectomy for removal of their breast carcinoma, and some of them received adjuvant chemotherapy before TALL-104 cell therapy. Most cats had lymph node metastases. TALL-104 cell therapy consisted of 5 consecutive day infusions at 10^8/kg, followed by 2-day monthly boosts. At the time of this writing, seven cats (50%) are still alive with no evidence of disease up to 27 months from start of cell therapy; one cat (7%) is alive with disease at 32 months, and six (43%) died of disease at intervals ranging from 5 to 27 months.

5.1.4.3. Phase I Trial of TALL-104 Cells in Patients with Refractory Metastatic Breast Cancer.
We have recently completed a phase I trial to evaluate dose-related toxicities of TALL-104 cells in women with metastatic breast cancer resistant to at least two forms of conventional therapy (including stem cell transplantation) *(56)*. The trial was designed as a single-center, open-label, dose-escalation study. It was conducted at the Cancer Center of the Hospital of the University of Pennsylvania by Drs. E. Stadtmauer, D. Porter, and M. Torosian. Fifteen patients with metastatic infiltrating ductal or lobular carcinoma (12 and 2 patients) or medullary carcinoma (1 patient) received escalating doses of lethally irradiated TALL-104 cells intravenously (10^6, 3×10^6, 10^7, 3×10^7, and 10^8 cells/kg) for 5 consecutive days (induction course). Patients without progressive disease to induction received monthly maintenance 2-day infusions at the same dose level. Nine patients progressed in the month after the induction course, five patients had disease stablization lasting for 2–6 months, and 1 patient (at 3×10^7 cells/kg) had a marginal response consisting of decrease in size of liver metastases and ascites.

The first patient enrolled (at 10^6 cells/kg) experienced temporary relief in bone pain. Mild (grade I/II) clinical toxicities developed in 11 patients during infusions. One grade IV toxicity consequent to hepatic tumor necrosis occurred in a patient at the highest dose level, 3 weeks after the induction course. Occasional hypo- or hyperglycemia, hypocalcemia, elevated SGOT, and alkaline phosphatases occurred regardless of cell dose. Most patients developed absolute and relative monocytosis and eosinophilia together with increases in peripheral blood natural killer activity, serum levels of IFN-γ, IL-10, and activation markers (sIL2-R and sICAM-1). Tumor biopsies (lymph node and chest wall) from five patients were killed effectively in vitro by TALL-104 cells and induced release of cytokines (IFN-γ, TNF-α, and TNF-β). Humoral and cellular immune responses against TALL-104 cells developed in only one and three patients, respectively. These results indicate that repeated injections of TALL-104 cells up to the dose of 10^8/kg are well tolerated by patients with advanced breast cancer; moreover, the disease stabilization and minor clinical responses observed suggest the potential efficacy of TALL-104 cells in an adjuvant setting. Phase I/II clinical trials evaluating the most effective regimen of TALL-104 cell administration have been planned in patients with metastatic melanoma under the direction of Drs. L. Schuchter, D. Guerry, C. June, and A. Alavi at the University of Pennsylvania Cancer Center.

5.2. Antigen-Specific Immunotherapy

Cytotoxic T cells specific for the protein core of the mucin and specifically lytic against tumor have been cultivated from breast and pancreatic tumor-draining lymph nodes *(58)*. Likewise, significant proliferative T-cell responses were observed against the HER-2 protein and peptide in the peripheral blood of patients with breast cancer. Several strategies have now been developed to isolate tumor or tumor-associated antigen-specific T cells from the lymph nodes, tumor, or peripheral blood of patients, and a number of tumor lytic T-cell clones or lines have been characterized *(59–61)*. Some groups have also investigated gene therapy procedures using chimeric TCRs to retarget the ability of naive T cells to recognize defined tumor targets *(62)*. In these strategies, gene segments encoding the variable regions of a specific antibody-binding domain have been fused with gene segments encoding constant effector regions of the TCR. When inserted into a T-cell hybridoma, these chimeric TCRs will specifically recognize and target cells bearing the antigen defined by the chosen antibody domain. Efforts to use chimeric TCRs to engineer naive T cells to recognize HER-2-positive breast tumors are currently under way. Major efforts are now being focused on procedures to isolate such tumor-specific T cells rapidly from a large number of patients to allow meaningful clinical testing of this mode of therapy. Currently, such T-cell therapies are planned in a variety of breast cancer therapeutic protocols, including those involving conventional or high-dose chemotherapy: the infused T cells would be used to reduce or eliminate minimal residual disease.

5.2.1. Mucin-Specific Immunotherapy

Polymorphic epithelial mucin (now termed MUC1) has been utilized as a target for the specific immunotherapy of breast cancer. MUC1 is a high molecular mass mucin-like glycoprotein that, unlike other mucins, is an integral membrane protein. The transmembrane and cytoplasmic tails show a high degree of homology between species, which suggests that they may have a basic function. The extracellular domain of MUC1 consists of tandemly repeated sequences of up to 20 amino acids, rich in serine, threonine, and proline, and could extend 150–500 nm above the cell membrane. The overexpression of MUC1 on malignant cells suggests that it may confer an advantage to the tumor by increasing metastatic potential. In addition, the physical size of MUC1 may prevent immune effector cells from binding to the tumor cell membrane.

Tumor-associated MUC1 has both tumorigenic and immunogenic potential and may be an effective immunogen for several reasons: its expression is upregulated in tumor cells; its normal apical distribution is lost in cancer cells; its aberrant glycosylation exposes peptide epitopes and novel carbohydrate antigens on cancer cells. Cellular and humoral immune responses to tumor-associated MUC1 have been demonstrated in cancer patients. T lymphocytes isolated from patients with breast or ovarian cancer specifically killed tumor cells expressing MUC1 *(58,59)*. The cellular response was specific for tumor-associated MUC1 and was TCR-dependent but was MHC-unrestricted. Serum IgM antibodies specific for MUC1 have been found in approximately 10–20% of patients with breast, pancreatic, or colon cancer *(62)*. The antibody response was directed against the same epitope on the mucin polypeptide core tandem repeat as the cellular response. There is evidence that an immune response to tumor-associated MUC1 may be associated with a better prognosis.

Several clinical trials are in progress to evaluate the immunogenicity of MUC1 and its suitability for immunotherapy of breast cancer. In a phase I trial, 13 patients were injected with a synthetic peptide from the human MUC1 tandem repeat conjugated to diphtheria toxoid *(63)*. Six patients generated antibody responses to both the peptide and MUC1, two developed a delayed-type hypersensitivity (DTH) response on rechallenge, and three developed proliferative T-cell responses to MUC1. Stable disease was reported in 6 of 12 evaluable patients during the study period *(63)*.

Others have used a 105-amino acid peptide (corresponding to five tandem repeats) admixed with bacille Calmette-Guérin as an immunogen in cancer patients *(64)*. Most patients developed a DTH reaction to rechallenge with the peptide; biopsy from these sites showed variable degrees of T-cell infiltration. In one-third of patients tested, the frequency of cytotoxic T-cell precursors specific for MUC1 rose more than twofold.

A recombinant VV carrying cDNA for MUC1 and for IL-2 (VV-MUC1/IL2) has been used in a phase I study of patients with advanced breast cancer. Immunization was not associated with significant toxicity, and immune responses were detected in some patients *(65)*. A phase II multicenter trial using the VV-MUC1/IL-2 construct in patients with metastatic breast cancer is in progress.

5.2.2. NOVEL CARBOHYDRATE ANTIGENS AS TARGETS FOR ACTIVE SPECIFIC IMMUNOTHERAPY

Alterations in the glycosylation of mucins result in novel oligosaccharides that are highly expressed in a variety of cancers, whereas in normal tissues they are weakly expressed and presumably masked by further oligosaccharide chain elongation *(66)*. Incomplete glycosylation in cancer is apparently caused by an alteration in glycosyl transferase activity, leading to shorter side chains and the exposure of O-linked core carbohydrate determinants that are normally hidden. Three different carbohydrate antigens (T antigens) have been identified in cancer cells *(66)*: 1) the Thompson-Friedenreich (TF) antigen, which is an O-linked disaccharide (βGal[1–3]αGalNAc-O-serine/threonine) found particularly in breast and colon cancer; 2) Tn, the monosaccharide precursor of TF (αGalNAc-O-serine); and 3) sialated Tn (STn). These carbohydrate epitopes may serve as tumor antigens against which antitumor immune responses could be induced; clinical studies using these antigens are in progress.

STn expression has been demonstrated in breast cancers and may be linked with a poor prognosis *(67)*. In multivariate analysis, STn positivity was associated with relative resistance to adjuvant chemotherapy *(68)*. A prospective, randomized clinical trial using STn as a target for active specific immunotherapy in patients with breast cancer has been reported *(69)*. The patients enrolled had locoregional relapse after appropriate primary therapy, or metastatic disease. All patients were immunized subcutaneously with STn conjugated to Keyhole limpet hemocyanin, (KLH), with DETOX adjuvant at various intervals. STn was detected in the circulation, and soluble antigens were demonstrated to induce tolerance or anergy, rather than an effective immune response. In mice, this apparent "suppressor" activity can be overcome by pretreatment with cyclophosphamide (CFM) *(70)*. Patients were therefore randomized to receive (before the first immunization) either 300 mg CFM intravenously on day –3, or 50 mg CFM orally on days –14 to –3, or no CFM pretreatment. The treatment had minimal toxicity. All patients generated an antibody response to STn, STn-positive mucin, and KLH. The median survival for the group pretreated with CFM intravenously was significantly longer than that for the other groups (19.7 versus 12.6 months). The patients receiving intravenous CFM were less likely to have progressive disease, and there was a negative correlation between the growth of measurable tumors and antibody titers to STn. There was no correlation between progression and antibody titers to KLH. These results suggested a therapeutic effect for pretreatment with intravenous CFM followed by immunization with STn-KLH. A similar association between antibody titers and survival has been demonstrated in patients with colorectal cancer immunized with STn-KLH *(71)*. A large multicenter trial comparing intravenous CFM and STn-KLH/DETOX-B with intravenous CFM and KLH/DETOX-B in the treatment of patients with breast cancer is now in progress.

6. CONCLUSIONS

Numerous questions remain to be answered in regard to the cell and gene therapy strategies proposed for the treatment of breast cancer. These include the phenotype and trafficking of the infused cells, the level and duration of gene expression, the therapeutic doses for efficacy, and the overall safety of these therapies. Surrogates for the efficacy of immunotherapy and gene therapy need to be defined, probably utilizing immunologic assays, to prevent these potentially useful treatments from being overlooked.

It is to be expected that both immunotherapy and gene therapy will be most useful as adjuvant treatments in the setting of minimal residual disease. Such approaches, if used alone, are unlikely to produce complete responses in patients with metastatic cancer; however, long-term stabilization of growth may be achievable. In addition, maximal therapeutic efficacy may require combinations of the above therapies with novel agents that are being developed such as growth factor receptor inhibitors and angiogenesis inhibitors. Large-scale clinical testing of these promising new strategies may ultimately result in the definition of optimal adjuvant therapies that could be customized for individual breast cancer patients based on the combination of biologic and prognostic factors.

REFERENCES

1. Kihara A, Pastan I (1995) Cytotoxic activity of chimeric toxins containing the epidermal growth factor-like domain of heregulins fused to PE38KDEL, a truncated recombinant form of *Pseudomonas exotoxin. Cancer Res.* **55,** 71–77.
2. Valone FH, Kaufman PA, Guyre PM, et al. (1995) Phase Ia/Ib trial of bispecific antibody MDX-210 in patients with advanced breast or ovarian cancer that overexpress the protooncogene HER-2/neu. *J. Clin. Oncol.* **13,** 2281–2292.
3. Zhang L, Chang C, Bacus SS, et al. (1995) Suppressed transformation and induced differentiation of HER-2/neu-overexpressing breast cancer cells by emodin. *Cancer Res.* **55,** 3890–3896.
4. Baselga J, Tripathy D, Mendelsohn J, et al. (1995) Phase II study of recombinant human anti-HER2 monoclonal antibody (rhu-Mab HER2) in stage IV breast cancer: HER2-shedding dependent pharmacokinetics and antitumor activity. *Proc. Am. Soc. Clin. Oncol.* **14,** 103.
5. Pegram M, Lipton A, Pietras R, et al. (1995) Phase II study of intravenous recombinant humanized anti-p185 HER-2 monoclonal antibody (rhuMab HER-2) plus cisplatin in patients with HER-2/neu overexpressing metastatic breast cancer. *Proc. Am. Soc. Clin. Oncol.* **14,** 106.
6. Folkman J (1990) What is the evidence that tumors are angiogenesis dependent? *J. Natl. Cancer Inst.* **82,** 4–6.
7. Kim KJ, Li B, Winer J, et al. (1993) Inhibition of vascular endothelial growth factor-induced angiogenesis suppresses tumour growth in vivo. *Nature* **362,** 841–844.
8. Kusaka M, Sudo K, Matsutani E, et al. (1994) Cytostatic inhibition of endothelial cell growth by the angiogenesis inhibitor TNP-470 (AGM-1470). *Br. J. Cancer* **69,** 212–216.
9. Taraboletti G, Garofalo A, Belotti D, et al. (1995) Inhibition of angiogenesis and murine hemangioma growth by Batimastat, a synthetic inhibitor of matrix metalloproteinases. *J. Natl. Cancer Inst.* **87,** 293–298.
10. Guerin C, Laterra J, Masnyk T, et al. (1992) Selective endothelial growth inhibition by tetracyclines that inhibit collagenase. *Biochem. Biophys. Res. Commun.* **188,** 740–745.
11. Brooks PC, Clark RAF, and Cheresh DA (1994) Requirement of vascular integrin $\alpha v \beta 3$ for angiogenesis. *Science* **264,** 569–571.
12. Boxhorn HKE, Eck SL (1998) Gene therapy for breast cancer. *Hematal. Oncol. Clin. North Am.* **12,** 665–675.
13. Nielsen LL, Dell J, Maxwell E, et al. (1997) Efficacy of p53 adenovirus-mediated gene therapy against human breast cancer xenografts. *Cancer Gene Ther.* **4,** 129–138.
14. Nielsen LL, Gurnani M, Syed J, et al. (1998) Recombinant E1-deleted adenovirus-mediated gene therapy for cancer: efficacy studies with p53 tumor suppressor gene and liver histology in tumor xenograft models. *Hum. Gene Ther.* **9,** 681–694.
15. Raper SE, Haskal ZJ, Ye X, et al. (1998) Selective gene transfer into the liver of non-human primates with E1 deleted, E2A-defective, or E1-E4 deleted recombinant adenoviruses. *Hum. Gene Ther.* **9,** 671–679.
16. Li Z, Shanmugam N, Katayose D, et al. (1997) Enzyme/prodrug gene therapy approach for breast cancer using a recombinant adenovirus expressing *Escherichia coli* cytosine deaminase. *Cancer Gene Ther.* **4,** 113–117.

17. Putzer BM, Bramson JL, Addison CL, et al. (1998) Combination therapy with interleukin-2 and wild-type p53 expressed by adenoviral vectors potentiates tumor regression in a murine model of breast cancer. *Hum. Gene Ther.* **9,** 707–718.

18. Topalian SL, Solomon D, Avis FP, et al. (1988) Immunotherapy of patients with advanced cancer using tumor-infiltrating lymphocytes and recombinant interleukin-2: a pilot study. *J. Clin. Oncol.* **6,** 839–853.

19. Hoover JC, Hanna MG Jr (1991) Immunotherapy by active specific immunization. In: (DeVita VT, Hellman S, Rosenberg SA (eds.) *Biological Therapy of Cancer* JB Lippincott, Philadelphia, p. 670.

20. Elder EM, Lotze MT, and Whiteside TL (1996) Successful culture and selection of cytokine gene-modified human dermal fibroblasts for the biologic therapy of patients with cancer. *Hum. Gene Ther.* **7,** 479–487.

21. Weitzman MD, Wilson JM, Eck SL (1995) Adenovirus vectors in cancer gene therapy. In: Sobol RE, Scanlon KJ (eds.) *The Internet Book of Gene Therapy: Cancer.* Appleton & Lange, Stamford CT, p. 17.

22. Marr RA, Addison CL, Snider D, et al. (1997) Tumour immunotherapy using an adenoviral vector expressing a membrane-bound mutant of murine TNF alpha. *Gene Ther.* **4,** 1181–1188.

23. Zhang JF, Hu C, Geng Y, et al. (1996) Treatment of a human breast cancer xenograft with an adenovirus vector containing an interferon gene results in rapid regression due to viral oncolysis and gene therapy. *Proc. Natl. Acad. Sci. USA* **93,** 4513–4518.

24. Hareuveni M, Gautier C, Kieny MP, et al. (1990) Vaccination against tumor cells expressing breast cancer epithelial tumor antigen. *Proc. Natl. Acad. Sci. USA* **87,** 9498–9502.

25. Bu D, Domenech N, Lewis J, et al. (1993) Recombinant vaccinia mucin vector: in vitro analysis of expression of tumor-associated epitopes for antibody and human cytotoxic T cell recognition. *J. Immunother.* **14,** 127–135.

26. Ding L, Lalani EN, Reddish M, et al. (1993) Immunogenicity of synthetic peptides related to the core peptide sequence encoded by the human MUC1 mucin gene: effect of immunization on the growth of murine mammary adenocarcinoma cells transfected with the human MUC1 gene. *Cancer Immunol. Immunother.* **36,** 9–17.

27. Pastan I, Gottesman MM (1991) Multidrug resistance. *Annu. Rev. Med.* **42,** 277–286.

28. Hanania EG, Fu S, Roninson I, et al. (1995) Resistance to taxol chemotherapy produced in mouse marrow cells by safety-modified retroviruses containing a human MDR-1 transcription unit. *Gene Ther.* **2,** 1–6.

29. Rosenberg S, Lotze M, Muul L, et al. (1987) A progress report on the treatment of 157 patients with advanced cancer using lymphokine-activated killer cells and interleukin-2 or high-dose interleukin-2 aone. *N. Engl. J. Med.* **316,** 889–897.

30. Law T, Motzer R, Mazumdar M, et al. (1995) Phase III randomized trial of interleukin-2 with or without lymphokine-activated killer cells in the treatment of patients with advanced renal cell cancer. *Cancer* **76,** 824–832.

31. Wei W-Z, Heppner G (1996) Breast cancer immunology. *Cancer Treat. Res.* **83,** 395–410.

32. Coventry B, Weeks S, Heckford S, et al. (1996) Lack of IL-2 cytokine expression despite IL-2 messenger mRNA transcription in tumor-infiltrating lymphocytes in primary breast carcinoma: selective expression of early activation markers. *J. Immunol.* **156,** 3486–3492.

33. Becker J, Czerny C, Brocker E (1994) Maintenance of clonal anergy by endogenously produced IL-10. *Int. Immunol.* **6,** 1605–1612.

34. Beissert S, Hosoi J, Grabbe S, et al. (1995) IL-10 inhibits tumor antigen presentation by epidermal antigen-presenting cells. *J. Immunol.* **154,** 1280–1286.

35. Sparano JA, Fisher RI, Weiss GR, et al. (1994) Phase II trials of high-dose interleukin-2 and lymphokine-activated killer cells in advanced breast carcinoma and carcinoma of the lung, ovary, and pancreas and other tumors. *J. Immunother.* **16,** 216–223.

36. Horowitz M, Gale R, Sondel P, et al. (1990) Graft-versus-leukemia reactions after bone marrow transplantation. *Blood* **75,** 555–562.

37. Porter D, Antin J (1997) Graft-versus-leukemia effect of allogeneic bone marrow transplantation and donor mononuclear cell infusions. In: Winter J (ed.) *Blood Stem Cell Transplantation* Kluwer, Norwell, MA, pp. 57–86.

38. Collins R, Shpilberg O, Drobyski W, et al. (1997) Donor leukocyte infusions in 140 patients with relapsed malignancy after allogeneic bone marrow transplantation. *J. Clin. Oncol.* **15,** 433–444.

39. Porter D, Connors J, VanDeerlin V, et al. (1999) Graft-versus-tumor induction with donor leukocyte infusions as primary therapy for patients with malignancies. *J. Clin. Oncol.* **17,** 1234–1243.

40. Giralt S, Estey E, Albitar M, et al. (1997) Engraftment of allogeneic hematopoietic progenitor cells with purine analog-containing chemotherapy: harnessing graft-versus-leukemia without myeloablative therapy. *Blood* **89,** 4531–4536.

41. Khouri I, Keating M, Korbling M, et al. (1988) Transplant-lite: induction of graft-vs-malignancy using fludarabine-based nonablative chemotherapy and allogeneic blood progenitor-cell transplantation as treatment for lymphoid malignancies. *J. Clin. Oncol.* **16,** 2817–2824.

42. Ueno N, Rondon G, Mirza N, et al. (1998) Allogeneic peripheral blood progenitor cell transplantation for poor risk patients with metastatic breast cancer. *J. Clin. Oncol.* **16,** 986–993.

43. Eibl B, Schwaighofer H, Nachbaur D, et al. (1996) Evidence for a graft-versus-tumor effect in a patient treated with marrow ablative chemotherapy and allogeneic bone marrow transplantation for breast cancer. *Blood* **88,** 1501–1508.

44. Or R, Ackerstein A, Nagler A, et al. (1998) Allogeneic cell-mediated immunotherapy for breast cancer after autologous stem cell transplantation: a clinical pilot study. *Cyto. Cell. Mol. Ther.* **4,** 1–6.

45. O'Connor R, Cesano A, Lange B, et al. (1991) Growth factor requirements of childhood acute T lymphoblastic leukemia: correlation between presence of chromosomal abnormalities and ability to grow permanently *in vitro. Blood* **77,** 1534–1545.

46. Cesano A, Visonneau S, Cioé L, Clark SC, Rovera G, and Santoli D (1994) Reversal of acute myelogenous leukemia in humanized SCID mice using a novel adoptive transfer approach. *J. Clin. Invest.* **94,** 1076 1084.

47. Cesano A, Visonneau S, and Santoli D (1995) Treatment of experimental glioblastoma with a human MHC non-restricted cytotoxic T-cell line. *Cancer Res.* **55,** 96–101.

48. Cesano A, Visonneau S, Cioé L, Clark SC, Santoli D (1995) Effects of lethal irradiation and cyclosporin A treatment on the growth and tumoricidal activity of a T cell clone potentially useful in cancer therapy. *Cancer Immunol. Immunother.* **40,** 139–151.

49. Cesano A, Visonneau S, Jeglum KA, et al. (1996) Phase I clinical trial with a human major histocompatibility complex nonrestricted cytotoxic T-cell line (TALL-104) in dogs with advanced tumors. *Cancer Res.* **56,** 3021–3029.

50. Cesano A, Visonneau S, Pasquini S, Rovera G, Santoli D (1996) Anti-tumor efficacy of a human MHC non-restricted cytotoxic T cell line (TALL-104) in immunocompetent mice bearing syngeneic leukemia. *Cancer Res.* **56,** 4444–4452.

51. Visonneau S, Cesano A, Torosian M, Santoli D (1997) Cell therapy of a highly invasive human breast carcinoma implanted in immunodeficient (SCID) mice. *Clin. Cancer Res.* **3,** 1491–1500.

52. Visonneau S, Cesano A, Tran T, Jeglum KA, Santoli D (1997) Successful treatment of canine malignant histiocytosis with the human MHC non-restricted cytotoxic T cell line TALL-104. *Clin. Cancer Res.* **3,** 1789–1797.

53. Cesano A, Visonneau S, Santoli D (1998) TALL-104 cell therapy of human solid tumors implanted in immunodeficient (SCID) mice. *Anticancer Res.* **18,** 2289–2295.

54. Cesano A, Visonneau S, Tran T, Santoli D (1999) Biodistribution of human MHC non-restricted TALL-104 killer cells in healthy and tumor bearing mice. *Int. J. Oncol.* **4,** 245–251.

55. Visonneau S, Cesano A, Jeglum KA, Santoli D (1999) Adjuvant treatment of canine osteosarcoma with the human cytotoxic T cell line TALL-104. *Clin. Cancer Res.* **5,** 1868–1875.

56. Visonneau S, Cesano A, Porter DL, et al. (2000) Phase I trial of TALL-104 cells in patients with refractory metastatic breast cancer. *Clin. Cancer Res.* **6,** 1744–1754.

57. Visonneau S, Cesano A, Jeglum KA, Santoli D (1999) Adoptive therapy of canine metastatic mammary carcinoma with the human MHC non-restricted cytotoxic T-cell line TALL-104. *Oncol. Rep.* **6,** 1181–1188.

58. Ioannides C, Fisk B, Jerome K, et al. (1993) Cytotoxic T cells from ovarian malignant tumors can recognize polymorphic epithelial mucin core peptides. *J. Immunol.* **151,** 3693–3703.

59. Jerome K, Barnd D, Bendt K, et al. (1991) Cytotoxic T-lymphocytes derived from patients with breast adenocarcinoma recognize an epitope present on the protein core of a mucin molecule preferentially expressed by malignant cells. *Cancer Res.* **51,** 2908–2916.

60. Barnd D, Lan M, Metzgar R, et al. (1989) Specific, major histocompatibility complex-unrestricted recognition of tumor-associated mucins by human cytotoxic T cells. *Proc. Natl. Acad. Sci. USA* **86,** 7159–7163.

61. Finn O, Jerome K, Henderson R, et al. (1995) MUC1 epithelial tumor mucin-based immunity and cancer vaccines. *Immunol. Rev.* **145,** 61–89.

62. Kotera Y, Fontenot J, Pecher G, et al. (1994) Humoral immunity against a tandem repeat epitope of human mucin MUC-1 in sera from breast, pancreatic and colon cancer patients. *Cancer Res.* **54,** 2856–2860.

63. Xing P-X, Michael M, Apostolopoulos V, et al. (1995) Phase I study of synthetic MUC1 peptides in breast cancer. *Int. J. Oncol.* **6,** 1283–1289.

64. Goydos J, Elder E, Whiteside T, et al. (1996) A phase I trial of a synthetic mucin peptide vaccine. Induction of specific immune reactivity in patients with adenocarcinoma. *J. Surg. Res.* **63,** 298–304.

65. Scholl SM, Balloul JM, Le Goc G, et al. (2000) Recombinant vaccinia virus encoding human MUC1 and IL2 as immunotherapy in patients with breast cancer. *J. Immunother.* **23,** 570–580.

66. Itzkowitz SH, Yuan M, Montgomery CK, et al. (1989) Expression of Tn, sialosyl-Tn and T antigens in human colon cancer. *Cancer Res.* **49,** 197–204.

67. Longenecker B, Reddish M, Miles D, et al. (1993) Synthetic tumor-associated sialyl-Tn antigen as an immunotherapeutic cancer vaccine. *Vaccine Res.* **2,** 151–162.

68. Miles D, Happerfield L, Smith P, et al. (1994) Expression of sialyl-Tn predicts the utility of adjuvant chemotherapy in node positive breast cancer. *Br. J. Cancer* **70,** 1272–1275.

69. MacLean G, Miles D, Rubens R, et al. (1996) Enhancing the effect of THERATOPE Stn-KLH cancer vaccine patients with metastatic breast cancer by pre-treatment with low-dose intravenous cyclophosphamide. *J. Immunother.* **19,** 309–316.

70. Fung P, Longenecker B (1991) Specific immunosuppressive activity of epiglycanin, a mucin-like glycoprotein secreted by a murine adenocarcinoma (TA3-HA). *Cancer Res.* **51,** 1170–1176.

71. MacLean G, Reddish M, Koganty R, et al. (1996) Antibodies against mucin-associated sialyl-Tn epitopes correlate with survival of metastatic adenocarcinoma patients undergoing active specific immunotherapy with synthetic STn vaccine. *J. Immunol. Emphasis Tumor Immunol.* **19,** 59–68.

Index

A

Adjuvant systemic therapy, 137–139,
  145–150, 166–169, 232
  chemotherapy, 145–150, 232
  hormonal therapy, 166–169, 232
  radiation therapy and, 137–139
Antiangiogenic therapy, 326–328
  angiogenic peptides, 327
  basement membrane of vessels, 327
  endothelial cell proliferation, 327
  extracellular matrix proteins, 327
  natural angiogenesis inhibitors, 327
Ataxia telangiectasia, 15
Autologous stem cell transplantation,
  313–324
  adjuvant therapy followed by, 321–322
  future directions, 318–320, 322–323
  high risk patients and, 320–323
  history of, 314–315, 320
  induction chemotherapy followed by,
  315–317
  introduction, 313
  metastatic disease and, 314–319
  tandem transplant, 317–318
Axillary adenopathy, 227–234
  adjuvant therapy, 232
  axillary dissection, 232
  breast conserving therapy, 231–232
  evaluation, 227–230
  mastectomy, 230–231
  prognosis, 232
Axillary node dissection, 285–294
  history, 285–286
  primary tumor characteristics and,
  287–288

radiologic evaluation, 288
sentinel lymph node mapping and
  biopsy, 289
staging, 286–287
therapeutic value, 290–291

B

BRCA1/BRCA2, 12–14, 198–205
Breast biopsy, 71–80, 90–91
  advanced breast biopsy instrumentation
  (ABBI), 75–76
  core needle biopsy, 72–75, 91
  excisional, 76–79
  fine needle aspiration, 72–75, 90–91,
  236
  incisional, 76
  nipple discharge, 79
  nonpalpable lesions, 73–78, 91
  palpable masses, 72–73, 76–78
  stereotactic biopsy, 73–75, 91
Breast conservation without radiation
  therapy, 273–283
  ductal carcinoma *in situ* (DCIS),
  276–279
  invasive/infiltrating cancer, 280–282
  lobular carcinoma *in situ* (LCIS),
  274–275
Breast conserving surgery, 89–97
  axillary adenopathy and, 231–232
  cystosarcoma phylloides, 95
  ductal carcinoma *in situ* (DCIS),
  89–91, 95
  invasive cancer, 92–93, 95
  lobular carcinoma *in situ* (LCIS), 91

From: *Current Clinical Oncology:*
Breast Cancer: A Guide Detection and Multidisciplinary Therapy
Edited by: M. H. Torosian © Humana Press Inc., Totowa, NJ

locally advanced cancer, 92–93
lumpectomy and axillary dissection, 93–94
neoadjuvant chemotherapy and, 95
Paget's disease, 96
radiation therapy, 95
regional cancer, 92–93
sentinel lymph node biopsy, 94
without radiation therapy, 273–283
Breast imaging, 19–69
computerized axial tomography (CT scan), 288
magnetic resonance imaging (MRI), 59–60, 229, 288
mammography, 10–11, 19–50, 62–67, 90–91, 228–229, 236
diagnostic, 21–22
digital, 62–67
screening, 19–21
positron emission tomography (PET), 229–230, 288
sestamibi scan, 61–62
ultrasound, 50–59, 91, 236

C

Chemotherapy, 145–159
adjuvant, 145–150
metastatic disease, 150–153
primary, 213–226
secondary malignancy and, 157
toxicity, 153–159
acute, 153–159
long-term, 156–157
Clinical classifications of breast cancer, 81–88
ductal carcinoma *in situ* (DCIS), 83–84
inflammatory cancer, 85–86
invasive/infiltrating cancer, 82–83
lobular carcinoma *in situ* (LCIS), 86–87
microinvasive carcinoma, 84–85
Paget's disease, 85
Core needle biopsy, 72–75, 91
Cowden's disease, 14–15
Cystosarcoma phylloides, 95, 264–265

D

Digital mammography, 62–67
Ductal carcinoma *in situ* (DCIS), 83–84, 89–90, 95, 169, 276–279

E

Epidemiology, 3–18
age, 3–4
benign breast disease, 9–10
diet, 7–9
environmental factors, 11–12
ethnicity, 4–5
genetic factors, 12–15
geography, 5
hormonal risk factors, 5–7
mammography, 10–11
occupational factors, 11
race, 4–5
radiation exposure, 9

F

Fine needle aspiration, 72–75, 90–91, 236

G

Gene therapy, 328–331
autologous transportation and, 330–331
immune response and, 329–330
signaling pathways and, 328–329

H

Hormonal therapy, 161–174, 188
adjuvant, 166–169
chemoprevention, 170–172
ductal carcinoma *in situ* (DCIS), 169
future directions, 172
male breast cancer and, 188
metastatic disease and, 161–166
postmenopausal, 162–165
premenopausal, 165–166

I

Immunotherapy, 325–342
adoptive immunotherapy, 331–339
allogenic cell, 332–333
antigen–specific 336–337
IL-2/LAK cell, 332
mucin-specific, 337–338
novel carbohydrate antigens, 338

TALL-104 cells, 333–336
 tumor infiltrating lymphocytes
 (TILs), 331–332
antiangiogenic therapy, 326–328
gene therapy and, 328–331
growth factor receptor inhibition,
 325–326
Inflammatory breast cancer, 85–86
Internal mammary lymph nodes, 295–311
 age of patient, 302
 axillary metastasis and, 298–300
 biopsy of, 308
 history, 295–296
 lymphatic drainage to, 296–297
 predictors of metastasis, 297–302
 primary tumor characteristics, 300–302
 biologic factors, 302
 histology, 302
 location, 300–301
 size, 302
 prognosis, 302
 radiation therapy, 305–307
 recurrence in, 307–308
 surgical dissection of, 303–305
Invasive/infiltrating cancer, 82–83, 89–90,
 95, 280–282

L

Li-Fraumeni syndrome, 14
Lobular carcinoma *in situ* (LCIS), 86–87,
 91, 274–275
Locally advanced breast cancer, 85, 92–93
Local–regional recurrence, 245–254
 axillary recurrence, 251–252
 breast conserving therapy and, 246–249
 incidence, 245
 mastectomy and, 249–251

M

Magnetic resonance imaging (MRI),
 59–60, 229, 288
Male breast cancer, 183–191
 chemotherapy, 188
 evaluation, 184–186
 histology, 186–187
 hormonal therapy, 188
 prevalence, 183

prognosis, 188–190
 radiation therapy and, 187–188
 risk factors, 184
 surgery, 187
Mammography, 10–11, 19–50, 62–67,
 90–91, 228–229, 236
 additional views, 21–22
 assessment categories, 30–31
 BI-RADS, 23–31
 breast cancer patient, evaluation of,
 45–50
 breast tissue type, 25–26
 calcifications, 40–45
 benign, 40–44
 malignant, 40–42, 45
 diagnostic, 21–22
 additional views, 21–22
 digital, 62–67
 masses, 33–40
 benign, 33–37
 malignant, 33–34, 37–40
 normal breast, 32–33
 screening, 19–21
 standard views, 20–21
 significant findings, 26–30
 standard views, 20–21
Mastectomy, 99–109
 history, 99–100
 indications, 100–101
 local regional recurrence, 249–251
 male breast cancer, 187
 modified radical mastectomy,
 104–107
 radical mastectomy, 107
 skin-sparing mastectomy, 107–108
 total mastectomy, 101–104
Metastatic disease, 141–142, 150–153,
 161–166, 175–182
 brain, 178–180
 liver, 177–178
 pulmonary, 175–177
 surgical resection of, 175–182
Microinvasive breast cancer, 84–85

N

Neoadjuvant chemotherapy (*see* Primary
 chemotherapy)

Nipple discharge, 79, 255–262
  classifications of, 255–256
  endocrine-mediated, 256–257
  evaluation, 259–260
  future directions, 260–261
  intrinsic etiologies, 257–259
  physiology, 256

O

Oncogene, 193–209
  bcl-2, 195–198, 205
  BRCA1 and *BRCA2*, 198–205
  HER-2/*neu*, 193–195, 205, 325–326, 328
  p53, 198, 203–206, 328–329

P

Paget's disease, 85, 96
Percutaneous biopsy, 72–76, 90–91
  advanced breast biopsy instrumentation
    (ABBI), 75–76
  core needle biopsy, 72–75
  fine needle aspiration, 72–75, 90–91, 236
  nonpalpable lesions, 73–75, 91
  palpable masses, 72–73
  stereotactic biopsy, 73–75, 91
Pregnancy and breast cancer, 235–243
  biopsy, 236
  chemotherapy, 238–239
  diagnosis, 235–236
  incidence, 235
  prognosis, 239–240
  radiation therapy, 237–238
  therapeutic abortion, 240
Primary chemotherapy, 95, 213–226
  chemosensitivity and, 214–215
  downstaging of primary tumor, 214
  future directions, 223–224
  Goldie-Coldman hypothesis, 215
  nonrandomized trials, 221–223
  operable breast cancer and, 218–221
  prognostic information and, 216–218

R

Radiation therapy, 129–143
  adjuvant systemic therapy and, 137–139
  complications, 139–140
  ductal carcinoma *in situ* (DCIS),
    129–133

breast conserving therapy and, 95,
    133–136
  internal mammary lymph nodes,
    305–307
  local recurrence after, 140–141
  locally advanced disease, 137–139
  male breast cancer, 187–188
  mastectomy and, 136–137
  palliation of metastatic disease, 141–142
  pregnancy and, 237–238
Reconstruction of the breast, 111–128
  alternative choices, 125
  consultation, 111–114
  controversies, 125–127
  latissimus dorsi flap, 116–119
  skin-sparing mastectomy, 107–108
  tissue expander and implant, 114–116
  transverse rectus abdominis
    myocutaneous flap, 119–125

S

Sarcomas of breast, 263–266
  angiosarcomas, 266
  cystosarcoma phylloides, 264–265
  etiology, 263
  incidence, 263
  lymphangiosarcoma (Stewart-Treves
    syndrome), 265–266
  radiation–induced, 265–266
Sentinel lymph node biopsy, 85, 94, 289
Sestamibi scan, 61–62
Stereotactic biopsy, 73–75, 91
Stewart-Treves syndrome, 265–266
Surgical biopsy, 76–79, 91
  excisional, 76–79
  incisional, 76
  nipple discharge, 79
  nonpalpable lesions, 76–78, 91
  palpable masses, 76–78

U

Ultrasound, 50–59
  analysis, 55–59
  equipment, 52
  indications, 52
  lesions, 55–59
  normal anatomy, 53–55
  technique, 52
  vascular imaging, 59

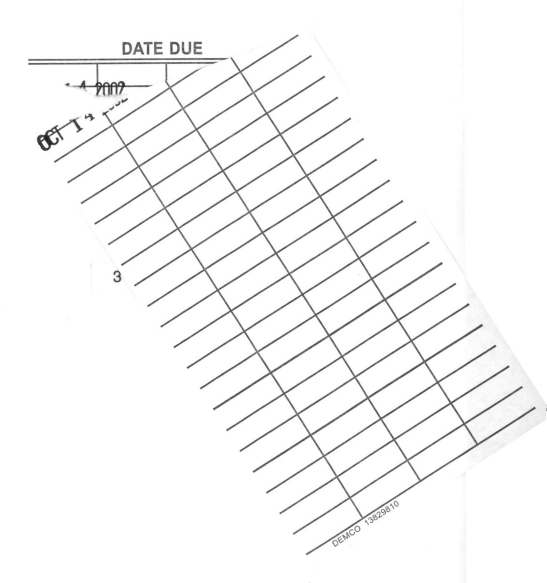